Neuroanatomy

An Atlas of Structures,
Sections, and Systems

Fourth Edition

Neuroanatomy

An Atlas of Structures, Sections, and Systems

Fourth Edition

Duane E. Haines, Ph.D.

Professor and Chairman
Department of Anatomy
The University of Mississippi Medical Center
Jackson, Mississippi

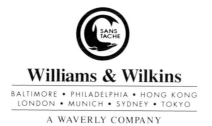

Williams & Wilkins

BALTIMORE • PHILADELPHIA • HONG KONG
LONDON • MUNICH • SYDNEY • TOKYO

A WAVERLY COMPANY

Editor: Patricia Coryell
Copy Editor: John M. Daniel
Designer: Norman W. Och
Illustration Planner: Ray Lowman
Production Coordinator: Charles E. Zeller
Cover Designer: Dan Pfisterer

Copyright © 1995
Williams & Wilkins
428 East Preston Street
Baltimore, Maryland 21202, USA

1st Edition, 1983
2nd Edition, 1987
3rd Edition, 1991
Portuguese Edition, 1991

Library of Congress Cataloging-in-Publication Data

Haines, Duane E.
    Neuroanatomy : an atlas of structures, sections, and systems /
Duane E. Haines.—4th ed.
      p. cm.
    Includes bibliographical references and index.
    ISBN 0-683-03817-6
    1. Neuranatomy—Atlases. I. Title.
    [DNLM: 1. Central Nervous System—anatomy & histology—atlases.
WL 17 H153n 1994]
QM451.H18   1994
611'.8—dc20
DNLM/DLC
for Library of Congress   94-4194
                                     CIP

                                  98
                      5 6 7 8 9 10

Preface to the Fourth Edition

The philosophy of making every attempt to provide *useful* material, organized in an integrated manner, has guided the previous editions of this book. It continues to be the primary goal of this new edition of *Neuroanatomy* to provide material that is contemporary, informative, and relevant to the educational needs of the user. The constructive suggestions I have received have been incorporated into this fourth edition.

In Chapter 2 some of the vascular drawings have been slightly modified to clarify minor points. In addition, five gross brain photographs have been replaced with new, significantly better, prints.

Chapter 5 has been *completely* modified based not only on my appreciation of what may constitute a better approach, but, more importantly, on the valuable comments and suggestions of my colleagues. The original stained sections (that appeared in previous editions) were used in this revision of Chapter 5. In this new version, the full stained section appears on the right-hand page and a complete drawing of the same section appears on the left-hand page. These new drawings are somewhat simplified from the more complex versions of the third edition and they are labeled with full words. To enhance the difference between the drawing of the section and the labels and leader lines, the section is printed in gray and the labels and leaders are printed at 100% black. This clearly differentiates the base art from the leader/labels, gives the image the appearance of depth, and significantly reduces competition between the various lines. Additional explanatory material has been added to this chapter.

Important modifications have also been made in Chapter 7. The *Neurotransmitter* information has been revised/updated where applicable. Recognizing the intrinsic value of clinical/anatomical integration, brief *Clinical Correlations* have been added to the description of each drawing. Consequently, each pathway drawing now contains the following information: 1) the trajectory of fibers [printed in color] making up the pathway, 2) the neuroactive substances associated with these various fibers, 3) clinical correlations highlighting some of the deficits seen following injury at representative levels, and 4) a summary of the blood supply to the pathway at all levels.

Chapter 8 has also been significantly revised. New angiograms (arterial and venous phases) have been added in standard and digital subtraction views. In addition, representative Magnetic Resonance Angiography (MRA) images are also included; a drawing, in color, accompanies one MRA. This non-invasive technique simultaneously shows arteries, veins, and venous sinuses.

Other minor, but equally important, changes have been made in all chapters. Many of these are in response to suggestions I have received from students and colleagues. It is hoped that the incorporation of these improvements will create a more useful book for medical, osteopathic, dental, graduate, and allied health students. I trust that this new edition will continue to meet the educational needs and expectations of these, and other, students.

I am solely responsible for any inconsistencies that may have found their way into this work. Suggestions, comments, and corrections from students and from my colleagues are always welcome.

Duane E. Haines
Jackson, Mississippi

Preface to the First Edition

This atlas is a reflection of, and a response to, suggestions from professional and graduate students over the years I have taught human neurobiology. Admittedly, some personal philosophy, as regards teaching, has crept into all parts of the work.

The goal of this atlas is to provide a maximal amount of useful information, in the form of photographs and drawings, so that the initial learning experience will be pleasant, logical, and fruitful, and the review process effective and beneficial to longterm professional goals. To this end several guiding principles have been followed. First, the entire anatomy of the central nervous system (CNS), external and internal, has been covered in appropriate detail. Second, a conscientious effort has been made to generate photographs and drawings of the highest quality: illustrations that clearly relay information to the reader. Third, complementary information always appears on the facing page. This may take the form of two views of related structures such as brainstem or successive brain slices or a list of abbreviations and description for a full-page figure. Fourth, illustrations of blood supply have been included *and* integrated into their appropriate chapters. When gross anatomy of the brain is shown, the patterns of blood vessels and relationships of sinuses appear on facing pages. The distribution pattern of blood vessels to internal CNS structures is correlated with internal morphology as seen in stained sections. Including information on external vascular patterns represents a distinct departure from what is available in most atlases, and illustrations of internal vessel distribution are unique to this atlas.

There are other features which, although not unique in themselves, do not usually appear in atlas format. In the chapter containing cross-sections, special effort has been made to provide figures that are accurate, clear, and allow considerable flexibility in how they can be used for both teaching and learning. The use of illustrations that are one-half photograph and one-half drawing is not entirely novel. In this atlas, however, the sections are large, clearly labeled, and the drawing side is a mirror-image of the photograph side. One section of the atlas is devoted to summaries of a variety of major pathways. Including this material in a laboratory atlas represents a distinct departure from the standard approach. However, feedback over the years strongly indicates that this type of information in atlas format is extremely helpful to students in the laboratory and greatly enhances their ability to grasp and retain information on CNS connections. While this atlas does not attempt to teach clinical concepts, a chapter correlating selected views of angiograms and CT scans with the morphological relationships of cerebral arteries and internal brain structures is included. These examples illustrate that a clear understanding of normal morphological relationships, as seen in the laboratory, can be directly transposed to clinical situations.

This atlas was not conceived with a particular audience in mind. It was designed to impart a clear and comprehensive understanding of CNS morphology to its readers, whoever they may be. It is most obviously appropriate for human neurobiology courses as taught to medical, dental, and graduate students. In addition, students in nursing, physical therapy, and other allied health curricula, and psychology as well, may also find its contents helpful and applicable to their needs. Inclusion and integration of blood vessel patterns, both external and internal, and the summary pathway drawings may be useful to the individual requiring a succinct, yet comprehensive review before taking board exams in the neurological, neurosurgical, and psychiatric specialties.

The details in some portions of this atlas may exceed that found in comparable parts of other atlases, If one is to err, it seems more judicious to err on the side of greater detail than on the side of inadequate detail. If the student is confronted with more information on a particular point than is needed during the initial learning process, he or she can simply bypass the extra information. However, once the initial learning is completed, the additional information will be there to enhance the review process. If students have inadequate information in front of them it may be difficult, or even impossible, to fill in missing points that may not be part of their repertoire of knowledge. In addition, information may be inserted out of context, and, thereby, hinder the learning experience.

A work such as this is bound to be subject to oversights, and for such foibles I am solely responsible. I welcome comments, suggestions, and corrections from my colleagues and from students.

Duane E. Haines

Acknowledgments

Many of my colleagues have offered suggestions or comments that have proven essential to the development of this fourth edition. I am deeply indebted to them for their time and interest. Students are also an unending source of helpful input and I greatly appreciate their ideas as to how this book can be improved.

I would like to thank my colleagues in the Department of Anatomy at The University of Mississippi Medical Center (UMC) (Drs. March Ard, Ben Clower, Pat Hardy, Jim Hutchins, Jim Lynch, Paul May, Tere Ma, Greg Mihailoff, John Naftel, and Susan Warren) for their helpful suggestions and especially for their good-natured patience with my repeated questions about new ideas as they emerged. My colleagues in Neurosurgery (Drs. Lon Alexander, Louis Harkey, and Bob Smith, Chair of Neurosurgery, UMC) have also offered valuable input. I am also *very* grateful to the following individuals for their constructive comments and fine cooperation: Drs. Conwell Anderson, Bill Anderson, Ron Baisden, Rosemary Borke, Patricia Brown, Paul Brown, Tony Castro, Bob Chronister, Art Craig, Jim Culberson, Espen Dietrichs, Jim Evans, Bill Falls, Cynthia Forehand, Rich Frederickson, Edgar Garcia-Rill, Gerald Grunwald, Jim King, Albert Lamperti, George Leichnetz, George Martin, Kenna Peusner, Christopher Phelps, Alan Rosenquist, Michael Schwartz, John Scott, Virginia Seybold, Diane Smith, Suzanne Stensaas, Dan Tolbert, Fred Walberg, Steve Walkley, Mike Woodruff, Mike Wyss, and Bob Yezierski. The stained sections used in this atlas are from the teaching collection at West Virginia.

The clinical correlations were critically reviewed by several individuals, especially Drs. Culberson and Mihailoff. However, I am particularly indebted to Dr. Jim Corbett (Chair of Neurology, UMC) and Mr. Jay Wellons, an M4 and wannabe clinical neuroscientist, for their critical review and suggestions on these clinical vignettes. All of these individuals held my feet to the fire for accuracy as to fact and appropriateness to the audience.

Dr. Brent Harrison (Chair of Radiology, UMC) and Dr. Bill Russell (Neuroradiology) generously gave me full access to all their facilities. I express a special thanks to Dr. Frank Raila for his interest in this project, his persistent attempts to locate good images, and for checking the labeling on the angiograms and MRAs and to Mr. Allen Terrell, RT, for his outstanding cooperation and his unrelenting efforts to generate truly fine images.

The excellent final renderings of the drawings in Chapter 5, modifications to the illustrations in Chapters 2 and 7, and the mounting and/or labeling of the new halftones in Chapters 2, 5 and 8 were the work of Mr. Michael Schenk (Director of Biomedical Illustration) and his co-workers Ms. Myriam Kirkman, Ms. Diane Johnson, and Mr. Ricky Manning, Mr. William deVeer and Mr. Bill Armstrong, Director and Assistant Directors, respectively, of Biomedical Photography, produced outstanding photographs of gross brain specimens, stained sections, angiograms, MRIs, and MRAs. I am *very* appreciative of the time, effort, and dedication of these individuals to create the very best artwork and photographs for this project. All of the typing for the fourth edition was done by Ms. Gail Rainer. Her good natured cooperation and patience with the author were key elements in getting the final draft done in a timely manner.

Some of the new photographs of gross brain in Chapter 2 and stained sections in Chapter 5 are also being used in a book that will be published by Churchill Livingstone. The author appreciates the agreement between C-L and W&W allowing these few images to be used in both projects.

This fourth edition would not have been possible without the interest and support of the publisher, Williams & Wilkins. I want to express thanks to Ms. Sara Finnegan, past President, Professional and Reference Group, Mr. Timothy Satterfield, Editor-in-Chief, my editor Ms. Patricia Coryell (Senior Editor), Mr. Charles Zeller, Book Production Coordinator, and Ms. Mary Finch, Marketing Manager for their encouragement, continuing interest, and confidence in this project. Their cooperation has given me the opportunity to make the improvements seen herein.

Last, but certainly not least, I would like to express a special thanks to my wife Gretchen. She put up with me while these revisions were in progress, helped with some parts of the project, and was a tangible factor in getting everything done. I dedicate this edition to her.

Contents

Chapter 1

Introduction and Reader's Guide

At a time when increasing numbers of atlases and textbooks are becoming available to students and instructors, it is appropriate to briefly outline the approach used in this volume. Most books are the result of two general forces. First, there is the philosophic approach of the author/instructor to the subject matter. Second, there are the needs of the students, as they may perceive them, and their suggestions and opinions based on their educational experiences. The present atlas is no exception and, as a result, several factors have guided its development. These include an appreciation of what enhances learning in the laboratory and classroom, the importance of integrating structure with function, and the great value of understanding the blood supply to the central nervous system (CNS). The goal is to make it obvious to the user that structure and function in the CNS are integrated elements and not separate entities.

Most neuroanatomic atlases approach the study of the CNS from fundamentally similar viewpoints. They present CNS anatomy as photographs or drawings of gross brain followed by illustrations of stained sections, in one or more planes, with the important structures labeled. Although there are some variations on this theme, the *basic* approach is similar. In addition, most atlases either omit information on the brain blood-vascular system or place it in a section of its own and make no effort to correlate vascular patterns with the organization of tracts and/or nuclei. Also, the vast majority of atlases include little or no information on neurotransmitters and make no effort to integrate clinical correlations with the study of functional systems.

Understanding CNS structure is the basis for learning pathways and, ultimately, neural function. Following a brief period devoted to the study of CNS morphology, a significant portion of many courses is spent learning functional systems. This learning experience may take place in the laboratory, since it is here that the student deals with slides (actual sections and/or 2 × 2 slides) of representative levels of the entire neuraxis. However, few attempts have been made to provide the student with a comprehensive guide—one that contains gross CNS anatomy and stained sections (both correlated with their vas-

cular supplies), summaries of clinically relevant pathways (all containing neurotransmitter and clinical correlations), and a variety of clinical images (angiogram, computed tomography [CT], magnetic resonance imaging [MRI], and magnetic resonance angiography [MRA]).

The present atlas attempts to address these points. The goal is not only to show external and internal structure per se, but also to show that the blood supply to specific areas of the CNS and the arrangement of pathways located therein, the neuroactive substances associated with pathways, and examples of clinical deficits are inseparable components of the learning experience. An effort has been made to provide a format that is dynamic and flexible and that makes the learning experience an interesting exercise.

Before describing some of the unique features of this atlas, a few general comments are appropriate. Even though the anatomy of the CNS is described in many textbooks, it is appropriate to provide this information in an atlas, since it is the gross brain and spinal cord that first confront the student in the laboratory. The relationship between blood vessels and specific brain regions (external and/or internal) is extremely important in light of the fact that about 50% of what goes wrong inside the skull, to produce clinical deficits, is vascular related. To emphasize the value of this information, the distribution pattern of blood vessels is correlated with external brain anatomy (Chapter 2) and with internal structures such as tracts and nuclei (Chapter 5), reviewed in each pathway drawing (Chapter 7), and shown in angiograms and MRAs (Chapter 8). This approach has several advantages: (1) the vascular pattern is *immediately* related to the structures just learned, (2) vascular patterns are shown in the sections of the atlas where they belong, (3) the reader cannot proceed from one part of the atlas to the next without being reminded of blood supply, and (4) the conceptual importance of the distribution pattern of blood vessels in the CNS is repeatedly reinforced.

Although the study of CNS pathways accounts for a significant portion of most neurobiology courses, this type of information is not available in most atlases. Consequently, the student may be required to page through 30, 40, or even 50 pages to follow a *single* tract, say the anterolateral system, from the cervical spinal cord to the thalamus. To the individual just becoming acquainted with the dynamics of neural pathways, this approach may be very confusing and quite frustrating, especially when the *overall* features of the pathway are not immediately obvious. Chapter 7 provides a series of semidiagrammatic illustrations of a variety of clinically relevant pathways. *Each figure* shows the trajectory of fibers making up the entire pathway, the positions and somatotopy of fibers composing each pathway at relevant levels, a review of their blood supply, important neurotransmitters associated with fibers of the pathway, and examples of deficits seen following lesions of the pathway at various levels. This chapter can be used by itself or integrated with other sections of the atlas and is designed to provide the reader with the *essentials of a given pathway in a single illustration*.

In addition to a variety of standard views of the gross and internal anatomy of the human brain, Chapters 3, 4, and 6 provide additional perspectives. Chapter 3 contains representative views of dissected brains, emphasizing structures and/or relationships commonly taught in many neurobiology courses. Chapter 4 shows the brain in coronal and axial (horizontal) slices, and Chapter 6 uses a correlated series of stained axial and sagittal sections to illustrate internal brain structures. These later photographs provide basic information on internal brain morphology and allow the user to identify three-dimensional relationships by comparing the images on facing pages.

The ensuing discussion briefly outlines the salient features of individual chapters. In some sections, considerable flexibility has been designed into the format; at these points, some suggestions are made as to how the atlas can be used.

Chapter 2   In the study of human neurobiology, one must become acquainted with basic structure prior to a consideration of functional systems. Chapter 2 presents the morphology of the CNS in two sections: the gross anatomy of the spinal cord and its principal arteries, and the gross external morphology of the brain. Classic views are included, followed immediately by illustrations showing the distribution of blood vessels from the same perspective. The patterns of vessels on external aspects of the spinal cord, all areas of the cerebral cortex, and on all aspects of the brainstem are correlated with surface anatomic landmarks. Details of brainstem and cerebellum are also included.

Chapter 3   The dissections in Chapter 3 offer detailed views of those brain structures introduced in Chapter 2. Certain structures and/or structural relationships—for example, the orientation of the larger association bundles,

the topography of the insular cortex and associated areas, and the gross relationships of brainstem and forebrain structures—are particularly suited to such a presentation. This chapter uses a representative series of dissected views to provide a broader basis for learning human neuroanatomy. Since it is not feasible to illustrate every anatomic feature, the views and structures selected are those usually emphasized in medical neurobiology courses. These views provide basic information necessary to make more detailed dissections, if appropriate, in a particular learning situation.

Chapter 4   The study of general morphology is continued in the three sections of Chapter 4. The first reviews the general features and relationships of meninges and illustrates ventricles and their relationships to adjacent structures. This section is intentionally short, emphasizes general concepts, and does not attempt to reiterate details available in standard textbooks. The second section contains a representative series of unstained coronal slices of brain, whereas the third section contains a series of unstained brain slices cut in a plane approximately corresponding to that seen in CT and MRI preparations. Since the brain, as sectioned at autopsy or in clinical pathologic conferences, is viewed in the form of unstained specimens, the preference here is to present the material in a format that will most closely parallel what is seen in these clinical situations.

Chapter 5   As noted in the Preface, Chapter 5 has been completely revised. However, the same stained sections that were used to generate the images for this chapter in previous editions are used in this revision.

As in earlier editions, this chapter consists of six sections covering, in sequence, the Spinal Cord, Medulla Oblongata, Cerebellar Nuclei, Pons, Midbrain, and Diencephalon and Basal Ganglia with MRI. In this new format, the right-hand page contains a complete image of the stained section. The left-hand page contains a labeled line drawing of the stained section, accompanied by a figure description and, for the brain sections, a small orientation drawing. These line drawings have been somewhat simplified from the more detailed style of earlier editions. In an effort to make it easy to differentiate lines belonging to the section from leader lines, the section part of this artwork is printed in gray (a 60% screen of black), whereas the leader lines and labels are printed at 100% black. This gives the illustration a sense of depth and texture, reduces competition between lines, and makes the illustration easy to read at a glance.

Semidiagrammatic representations of the internal blood supply to the spinal cord, brainstem, and forebrain follow-each set of stained sections in these parts of this chapter. This allows the immediate, and convenient, correlation of structure with its blood supply as one is studying the internal anatomy of the neuraxis. It is essential to develop a good understanding of what structure is served by what vessel, since so much of what goes wrong inside the cranial cavity is vascular related.

The Diencephalon and Basal Ganglia section of this chapter uses 10 cross-sections to illustrate internal anatomy. It should be emphasized that 8 of these 10 sections (those parallel to each other) are all from the same brain.

The use of MRIs (or CTs) in the teaching situation is now commonplace. It is, therefore, appropriate to use representative examples of such images in a format that allows a direct comparison with internal brain anatomy. Consequently, 7 of the 10 cross-sections in the Diencephalon and Basal Ganglia part of this chapter have correlated MRIs. *Many* of the anatomic features seen in the stained section are easy to recognize in the adjacent MRI. The MRIs are not labeled for two reasons. First, labeling these images in a book of this type would clutter the picture and reduce their instructional value. Second, when the student or physician sees MRIs in the clinical setting, they are unlabeled. It seems appropriate to give the user an opportunity to learn what can be seen in the MRI by juxtaposing it with an actual stained section at a comparable level. The labeled drawing on the facing page provides a framework for correlating structures in the MRIs with those in the stained sections. Consequently, the subsections of Chapter 5 can be used in a variety of ways and will accommodate a wide range of student and/or instructor preferences.

Chapter 6 The three-dimensional anatomy of internal structures in the CNS can be studied in dissected views (Chapter 3) *and* in photographs of stained sections that correlate similar structures in different planes. The photographs of stained axial (horizontal) and sagittal sections and of MRIs in Chapter 6 are organized to provide four important levels of information. First, the *general* internal anatomy of brain structures can be easily identified in each photograph. Second, axial photographs are on left-hand pages and arranged from dorsal to ventral (Figs. 6-1 to 6-9), whereas sagittal photographs are on right-hand pages and arranged from medial to lateral (Figs. 6-2 to 6-10). This, in essence, provides complete representations of the brain in *both* planes for use as independent study sets (axial only, sagittal only) or as integrated/correlated sets (compare facing pages). Third, because axial and sagittal sections are on facing pages *and* the plane of section of each is indicated on its companion by a heavy line, the

user is easily able to visualize the positions of internal structures in more than one plane and to develop a clear concept of three-dimensional topography. In other words, one can identify structures dorsal or ventral to the axial plane by comparing it with the sagittal, and structures medial or lateral to the sagittal plane by comparing it with the axial. This yields more usable information from individual photographs and, in the end, leads to a fuller understanding of internal three-dimensional relationships in the brain. Fourth, the inclusion of MRIs with representative axial (horizontal) and sagittal stained sections provides excellent examples of the fact that structures seen in the teaching laboratory are easy to recognize in clinical images. The term *axial* for *horizontal* is preferred in this book, since "axial" is used in the clinical setting to describe this plane of section. These MRIs are not labeled for the same reasons noted above (see notes on Chapter 5) but are located *adjacent* to their respective sections.

Chapter 7 This chapter provides summaries of a variety of clinically relevant CNS tracts and/or pathways and has four features that enhance student understanding. First, the inclusion of pathway information in atlas format broadens the basis one can use to teach functional neurobiology in the laboratory setting. Such summaries are not available in most other atlases. Second, each drawing illustrates, in line color, a given pathway completely, showing its longitudinal extent and course throughout the neuraxis; its position in representative cross-sections; and the somatotopic organization of fibers within the pathway, if applicable. Blood supply to each pathway is reviewed on the facing page. Third, a brief summary mentions the main neuroactive substances associated with cells and fibers composing particular segments of the pathway under consideration. The action of the substance, if widely agreed on, is indicated as excitatory "(+)" or inhibitory "(−)." *This allows the user to closely correlate a particular neurotransmitter with a specific population of projection neurons and their terminals.* The limitations of this approach, within the confines of an atlas, are self-evident. The transmitters associated with some pathways are not well-known; consequently, such information is not provided for some connections. Also, no attempt is made to differentiate neurotransmitters from neuromodulators, to identify substances that may be co-localized, to discuss their synthesis or degradation, or to mention *all* neurotransmitters associated with a particular cell group. All of these issues are well beyond the scope of this book. The goal here is to introduce the student to selected neurotransmitters and to *integrate* and *correlate* this information with a particular pathway, circuit, or connection. Fourth, the clinical correlations that accompany each pathway drawing provide examples of deficits resulting from lesions, at various levels in the neuraxis, of the fibers composing the pathway. Also, examples are given of syndromes or diseases in which these deficits are seen. The variety of ways in which these clinical correlations can be used to enrich the learning process are described in Figure 7-3 on p. 162.

The drawings in this section were designed to provide the maximum amount of information, to keep the extraneous points to a minimum, and to do it all in a single, easy-to-follow figure. A complete range of relevant information is contained in each drawing and in its description, including the complete organization of fibers composing the pathway, neurotransmitters associated with these fibers, clinical examples of lesions involving portions of the pathway, and a review of the blood supply to all parts of the pathway.

Since it is not possible to anticipate *all* pathways that may be taught in a wide range of neurobiology courses, flexibility has been designed into Chapter 7. The last figure in each section of this chapter is a blank master drawing that follows the same general format as the preceding figures. Photocopies of these blank master drawings can be used by the student for learning and/or review of any pathway or by the instructor to teach additional pathways not included in the atlas or as a substrate for examination

questions. The flexibility of information as presented in Chapter 7 extends equally to student and instructor.

Chapter 8 This chapter consists of two sections. The first contains a series of angiograms (arterial and venous phases) in lateral and anterior-posterior projections. These are shown as standard views and as corresponding digital subtraction images. In addition, MRA images are included and are shown in three-dimensional phase contrast and in inverted video image modes. This noninvasive method allows for simultaneous visualization of arteries, veins, and venous sinuses. Use of MRAs is becoming common, and this technology is an important diagnostic tool.

In the second section, photographs of slices through a normal brain appear on pages facing reproductions of normal and abnormal CT scans and MRIs taken at corresponding levels. Structures that can be identified in normal CT scans or MRIs are labeled on the appropriate brain slices; abnormal CT scans and MRIs illustrate how internal morphology is altered in pathologic states. The normal MRIs are T1 images, since these show normal internal brain structures most clearly. Abnormal MRIs are T2 images, which show pathologic changes, such as edema, to better advantage. These illustrations are examples of how information gleaned in the neuroanatomy laboratory can be directly translated to, and used in, the clinical setting.

Rationale for Abbreviations

There is no universally accepted way to identify specific features or structures in drawings or photographs. The variety of methods seen in currently available books and atlases reflects personal preferences of the authors. Such is the case in the present endeavor. The goal of this atlas is to present basic neuroanatomy in the most understandable manner, and therefore it is appropriate to explain the rationale behind the labeling style used.

Among currently available atlases, most plates are labeled with full names of structures on the plate or with numbers or letters on the plates keyed to a matching list of the full names. The first method immediately imparts the greatest amount of information; the second method is the most succinct. The present atlas uses an approach that incorporates the advantages of both. The use of full names immediately relays maximum information to the user. However, care must be exercised not to compromise on the quality, or size, of the illustration, on the number of structures labeled, or on the size of labels used. The use of single letters or numbers, although producing minimal clutter on the figure, has one primary drawback. The same number or letter may appear on several different plates and designate different structures in all cases. Consequently, there is no consistency between numbers and letters and their corresponding meanings as the reader moves from figure to figure. In consideration of all of these factors, this atlas uses a combination of full words and abbreviations that are clearly recognized versions of the full word. The quality and size of photographs and labels is not compromised, and an appropriate number of structures are labeled. On some drawings (i.e., blood vessel drawings in Chapter 2; cross-sectional drawings in Chapter 5), the use of full words is appropriate, because they do not compromise or clutter the drawings. However, on other illustrations, such as the pathway drawings in Chapter 7, the use of full words would seriously compromise the quality of the artwork; in most cases, the full words would simply not fit. Consequently, abbreviations are used on these, and some other, figures as appropriate.

The abbreviations used in this atlas are large and easy to read, even across the table or over a specimen in the laboratory (as for gross brain specimens and brain slices in the laboratory—see Chapters 2, 3, and 4). They do not clutter the illustration, they permit labeling of all relevant structures, and they are adequately informative while stimulating the thinking-learning process. The abbreviations are, in a very real sense, mnemonics. As the student begins to learn terminology given in the lecture and reads a text, the meanings of most abbreviations will be recognized easily. When learning gyri and sulci of the occipital lobe, for example, the abbreviation ''LinGy'' in the atlas could only mean ''Lingual Gyrus.'' It could not be confused with other structures in other parts of the nervous system. When pathways are being studied, ''RuSp'' could mean only ''Rubrospinal Tract'' and ''LenFas'' the ''Lenticular Fasciculus.'' As the student learns more and more terminology from lectures and readings, he or she will be able to use the atlas with minimal reference to the lists of abbreviations. Each figure, however, always has its accompanying list of abbreviations. In addition, a subtle advantage of this method of labeling is that, as the user looks at the abbreviation and momentarily pauses to think about its meaning, he or she may form a mental image of the structure *and* the full word. Since neuroanatomy requires one to conceptualize and form mental images so as to more clearly understand CNS relationships, this method seems especially appropriate.

Chapter 2

External Morphology of the Central Nervous System

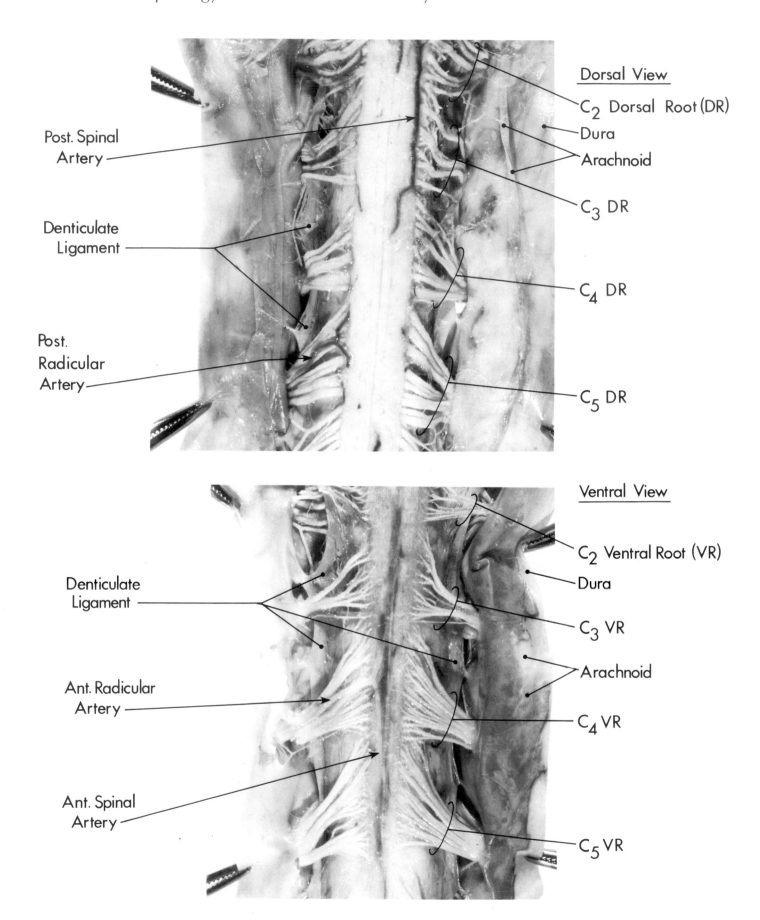

Post. Spinal Artery

Denticulate Ligament

Post. Radicular Artery

Dorsal View

C₂ Dorsal Root (DR)

Dura

Arachnoid

C₃ DR

C₄ DR

C₅ DR

Denticulate Ligament

Ant. Radicular Artery

Ant. Spinal Artery

Ventral View

C₂ Ventral Root (VR)

Dura

C₃ VR

Arachnoid

C₄ VR

C₅ VR

2–1   Dorsal (upper) and ventral (lower) views showing the general features of the spinal cord as seen at levels C₂–C₅. The dura and arachnoid are reflected, and the pia is intimately adherent to the spinal cord and rootlets. Posterior and anterior radicular arteries follow their respective roots. The posterior spinal artery is found medial to the entering dorsal rootlets (and the dorsolateral sulcus), while the anterior spinal artery is in the ventral median fissure (see also Fig. 2–2, facing page).

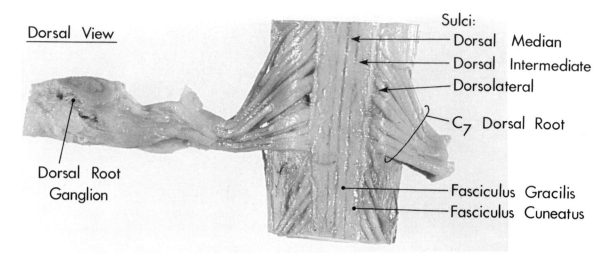

Dorsal View

Dorsal Root
Ganglion

Sulci:
Dorsal Median
Dorsal Intermediate
Dorsolateral
C₇ Dorsal Root
Fasciculus Gracilis
Fasciculus Cuneatus

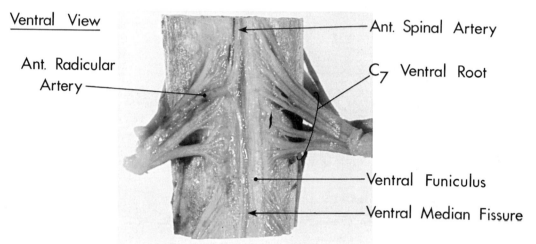

Ventral View

Ant. Radicular
Artery

Ant. Spinal Artery
C₇ Ventral Root
Ventral Funiculus
Ventral Median Fissure

2–2 Dorsal (upper) and ventral (lower) views showing details of the spinal cord as seen in the C₇ segment. The dorsal root ganglion is partially covered by dura.

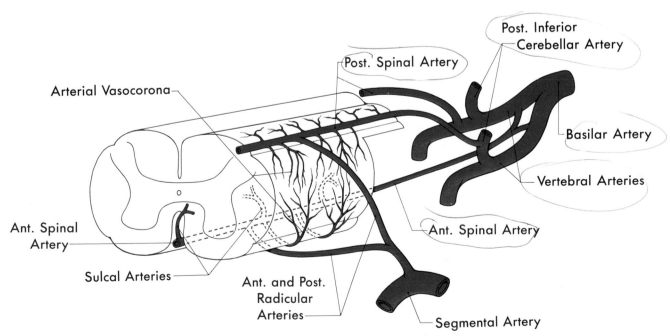

Arterial Vasocorona

Post. Inferior
Cerebellar Artery

Post. Spinal Artery

Basilar Artery

Vertebral Arteries

Ant. Spinal Artery

Ant. Spinal
Artery

Sulcal Arteries

Ant. and Post.
Radicular
Arteries

Segmental Artery

2–3 Semi-diagrammatic representation showing the origin and general location of principal arteries supplying the spinal cord. The arterial vasocorona is a diffuse anastomotic plexus covering the cord surface.

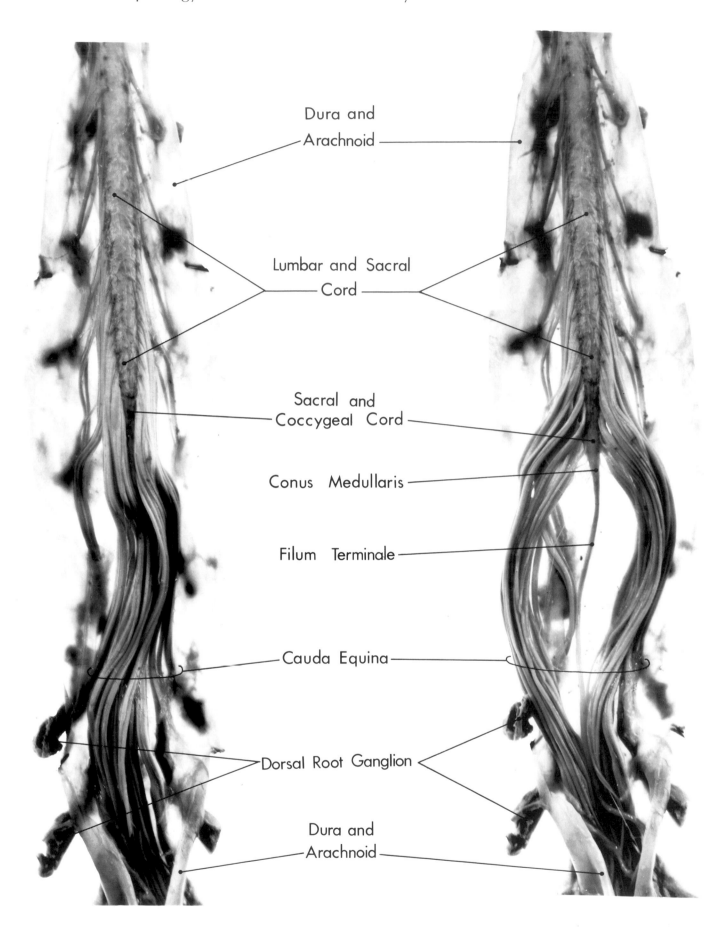

Dura and
Arachnoid

Lumbar and Sacral
Cord

Sacral and
Coccygeal Cord

Conus Medullaris

Filum Terminale

Cauda Equina

Dorsal Root Ganglion

Dura and
Arachnoid

2–4 Overall dorsal view of lumbar, sacral, and coccygeal cord
and the cauda equina. The dura and arachnoid are retracted. The cauda
equina is shown *in situ* on the left, while on the right nerve rootlets
have been spread laterally to expose the conus medullaris and filum
terminale (internum).

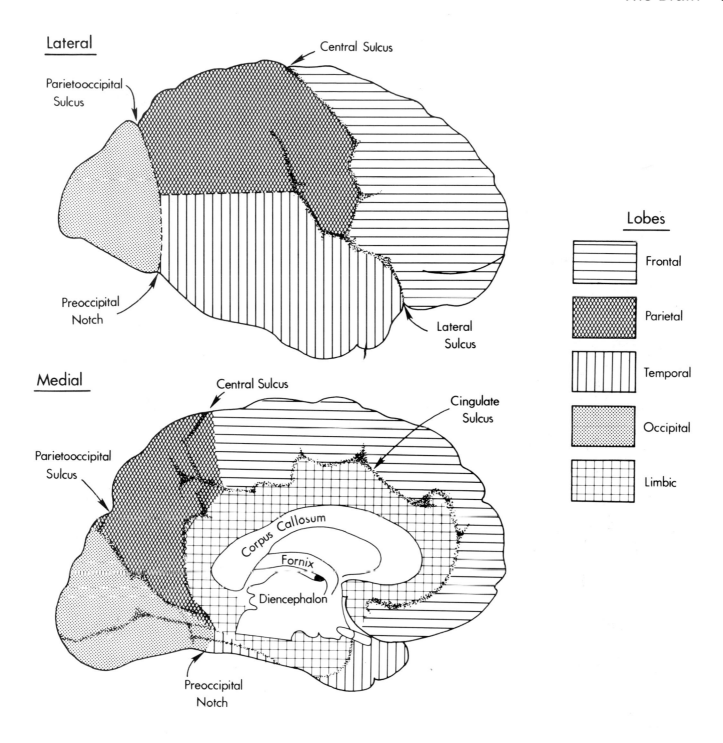

2–5 Lateral (upper) and medial (lower) views of the cerebral hemisphere showing the landmarks used to divide the cortex into its main lobes.

On the lateral aspect the central sulcus (of Rolando) separates frontal and parietal lobes. The lateral sulcus (of Sylvius) forms the border between frontal and temporal lobes. The occipital lobe is located caudal to an arbitrary line drawn between the terminus of the parieto-occipital sulcus and the preoccipital notch. A horizontal line drawn from the upper two-thirds of the lateral fissure to the rostral edge of the occipital lobe represents the border between parietal and temporal lobes. The insular cortex (see Figure 3–1 on page 38) is located deep to the lateral sulcus. On the medial aspect the cingulate sulcus separates medial portions of frontal and parietal lobes from the limbic lobe. An imaginary continuation of the central sulcus intersects with the cingulate sulcus and forms the border between frontal and parietal lobes. The parieto-occipital sulcus and an arbitrary continuation of this line to the preoccipital notch separates parietal, limbic, and temporal lobes from the occipital lobe.

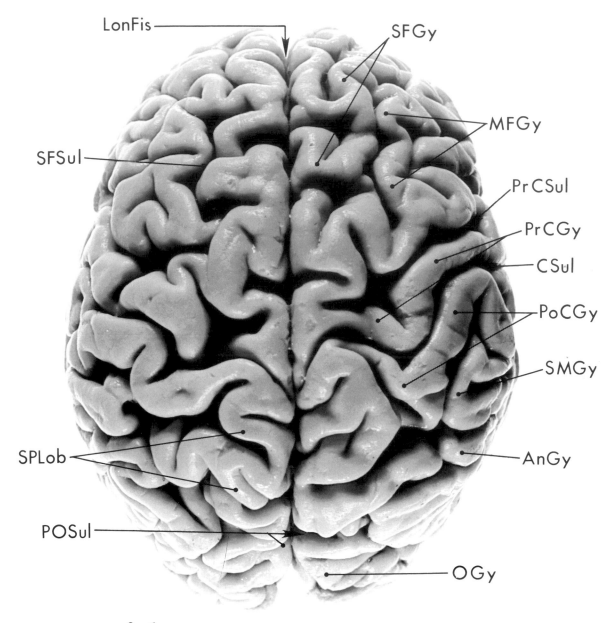

2–6 Dorsal view of the cerebral hemispheres showing the principal gyri and sulci.

Abbreviations

AnGy	Angular Gyrus
CSul	Central Sulcus (of Rolando)
LonFis	Longitudinal Fissure
MFGy	Middle Frontal Gyrus
OGy	Occipital Gyri
PoCGy	Postcentral Gyrus
POSul	Parieto-occipital Sulcus
PrCGy	Precentral Gyrus
PrCSul	Precentral Sulcus
SFGy	Superior Frontal Gyrus
SFSul	Superior Frontal Sulcus
SMGy	Supramarginal Gyrus
SPLob	Superior Parietal Lobule

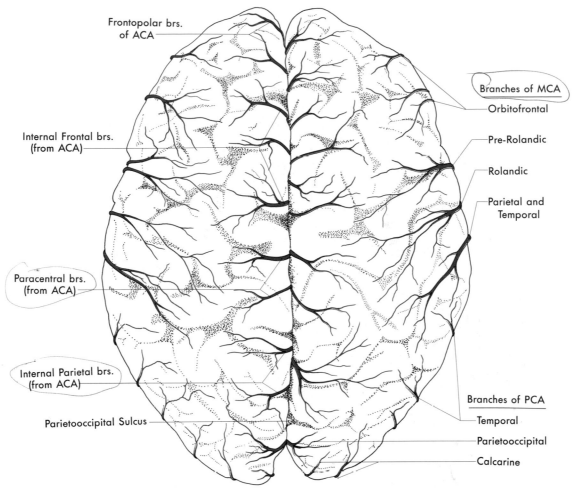

Frontopolar brs.
of ACA

Branches of MCA

Orbitofrontal

Internal Frontal brs.
(from ACA)

Pre-Rolandic

Rolandic

Parietal and
Temporal

Paracentral brs.
(from ACA)

Internal Parietal brs.
(from ACA)

Branches of PCA

Temporal

Parietooccipital Sulcus

Parietooccipital

Calcarine

2–7 Dorsal view of the cerebral hemispheres showing the location and general branching patterns of the terminal ramifications of anterior (ACA), middle (MCA), and posterior (PCA) cerebral arteries. Gyri and sulci can be easily identified by comparison with Figure 2–6 (facing page).

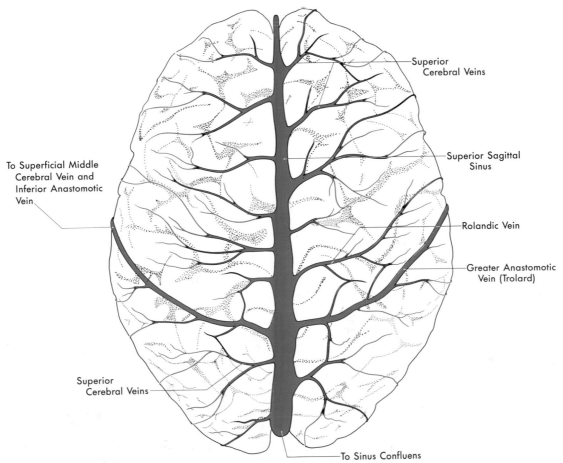

Superior
Cerebral Veins

Superior Sagittal
Sinus

To Superficial Middle
Cerebral Vein and
Inferior Anastomotic
Vein

Rolandic Vein

Greater Anastomotic
Vein (Trolard)

Superior
Cerebral Veins

To Sinus Confluens

2–8 Dorsal view of the cerebral hemispheres showing the location of the superior sagittal sinus and the locations and general branching patterns of veins. Gyri and sulci can be easily identified by comparison with Figure 2–6 (facing page).

Station II

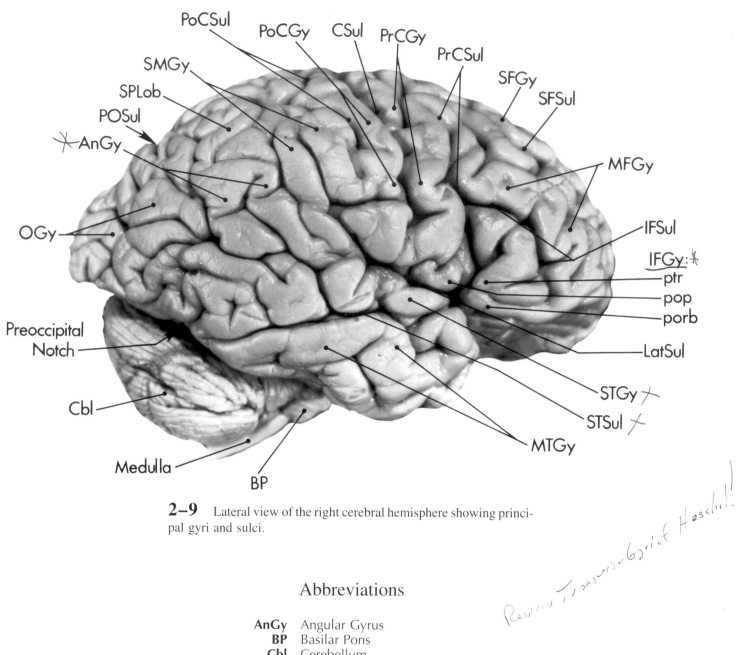

Revino Transverio Gyri of Heschl!

2–9   Lateral view of the right cerebral hemisphere showing principal gyri and sulci.

Abbreviations

AnGy	Angular Gyrus
BP	Basilar Pons
Cbl	Cerebellum
CSul	Central Sulcus (of Rolando)
IFGy	Inferior Frontal Gyrus
pop	pars opercularis
porb	pars orbitalis
ptr	pars triangularis
IFSul	Inferior Frontal Sulcus
LatSul	Lateral Sulcus (of Sylvius)
MFGy	Middle Frontal Gyrus
MTGy	Middle Temporal Gyrus
OGy	Occipital Gyri
PoCGy	Postcentral Gyrus
PoCSul	Postcentral Sulcus
POSul	Parieto-occipital Sulcus
PrCGy	Precentral Gyrus
PrCSul	Precentral Sulcus
SFGy	Superior Frontal Gyrus
SFSul	Superior Frontal Sulcus
SMGy	Supramarginal Gyrus
SPLob	Superior Parietal Lobule
STGy	Superior Temporal Gyrus
STSul	Superior Temporal Sulcus

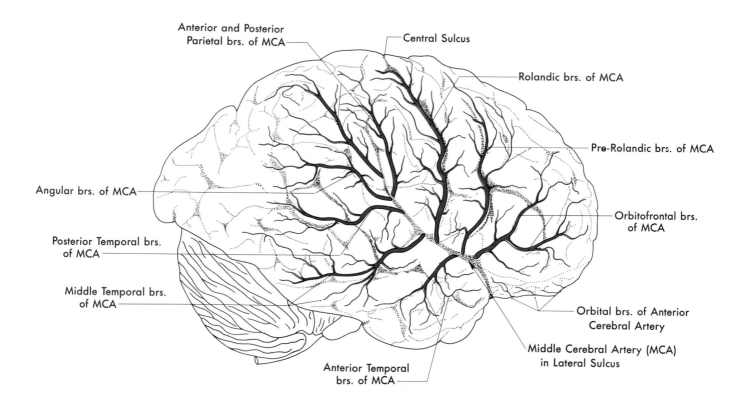

Labels in figure 2-10:
- Anterior and Posterior Parietal brs. of MCA
- Central Sulcus
- Rolandic brs. of MCA
- Pre-Rolandic brs. of MCA
- Angular brs. of MCA
- Orbitofrontal brs. of MCA
- Posterior Temporal brs. of MCA
- Middle Temporal brs. of MCA
- Orbital brs. of Anterior Cerebral Artery
- Middle Cerebral Artery (MCA) in Lateral Sulcus
- Anterior Temporal brs. of MCA

2–10 Lateral view of the right cerebral hemisphere showing the location and general branching pattern of the middle cerebral artery. Gyri and sulci can be easily identified by comparison with Figure 2–9 (facing page). The middle cerebral artery branches in the depths of the lateral sulcus. Terminal branches of the posterior and anterior cerebral arteries course over the edges of the temporal and occipital lobes, and parietal and frontal lobes, respectively (see Figure 2–7 on page 15).

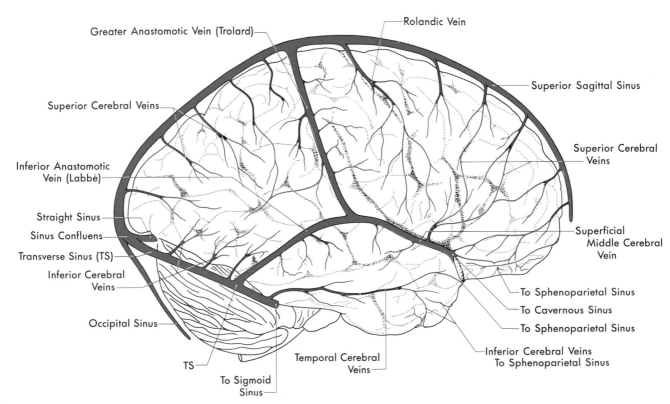

Labels in figure 2-11:
- Greater Anastomotic Vein (Trolard)
- Rolandic Vein
- Superior Sagittal Sinus
- Superior Cerebral Veins
- Superior Cerebral Veins
- Inferior Anastomotic Vein (Labbé)
- Straight Sinus
- Sinus Confluens
- Transverse Sinus (TS)
- Inferior Cerebral Veins
- Occipital Sinus
- Superficial Middle Cerebral Vein
- To Sphenoparietal Sinus
- To Cavernous Sinus
- To Sphenoparietal Sinus
- Inferior Cerebral Veins To Sphenoparietal Sinus
- TS
- To Sigmoid Sinus
- Temporal Cerebral Veins

2–11 Lateral view of the right cerebral hemisphere showing the locations of sinuses and the locations and general branching patterns of veins. Gyri and sulci can be easily identified by comparison with Figure 2–9 (facing page). Communications between veins and sinuses or between sinuses are so indicated.

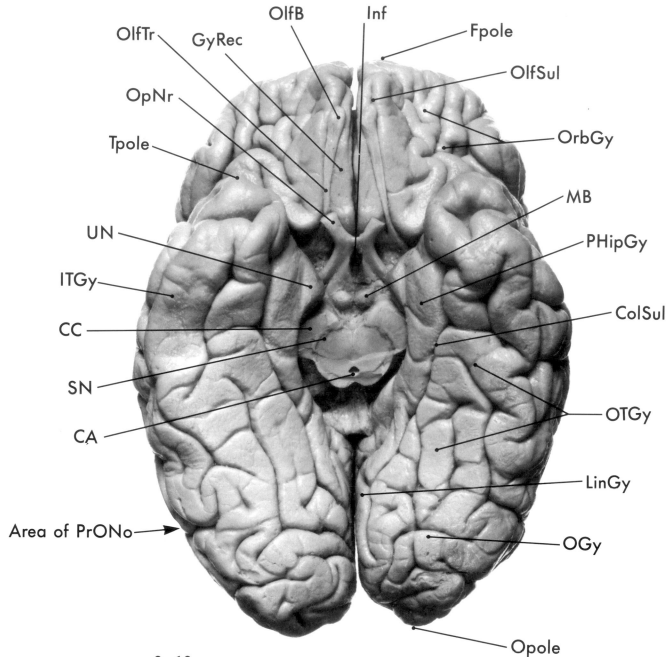

2–12   Ventral view of the cerebral hemispheres and diencephalon with brainstem caudal to midbrain removed.

Abbreviations

CA	Cerebral Aqueduct		**OlfSul**	Olfactory Sulcus
CC	Crus Cerebri		**OlfTr**	Olfactory Tract
ColSul	Collateral Sulcus		**OpNr**	Optic Nerve
Fpole	Frontal Pole		**Opole**	Occipital Pole
GyRec	Gyrus Rectus (Straight Gyrus)		**OrbGy**	Orbital Gyri
Inf	Infundibulum		**OTGy**	Occipitotemporal Gyri
ITGy	Inferior Temporal Gyrus		**PHipGy**	Parahippocampal Gyrus
LinGy	Lingual Gyrus		**PrONo**	Preoccipital Notch
MB	Mammillary Body		**SN**	Substantia Nigra
OGy	Occipital Gyri		**Tpole**	Temporal Pole
OlfB	Olfactory Bulb		**Un**	Uncus

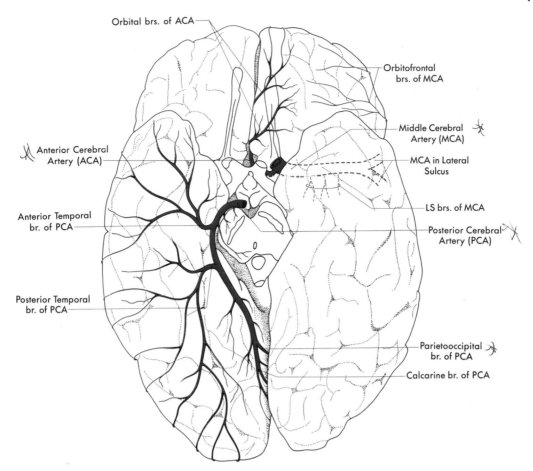

Orbital brs. of ACA

Orbitofrontal brs. of MCA

Anterior Cerebral Artery (ACA)

Middle Cerebral Artery (MCA)

MCA in Lateral Sulcus

Anterior Temporal br. of PCA

LS brs. of MCA

Posterior Cerebral Artery (PCA)

Posterior Temporal br. of PCA

Parietooccipital br. of PCA

Calcarine br. of PCA

2–13 Ventral view of the cerebral hemisphere with brainstem removed showing the branching pattern of the posterior cerebral artery and the general locations and some branches of anterior and middle cerebral arteries. Gyri and sulci can be easily identified by comparison with Figure 2–12 (facing page).

Abbreviation: **LS** Lenticulostriate

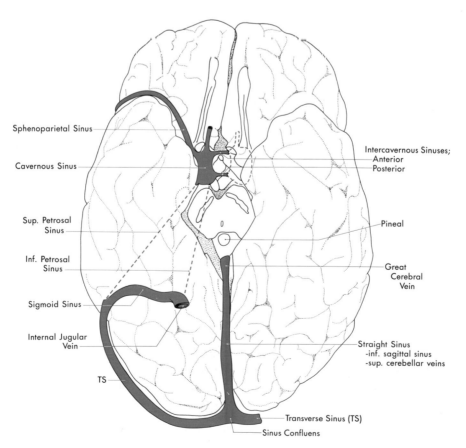

Sphenoparietal Sinus

Intercavernous Sinuses; Anterior Posterior

Cavernous Sinus

Sup. Petrosal Sinus

Pineal

Inf. Petrosal Sinus

Great Cerebral Vein

Sigmoid Sinus

Internal Jugular Vein

Straight Sinus -inf. sagittal sinus -sup. cerebellar veins

TS

Transverse Sinus (TS)

Sinus Confluens

2–14 Ventral view of the cerebral hemisphere with brainstem removed showing the locations and relationships of the main sinuses. Gyri and sulci can be easily identified by comparison with Figure 2–12 (facing page). The listings preceded by a hyphen (-) under principal sinuses are the main tributaries of that sinus.

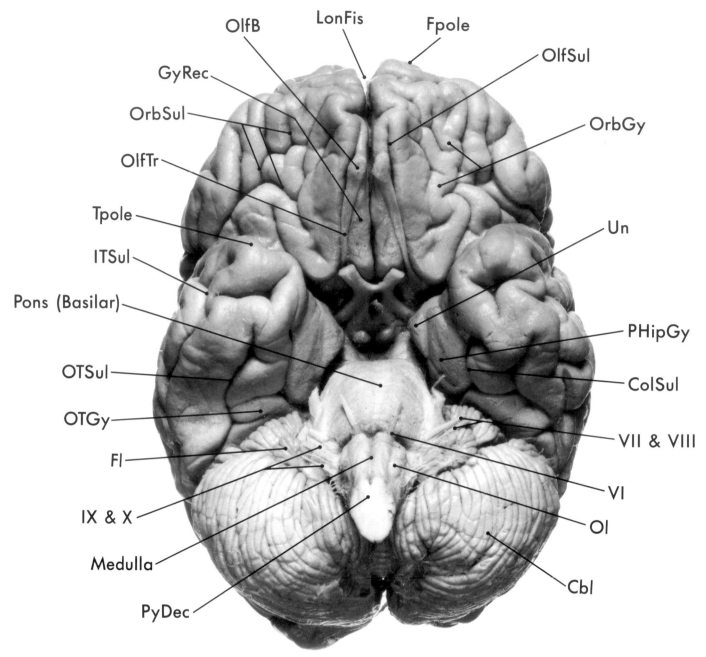

2–15   Ventral view of the cerebral hemispheres, diencephalon, brainstem, and cerebellum. For details of the brainstem and diencephalon see Figure 2–18 on page 22.

Abbreviations

Cbl	Cerebellum	**OrbSul**	Orbital Sulci
ColSul	Collateral Sulcus	**OTGy**	Occipitotemporal Gyri
Fl	Flocculus	**OTSul**	Occipitotemporal Sulcus
Fpole	Frontal Pole	**PHipGy**	Parahippocampal Gyrus
GyRec	Gyrus Rectus (Straight Gyrus)	**PyDec**	Pyramidal Decussation
ITSul	Inferior Temporal Sulcus	**Tpole**	Temporal Pole
LonFis	Longitudinal Fissure	**Un**	Uncus
Ol	Olive (Inferior)	**VI**	Sixth (Abducens) Cranial Nerve
OlfB	Olfactory Bulb	**VII**	Seventh (Facial) Cranial Nerve
OlfSul	Olfactory Sulcus	**VIII**	Eighth (Vestibulocochlear) Cranial Nerve
OlfTr	Olfactory Tract	**IX**	Ninth (Glossopharyngeal) Cranial Nerve
OrbGy	Orbital Gyri	**X**	Tenth (Vagus) Cranial Nerve

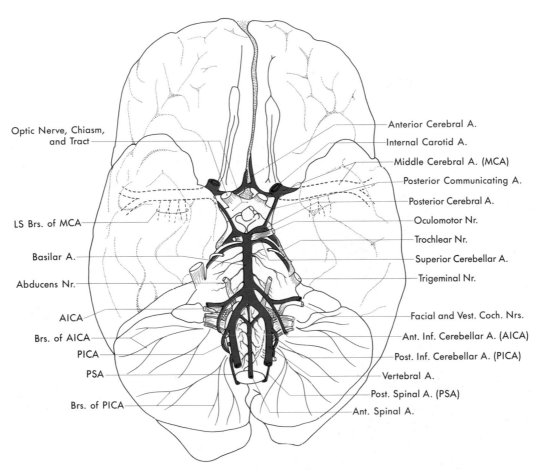

Optic Nerve, Chiasm, and Tract

Anterior Cerebral A.

Internal Carotid A.

Middle Cerebral A. (MCA)

Posterior Communicating A.

Posterior Cerebral A.

Oculomotor Nr.

LS Brs. of MCA

Trochlear Nr.

Basilar A.

Superior Cerebellar A.

Abducens Nr.

Trigeminal Nr.

AICA

Facial and Vest. Coch. Nrs.

Brs. of AICA

Ant. Inf. Cerebellar A. (AICA)

PICA

Post. Inf. Cerebellar A. (PICA)

PSA

Vertebral A.

Post. Spinal A. (PSA)

Brs. of PICA

Ant. Spinal A.

2–16   Ventral view of the cerebral hemispheres, diencephalon, brainstem, and cerebellum showing the arterial patterns created by the internal carotid and vertebrobasilar systems. Note the circle of Willis. Gyri and sulci can be identified by comparison with Figure 2–15 (facing page). Details of the vertebrobasilar arterial pattern are shown in Figure 2–20 on page 24.

Abbreviation: **LS**   Lenticulostriate

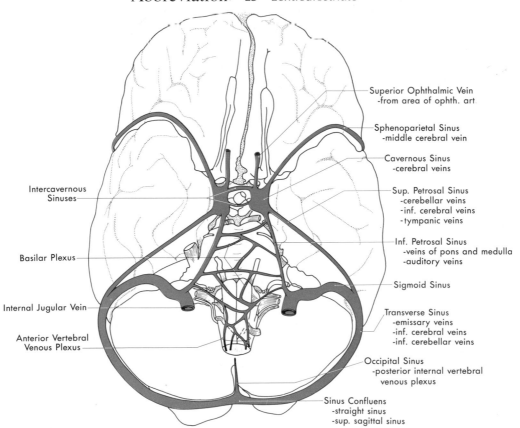

Superior Ophthalmic Vein
-from area of ophth. art.

Sphenoparietal Sinus
-middle cerebral vein

Cavernous Sinus
-cerebral veins

Intercavernous Sinuses

Sup. Petrosal Sinus
-cerebellar veins
-inf. cerebral veins
-tympanic veins

Inf. Petrosal Sinus
-veins of pons and medulla
-auditory veins

Basilar Plexus

Sigmoid Sinus

Internal Jugular Vein

Transverse Sinus
-emissary veins
-inf. cerebral veins
-inf. cerebellar veins

Anterior Vertebral Venous Plexus

Occipital Sinus
-posterior internal vertebral venous plexus

Sinus Confluens
-straight sinus
-sup. sagittal sinus

2–17   Ventral view of the cerebral hemispheres, diencephalon, brainstem, and cerebellum showing the locations and relationships of principal sinuses and veins. The listings preceded by a hyphen (-) under principal sinuses are the main tributaries of that sinus.

Abbreviation   **Ophth**   Ophthalmic

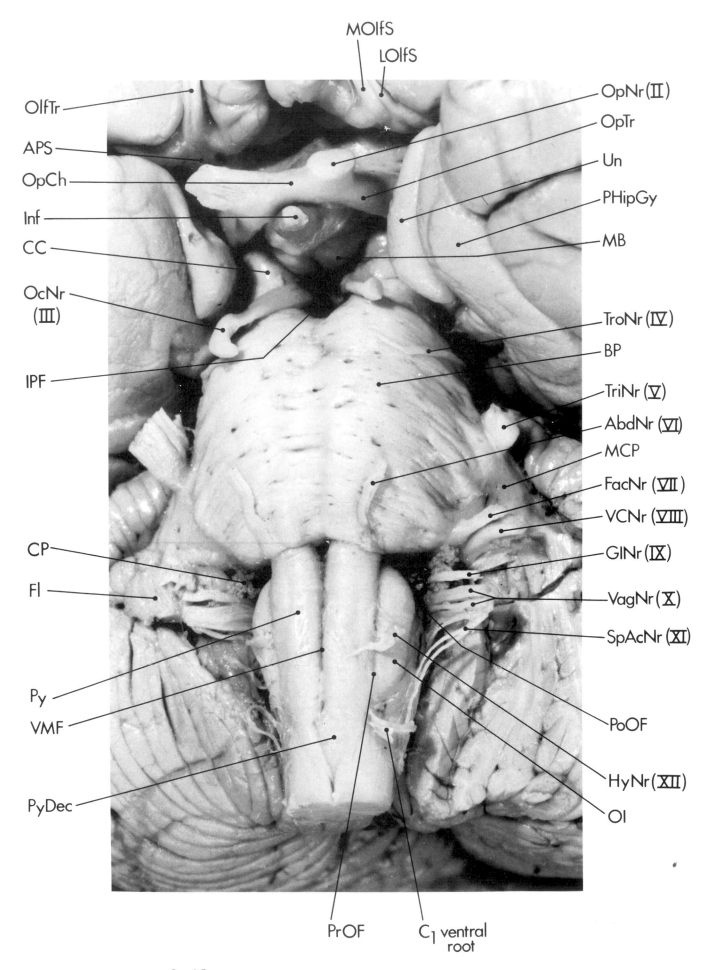

MOlfS

LOlfS

OlfTr

APS

OpCh

Inf

CC

OcNr (III)

IPF

CP

Fl

Py

VMF

PyDec

OpNr (II)

OpTr

Un

PHipGy

MB

TroNr (IV)

BP

TriNr (V)

AbdNr (VI)

MCP

FacNr (VII)

VCNr (VIII)

GlNr (IX)

VagNr (X)

SpAcNr (XI)

PoOF

HyNr (XII)

OI

PrOF

C₁ ventral root

2–18   Detailed ventral view of the diencephalon and brainstem with particular emphasis on cranial nerves and related structures.

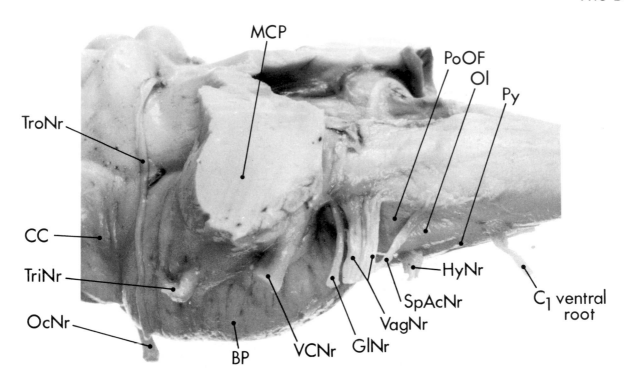

2–19 Lateral view of the left side of the brainstem showing a different perspective of those structures, mainly cranial nerves, labeled in Figure 2–18 (left page). Abbreviations for Figures 2–18 through 2–20 are listed below.

Abbreviations

AbdNr	Abducens Nerve (Cranial Nerve VI)
APS	Anterior Perforated Substance
BP	Basilar Pons
CC	Crus Cerebri
CP	Choroid Plexus
FacNr	Facial Nerve (Cranial Nerve VII)
Fl	Flocculus
GlNr	Glossopharyngeal Nerve (Cranial Nerve IX)
HyNr	Hypoglossal Nerve (Cranial Nerve XII)
Inf	Infundibulum
IntNr	Intermediate Nerve
IPF	Interpeduncular Fossa
LOlfS	Lateral Olfactory Stria
MB	Mammillary Body
MCP	Middle Cerebellar Peduncle (Brachium Pontis)
MOlfS	Medial Olfactory Stria
OcNr	Oculomotor Nerve (Cranial Nerve III)
Ol	Olive (Inferior)
OlfTr	Olfactory Tract
OpCh	Optic Chiasm
OpNr	Optic Nerve (Cranial Nerve II)
OpTr	Optic Tract
PHipGy	Parahippocampal Gyrus
PoOF	Postolivary Fissure
PrOF	Preolivary Fissure
Py	Pyramid
PyDec	Pyramidal Decussation
SpAcNr	Spinal Accessory Nerve (Cranial Nerve XI)
TriNr	Trigeminal Nerve (Cranial Nerve V)
TroNr	Trochlear Nerve (Cranial Nerve IV)
Un	Uncus
VagNr	Vagus Nerve (Cranial Nerve X)
VCNr	Vestibulocochlear Nerve (Cranial Nerve VIII)
VMF	Ventral Median Fissure

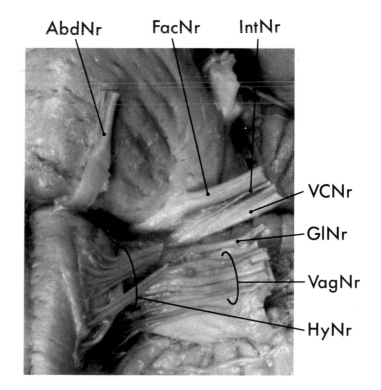

2–20 Cranial nerves at the pons-medulla junction showing the intermediate nerve located between facial and vestibulocochlear nerves. The intermediate nerve is, functionally, considered part of the VIIth (facial) nerve.

Vessels

Structures

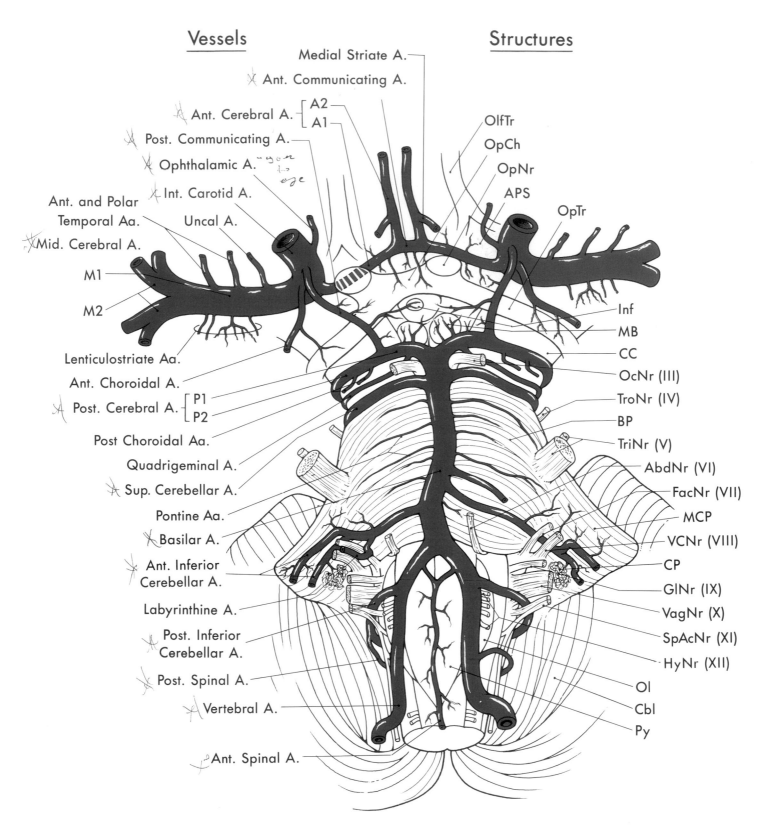

Medial Striate A.
Ant. Communicating A.
Ant. Cerebral A. — A2 / A1
Post. Communicating A.
Ophthalamic A. "ger to eye"
Int. Carotid A.
Ant. and Polar Temporal Aa.
Uncal A.
Mid. Cerebral A.
M1
M2
Lenticulostriate Aa.
Ant. Choroidal A.
Post. Cerebral A. — P1 / P2
Post Choroidal Aa.
Quadrigeminal A.
Sup. Cerebellar A.
Pontine Aa.
Basilar A.
Ant. Inferior Cerebellar A.
Labyrinthine A.
Post. Inferior Cerebellar A.
Post. Spinal A.
Vertebral A.
Ant. Spinal A.

OlfTr
OpCh
OpNr
APS
OpTr
Inf
MB
CC
OcNr (III)
TroNr (IV)
BP
TriNr (V)
AbdNr (VI)
FacNr (VII)
MCP
VCNr (VIII)
CP
GlNr (IX)
VagNr (X)
SpAcNr (XI)
HyNr (XII)
Ol
Cbl
Py

2–21 Ventral view of the brainstem showing the relationship of brain structures and cranial nerves to the arteries forming the vertebrobasilar system and the circle of Willis. The posterior spinal artery usually originates from the posterior inferior cerebellar artery (left), but it may arise from the vertebral (right). While the labyrinthine artery may occasionally branch from the basilar (right), it most frequently originates from the anterior inferior cerebellar artery (left). Many vessels that arise ventrally course around the brainstem to serve dorsal structures. The anterior cerebral artery consists of A_1 (between the internal carotid bifurcation and the anterior communicating artery) and A_2 (distal to the anterior communicator) segments. Lateral to the internal carotid bifurcation is the M_1 segment of the middle cerebral artery; M_2 indicates those more distal branches that serve the insular cortex and the lateral hemisphere surface. Between the basilar bifurcation and the posterior communicating artery is the P_1 segment of the posterior cerebral artery; P_2 is between the posterior communicator and the first temporal branches.

This view correlates with that of Figure 2–18 on p. 22.

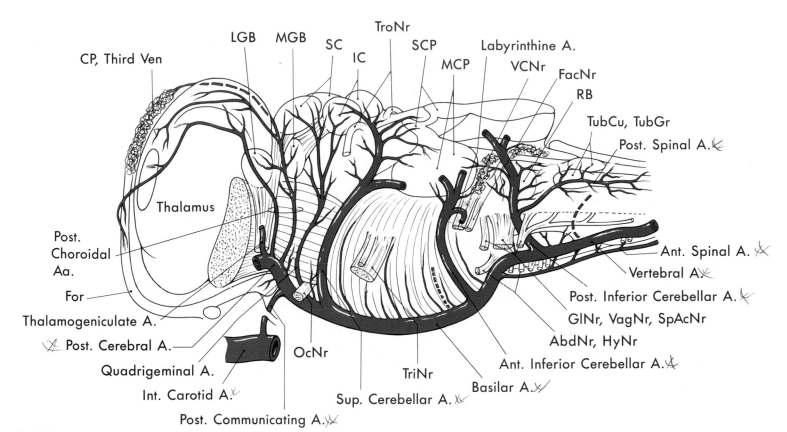

2–22   Lateral view of the brainstem and thalamus showing the relationship of structures and cranial nerves to arteries. Arteries that serve dorsal structures originate from ventrally located parent vessels. The approximate positions of the posterior spinal and labyrinthine arteries, when they originate from the vertebral and basilar arteries, respectively, are shown as dashed lines. This view and that in Figure 2–21 (left page) provide different perspectives on arteries that serve the brainstem. Abbreviations for both figures are listed below.

Abbreviations

A	Artery		**Ol**	Olive (Inferior)
Aa	Arteries		**OlfTr**	Olfactory Tract
AbdNr	Abducens Nerve (Cranial Nerve VI)		**OpCh**	Optic Chiasm
APS	Anterior Perforated Substance		**OpNr**	Optic Nerve (Cranial Nerve II)
BP	Basilar Pons		**OpTr**	Optic Tract
Cbl	Cerebellum		**Py**	Pyramid
CC	Crus Cerebri		**RB**	Restiform Body
CP	Choroid Plexus		**SC**	Superior Colliculus
FacNr	Facial Nerve (Cranial Nerve VII)		**SCP**	Superior Cerebellar Peduncle (Brachium Conjunctivum)
For	Fornix			
GlNr	Glossopharyngeal Nerve (Cranial Nerve IX)		**SpAcNr**	Spinal Accessory Nerve (Cranial Nerve XI)
HyNr	Hypoglossal Nerve (Cranial Nerve XII)		**TriNr**	Trigeminal Nerve (Cranial Nerve V)
IC	Inferior Colliculus		**TroNr**	Trochlear Nerve (Cranial Nerve IV)
Inf	Infundibulum		**TubCu**	Tuberculum Cuneatum (Cuneate Tubercle)
LGB	Lateral Geniculate Body			
LOlfS	Lateral Olfactory Stria		**TubGr**	Tuberculum Gracile (Gracile Tubercle)
MB	Mammillary Body		**VagNr**	Vagus Nerve (Cranial Nerve X)
MCP	Middle Cerebellar Peduncle (Brachium Pontis)		**VCNr**	Vestibulocochlear Nerve (Cranial Nerve VIII)
MGB	Medial Geniculate Body		**Ven**	Ventricle
OcNr	Oculomotor Nerve (Cranial Nerve III)			

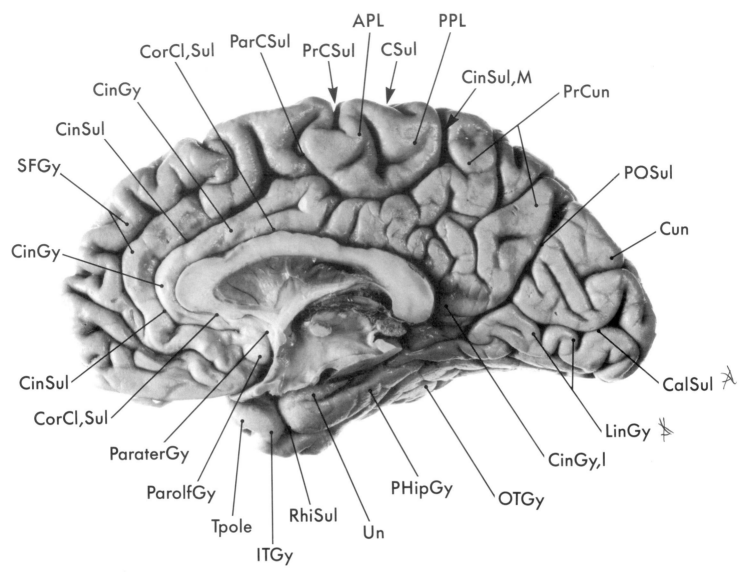

2–23   Mid-sagittal view of the right cerebral hemisphere and diencephalon, with brainstem removed, showing the principal gyri and sulci. For details of the diencephalon and brainstem see Figure 2–26 on page 29.

Abbreviations

APL	Anterior Paracentral Lobule	**ParolfGy**	Parolfactory Gyri
CalSul	Calcarine Sulcus	**ParaterGy**	Paraterminal Gyri
CinGy	Cingulate Gyrus	**ParCSul**	Paracentral Sulcus
CinGy, I	Cingulate Gyrus, Isthmus	**PHipGy**	Parahippocampal Gyrus
CinSul	Cingulate Sulcus	**POSul**	Parieto-occipital Sulcus
CinSul, M	Cingulate Sulcus, Marginal Branch	**PPL**	Posterior Paracentral Lobule
CorCl, Sul	Corpus Callosum, Sulcus	**PrCun**	Precuneus
CSul	Central Sulcus (of Rolando)	**PrCSul**	Precentral Sulcus
Cun	Cuneus	**RhiSul**	Rhinal Sulcus
ITGy	Inferior Temporal Gyrus	**SFGy**	Superior Frontal Gyrus
LinGy	Lingual Gyrus	**Tpole**	Temporal Pole
OTGy	Occipitotemporal Gyri	**Un**	Uncus

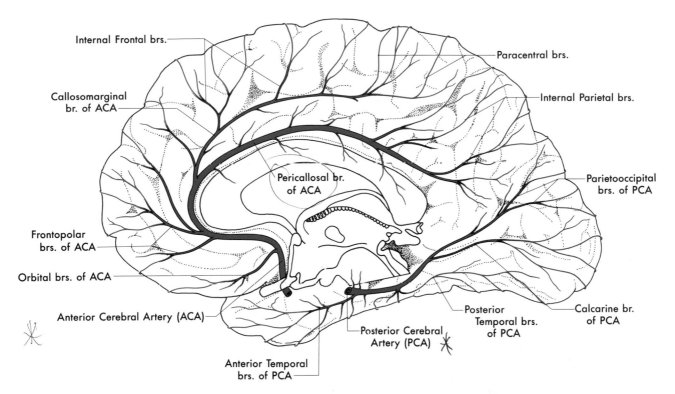

Internal Frontal brs.

Callosomarginal
br. of ACA

Pericallosal br.
of ACA

Frontopolar
brs. of ACA

Orbital brs. of ACA

Anterior Cerebral Artery (ACA)

Anterior Temporal
brs. of PCA

Posterior Cerebral
Artery (PCA)

Posterior
Temporal brs.
of PCA

Paracentral brs.

Internal Parietal brs.

Parietooccipital
brs. of PCA

Calcarine br.
of PCA

2–24 Mid-sagittal view of the cerebral hemisphere and diencephalon showing the locations and branching patterns of anterior and posterior cerebral arteries. The positions of gyri and sulci can be easily extrapolated from Figure 2–23 (facing page). Terminal branches of the anterior cerebral artery arch laterally over the edge of the hemisphere to serve medial aspects of the frontal and parietal lobes, while the same relationship is maintained for the occipital and temporal lobes by branches of the posterior cerebral artery.

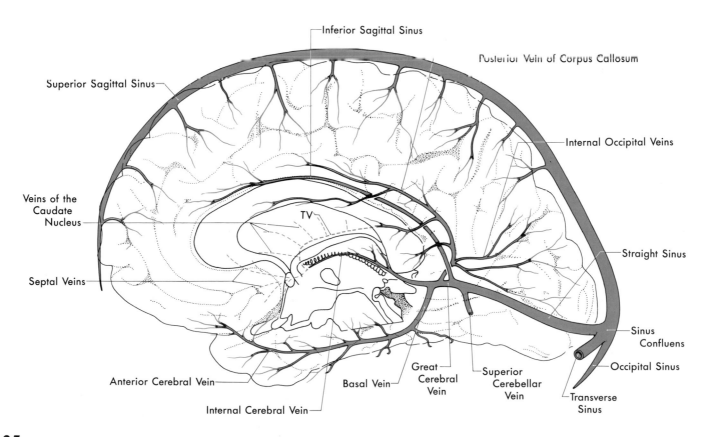

Inferior Sagittal Sinus

Posterior Vein of Corpus Callosum

Superior Sagittal Sinus

Internal Occipital Veins

Veins of the
Caudate
Nucleus

TV

Straight Sinus

Septal Veins

Sinus
Confluens

Anterior Cerebral Vein

Basal Vein

Great
Cerebral
Vein

Superior
Cerebellar
Vein

Occipital Sinus

Transverse
Sinus

Internal Cerebral Vein

2–25 Mid-sagittal view of the cerebral hemisphere and diencephalon showing the locations and relationships of sinuses and the locations and general branching patterns of veins. The position of gyri and sulci can be easily extrapolated from Figure 2–23 (facing page).

Abbreviation **TV** Terminal Vein

2–26 Details of the corpus callosum, diencephalon, brainstem, and adjacent structures as seen in a mid-sagittal view of the left side of the brain (upper) and in a normal magnetic resonance image (MRI) of the brain taken in the same orientation (lower). In this cardinal view of the brain, many of the structures labeled on the gross specimen can be easily identified in the MRI by comparing one with the other.

Abbreviations

AC	Anterior Commissure
AMV	Anterior Medullary Velum
BP	Basilar Pons
CA	Cerebral Aqueduct
Cbl	Cerebellum
CorCl, B	Corpus Callosum, Body
CorCl, G	Corpus Callosum, Genu
CorCl, R	Corpus Callosum, Rostrum
CorCl, Spl	Corpus Callosum, Splenium
CP	Choroid Plexus
DorTh	Dorsal Thalamus
For, B	Fornix, Body
For, Col	Fornix, Column
Hab	Habenula
HyTh	Hypothalamus
HyTh, Sul	Hypothalamic Sulcus
IC	Inferior Colliculus
IR	Infundibular Recess of Third Ventricle
LT	Lamina Terminalis
MB	Mammillary Body
MI	Massa Intermedia
OcNr	Oculomotor Nerve (Cranial Nerve III)
OpCh	Optic Chiasm
OpNr	Optic Nerve (Cranial Nervi II)
PC	Posterior Commissure
Pi	Pineal
PICA	Posterior Inferior Cerebellar Artery
Py	Pyramid
SC	Superior Colliculus
SMT	Stria Medullaris Thalami
SOR	Supraoptic Recess of Third Ventricle
Sep	Septum Pellucidum
SupCis	Superior Cistern
Ven	Ventricle

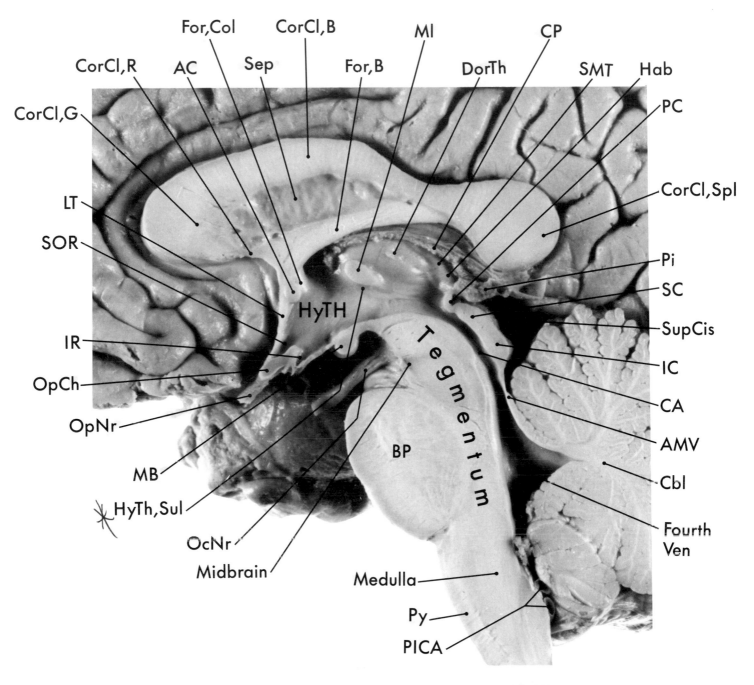

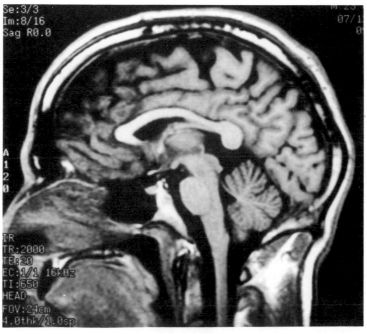

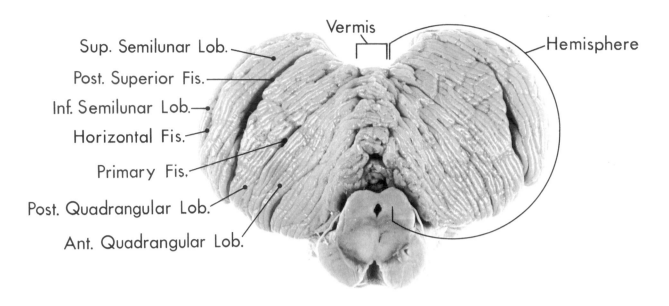

Vermis

Sup. Semilunar Lob.

Post. Superior Fis.

Inf. Semilunar Lob.

Horizontal Fis.

Primary Fis.

Post. Quadrangular Lob.

Ant. Quadrangular Lob.

Hemisphere

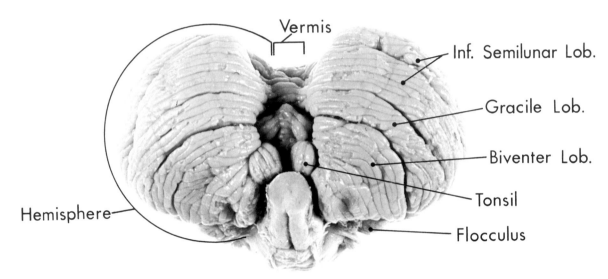

Vermis

Inf. Semilunar Lob.

Gracile Lob.

Biventer Lob.

Tonsil

Flocculus

Hemisphere

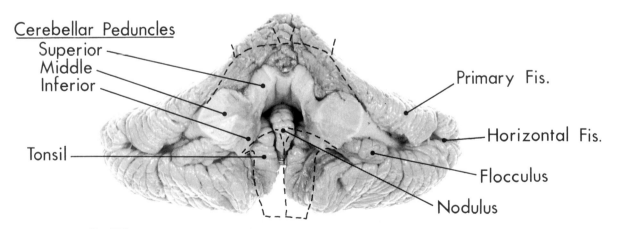

Cerebellar Peduncles

Superior

Middle

Inferior

Tonsil

Primary Fis.

Horizontal Fis.

Flocculus

Nodulus

2–27 Rostral (upper), caudal (middle), and ventral (lower, brain-stem removed) views of the cerebellum showing the hemisphere, vermis, and main lobules and fissures. Note the relative positions of the midbrain, pons, and medulla on the upper and middle photographs. The approximate positions of the medulla and pons are superimposed (dashed lines) on the ventral view. See Figure 2–30 on page 32 for the dorsal view of the brainstem, which correlates with the ventral view of the cerebellum.

Abbreviations   **Fis** Fissure **Lob** Lobule

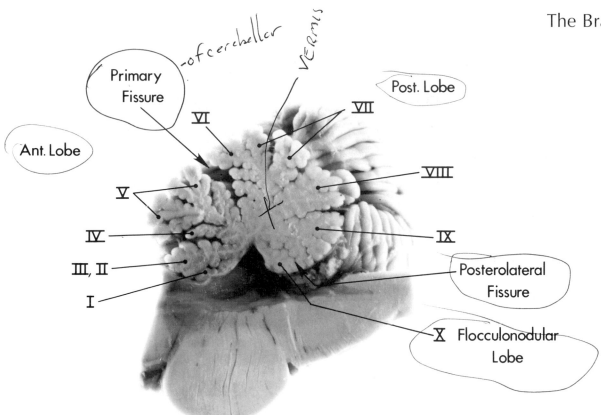

Primary Fissure

-of cerebellar

VERMIS

Post. Lobe

Ant. Lobe

VI

VII

VIII

V

IV

IX

III, II

I

Posterolateral Fissure

X Flocculonodular Lobe

2–28   Mid-sagittal view of the cerebellum showing the three main fissures and the vermis portion of the ten lobules. Designation of lobules after Larsell. Lobules I–V are the vermis parts of the anterior lobe, lobules VI–IX are the vermis parts of the posterior lobe, and lobule X (the nodulus) is the vermis part of the flocculonodular lobe.

Lobule Designations

I	lingual
II, III	central lobule
IV, V	culmen
VI	declive
VII	folium and tuber vermis
VIII	pyramis
IX	uvula
X	nodulus

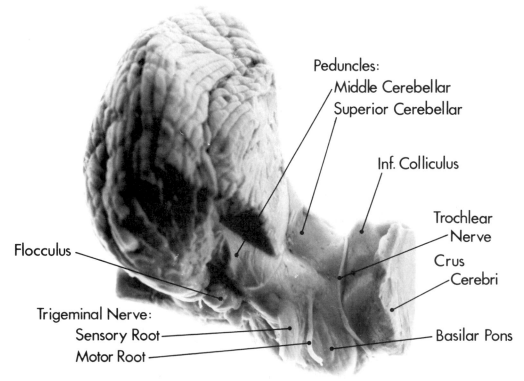

Peduncles:
Middle Cerebellar
Superior Cerebellar

Inf. Colliculus

Trochlear Nerve

Crus Cerebri

Flocculus

Trigeminal Nerve:
Sensory Root
Motor Root

Basilar Pons

2–29   Lateral and slightly rostral view of the cerebellum and brainstem with the middle and superior cerebellar peduncles exposed. Note the relationship of the trochlear nerve to the inferior colliculus and the relative positions of, and distinction between, motor and sensory roots of the trigeminal nerve.

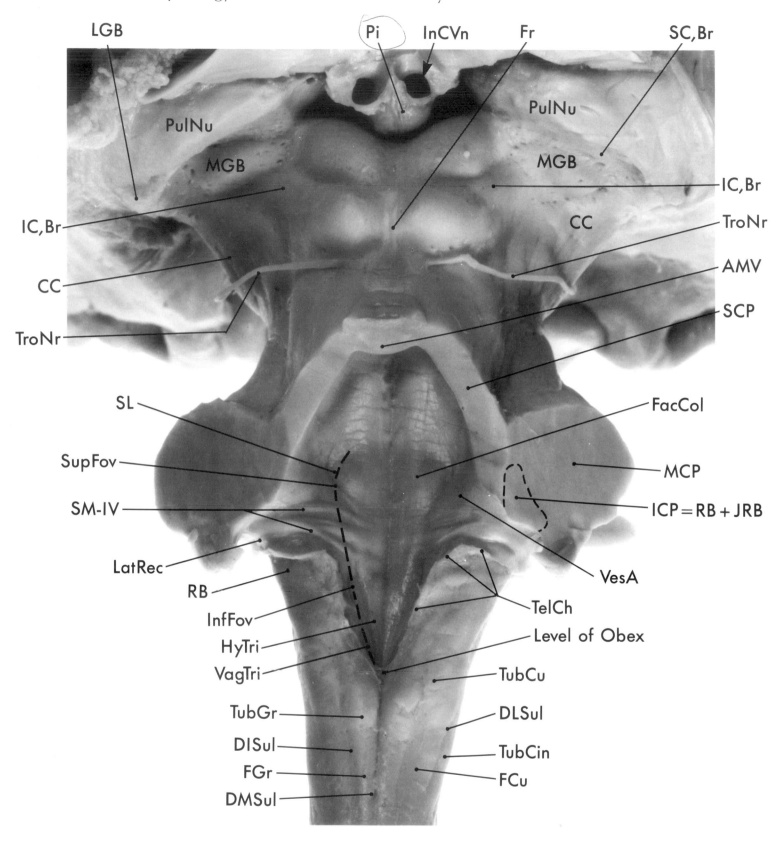

2–30 Detailed dorsal view of the brainstem, with cerebellum removed, providing a clear view of the rhomboid fossa and contiguous
parts of the caudal diencephalon. Figure 3–10 on page 43 also shows
a dorsal view of the brainstem and the caudal diencephalon.

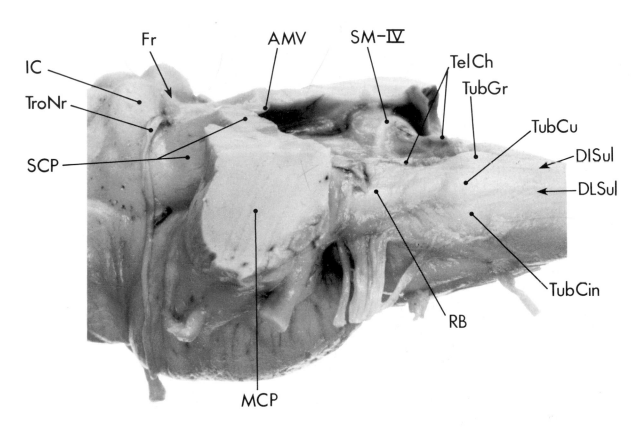

2–31 Lateral view of the left side of the brainstem showing a different perspective on many of those structures labeled in Figure 2–30 (left page). Abbreviations for both are listed below.

Abbreviations

AMV	Anterior Medullary Velum	**Pi**	Pineal
CC	Crus Cerebri	**PulNu**	Pulvinar Nuclear Complex
DISul	Dorsal Intermediate Sulcus	**RB**	Restiform Body (+ Juxtarestiform Body = Inferior Cerebellar Peduncle)
DLSul	Dorsolateral Sulcus		
DMSul	Dorsomedial Sulcus	**SC**	Superior Colliculus
FacCol	Facial Colliculus	**SC, Br**	Superior Colliculus, Brachium
FCu	Cuneate Fasciculus	**SCP**	Superior Cerebellar Peduncle (Brachium Conjunctivum)
FGr	Gracile Fasciculus		
Fr	Frenulum	**SL**	Sulcus Limitans
GlNr	Glossopharyngeal Nerve (Cranial Nerve IX)	**SM-IV**	Striae Medullares of Fourth Ventricle
HyTri	Hypoglossal Trigone	**SpAcNr**	Spinal Accessory Nerve (Cranial Nerve XI)
IC	Inferior Colliculus	**SupFov**	Superior Fovea
IC, Br	Inferior Colliculus, Branchium	**TelCh**	Tela Choroidea (cut edge is labeled)
ICP	Inferior Cerebellar Peduncle	**TroNr**	Trochlear Nerve (Cranial Nerve IV)
InCVn	Internal Cerebral Vein	**TubCin**	Tuberculum Cinerum
InfFov	Inferior Fovea	**TubCu**	Tuberculum Cuneatum (Cuneate Tubercle)
JRB	Juxtarestiform Body	**TubGr**	Tuberculum Gracile (Gracile Tubercle)
LatRec	Lateral Recess of Fourth Ventricle	**VagNr**	Vagus Nerve (Cranial Nerve X)
LGB	Lateral Geniculate Body	**VagTri**	Vagal Trigone
MCP	Middle Cerebellar Peduncle (Brachium Pontis)	**VesA**	Vestibular Area
MGB	Medial Geniculate Body		

Vessels

Structures

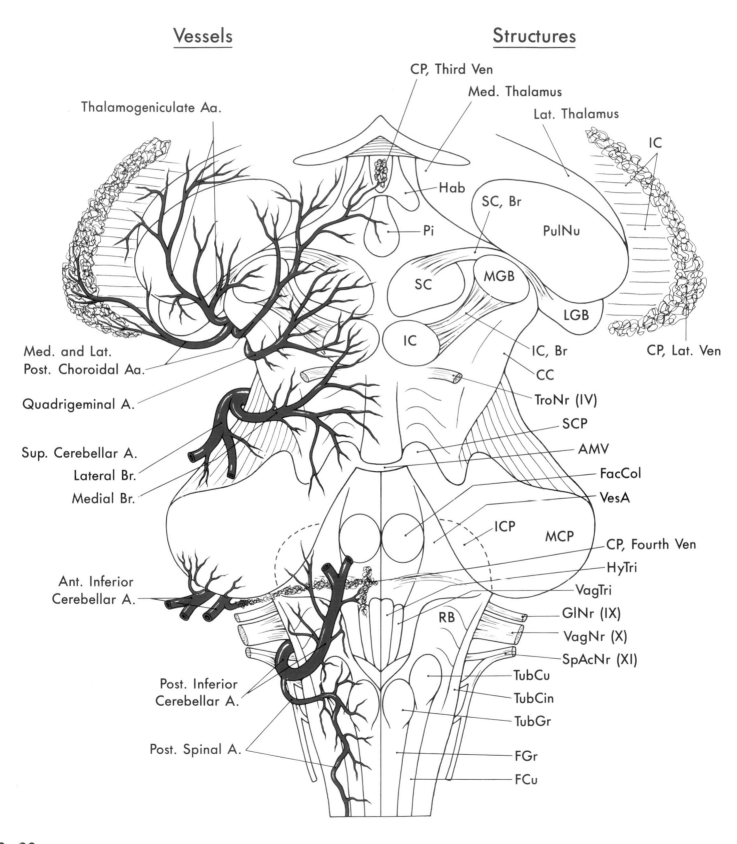

CP, Third Ven

Med. Thalamus

Lat. Thalamus

IC

Thalamogeniculate Aa.

Hab

SC, Br

PulNu

Pi

SC

MGB

LGB

IC

CP, Lat. Ven

Med. and Lat.
Post. Choroidal Aa.

IC, Br

CC

Quadrigeminal A.

TroNr (IV)

SCP

Sup. Cerebellar A.

AMV

Lateral Br.

FacCol

Medial Br.

VesA

ICP

MCP

CP, Fourth Ven

HyTri

VagTri

Ant. Inferior
Cerebellar A.

GlNr (IX)

RB

VagNr (X)

SpAcNr (XI)

TubCu

Post. Inferior
Cerebellar A.

TubCin

TubGr

Post. Spinal A.

FGr

FCu

2–32 Dorsal view of the brainstem and caudal diencephalon showing the relationship of structures and some of the cranial nerves to arteries. The vessels shown in this view (compare with figure on facing page) have originated ventrally and essentially wrapped around the brainstem to gain their dorsal positions. In addition to serving the medulla, branches of the posterior inferior cerebellar artery also supply the choroid plexus of the fourth ventricle. This view correlates with that of Figure 2–30 on p. 32.

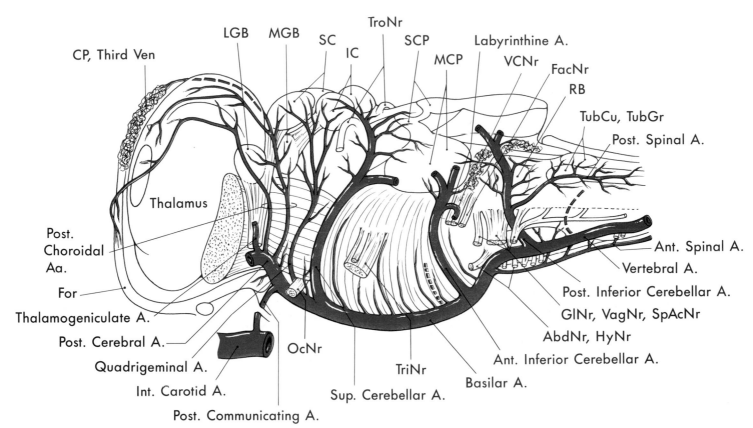

CP, Third Ven · LGB · MGB · SC · IC · TroNr · SCP · MCP · Labyrinthine A. · VCNr · FacNr · RB · TubCu, TubGr · Post. Spinal A. · Thalamus · Post. Choroidal Aa. · For · Thalamogeniculate A. · Post. Cerebral A. · Quadrigeminal A. · Int. Carotid A. · Post. Communicating A. · OcNr · TriNr · Sup. Cerebellar A. · Basilar A. · Ant. Inferior Cerebellar A. · AbdNr, HyNr · GlNr, VagNr, SpAcNr · Post. Inferior Cerebellar A. · Vertebral A. · Ant. Spinal A.

2–33 Lateral view of the brainstem and thalamus showing the relationship of structures and cranial nerves to arteries. The approximate positions of the labyrinthine and posterior spinal arteries, when they originate from the basilar and vertebral arteries, respectively, are shown as dashed lines. Arteries that distribute to dorsal structures originate from large ventral vessels. This view and that in Figure 2–32 (left page) provide different perspectives on arteries that serve the brainstem. Abbreviations for both figures are listed below.

Abbreviations

A	Artery
Aa	Arteries
AbdNr	Abducens Nerve (Cranial Nerve VI)
AMV	Anterior Medullary Velum
CC	Crus Cerebri
CP	Choroid Plexus
FacCol	Facial Colliculus
FacNr	Facial Nerve (Cranial Nerve VII)
FCu	Cuneate Fasciculus
FGr	Gracile Fasciculus
For	Fornix
GlNr	Glossopharyngeal Nerve (Cranial Nerve IX)
Hab	Habenula
HyNr	Hypoglossal Nerve (Cranial Nerve XII)
HyTri	Hypoglossal Trigone
IC	Inferior Colliculus
IC, Br	Inferior Colliculus, Brachium
ICP	Inferior Cerebellar Peduncle (= Restiform Body + Juxtarestiform Body)
LGB	Lateral Geniculate Body
MCP	Middle Cerebellar Peduncle (Brachium Pontis)
MGB	Medial Geniculate Body
OcNr	Oculomotor Nerve (Cranial Nerve III)
Pi	Pineal
PulNu	Pulvinar Nuclear Complex
RB	Restiform Body (+ Juxtarestiform Body = Inferior Cerebellar Peduncle)
SC	Superior Colliculus
SC, Br	Superior Colliculus, Brachium
SCP	Superior Cerebellar Peduncle (Brachium Conjunctivum)
SpAcNr	Spinal Accessory Nerve (Cranial Nerve XI)
TriNr	Trigeminal Nerve (Cranial Nerve V)
TroNr	Trochlear Nerve (Cranial Nerve IV)
TubCin	Tuberculum Cinerum
TubCu	Tuberculum Cuneatum (Cuneate Tubercle)
TubGr	Tuberculum Gracile (Gracile Tubercle)
VagNr	Vagus Nerve (Cranial Nerve X)
VagTri	Vagal Trigone
VcNr	Vestibulocochlear Nerve (Cranial Nerve VIII)
Ven	Ventricle
VesA	Vestibular Area

Chapter 3

Dissections of the
Central Nervous System

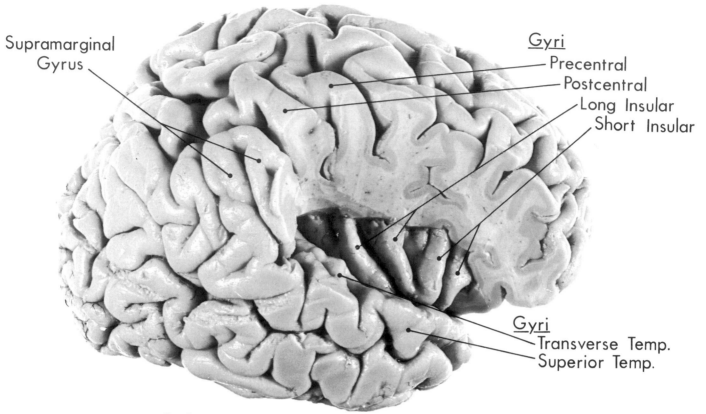

Supramarginal
Gyrus

<u>Gyri</u>
Precentral
Postcentral
Long Insular
Short Insular

<u>Gyri</u>
Transverse Temp.
Superior Temp.

3–1 Lateral view of the right cerebral hemisphere with the inferior and parts of the middle frontal gyri and pre- and post-central gyri removed to show the insular cortex, transverse temporal gyri, and related structures.

Abbreviation: **Temp** Temporal

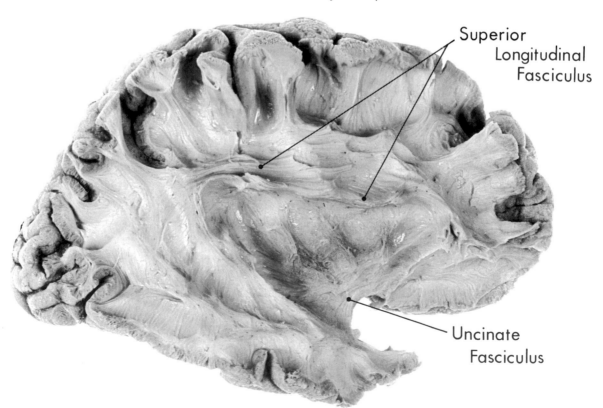

Superior
Longitudinal
Fasciculus

Uncinate
Fasciculus

3–2 Dissected view of the lateral aspect of the right cerebral hemisphere showing the locations and relationships of some of the main bundles of subcortical white matter. This dissection is deep to that shown in Figure 3-1 and superficial to that shown in Figure 3-3.

Superior
Longitudinal
Fasciculus

Corona Radiata

Lenticular
Nucleus

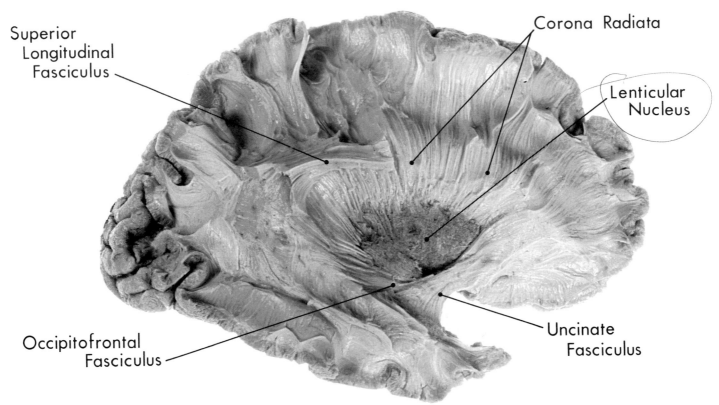

Occipitofrontal
Fasciculus

Uncinate
Fasciculus

3–3 Dissected view of the lateral aspect of the right cerebral hemisphere showing the relationship between fibers (corona radiata) radiating from the internal capsule and those of the superior longitudinal fasciculus. The lenticular nucleus is shown *in situ* lateral to the internal capsule. This is a deeper dissection of the specimen shown in Figure 3–2.

Internal Capsule (IC)
Posterior Limb
Genu
Anterior Limb

Optic
Radiations

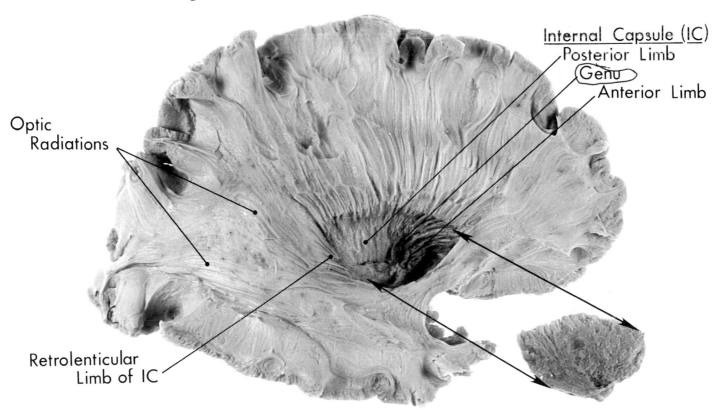

Retrolenticular
Limb of IC

3–4 Dissected view of the lateral aspect of the right cerebral hemisphere showing the internal capsule and the concavity left by removal of the lenticular nucleus. Note the other bundles of subcortical white matter. This is a deeper dissection of the specimen shown in Figure 3-3.

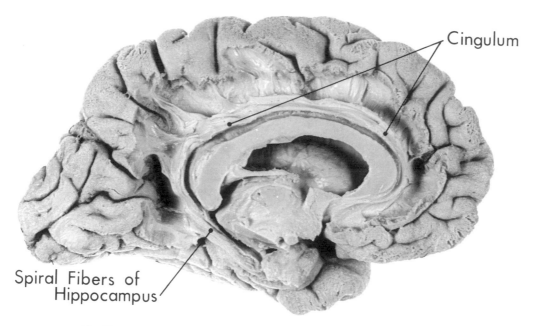

Cingulum

Spiral Fibers of
Hippocampus

3–5 Dissected view of the medial aspect of the left cerebral hemisphere showing the cingulum and spiral fibers of the hippocampus.

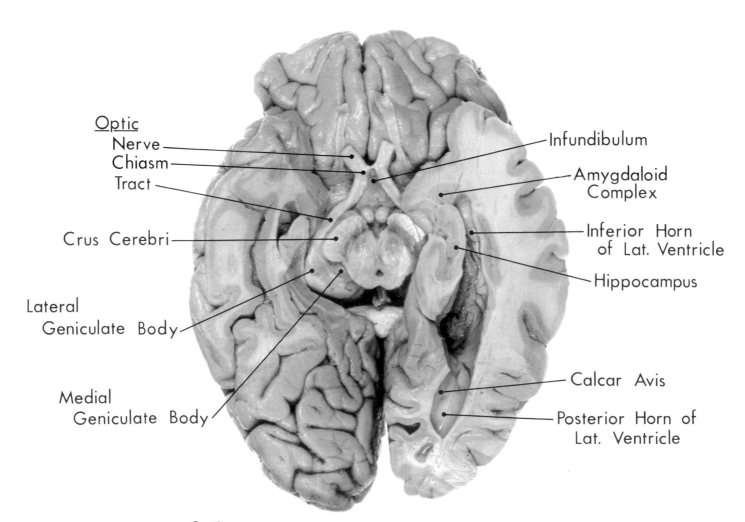

Optic
  Nerve
  Chiasm
  Tract

Crus Cerebri

Lateral
Geniculate Body

Medial
Geniculate Body

Infundibulum

Amygdaloid
Complex

Inferior Horn
of Lat. Ventricle

Hippocampus

Calcar Avis

Posterior Horn of
Lat. Ventricle

3–6 Overview of a dissection showing the ventral aspect of the cerebral hemispheres. Note the structures related to ventricular spaces and the structures located at the mesencephalon-diencephalon interface. A number of structures in addition to those labeled can be identified.

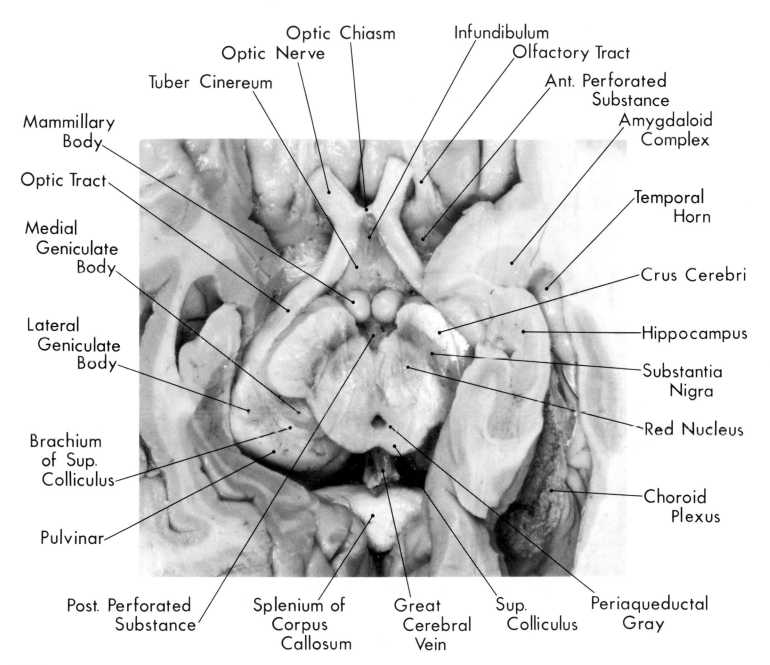

Optic Chiasm

Optic Nerve

Infundibulum

Olfactory Tract

Tuber Cinereum

Ant. Perforated
Substance

Mammillary
Body

Amygdaloid
Complex

Optic Tract

Temporal
Horn

Medial
Geniculate
Body

Crus Cerebri

Lateral
Geniculate
Body

Hippocampus

Substantia
Nigra

Brachium
of Sup.
Colliculus

Red Nucleus

Pulvinar

Choroid
Plexus

Post. Perforated
Substance

Splenium of
Corpus
Callosum

Great
Cerebral
Vein

Sup.
Colliculus

Periaqueductal
Gray

3–7 Detailed view of a dissection showing the ventral aspects of the cerebral hemispheres; this is of the same specimen shown in Figure 3-6. Note the continuum of optic nerve, chiasm, and tract to the lateral geniculate body, the relationship of the optic tract to the crus cerebri, and the relationship of hypothalamic structures on the ventral aspect of the brain. Other structures in addition to those labeled can be identified.

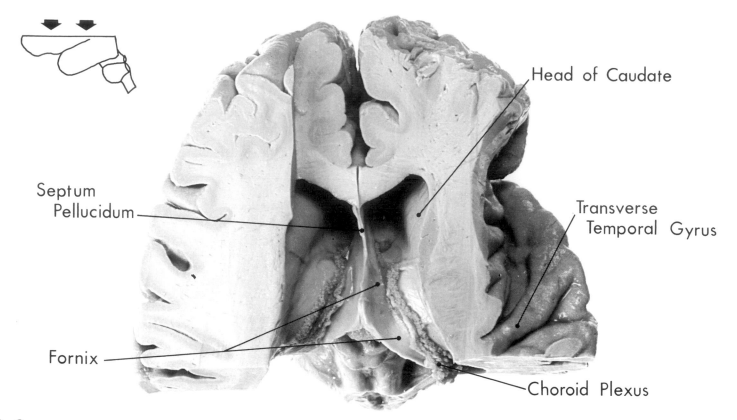

Septum
Pellucidum

Fornix

Head of Caudate

Transverse
Temporal Gyrus

Choroid Plexus

3-8 Dissected view of the brain from the dorsal aspect showing structures associated with the lateral ventricles. Note the appearance of insular and transverse temporal gyri, the fornix, and other structures in addition to those labeled.

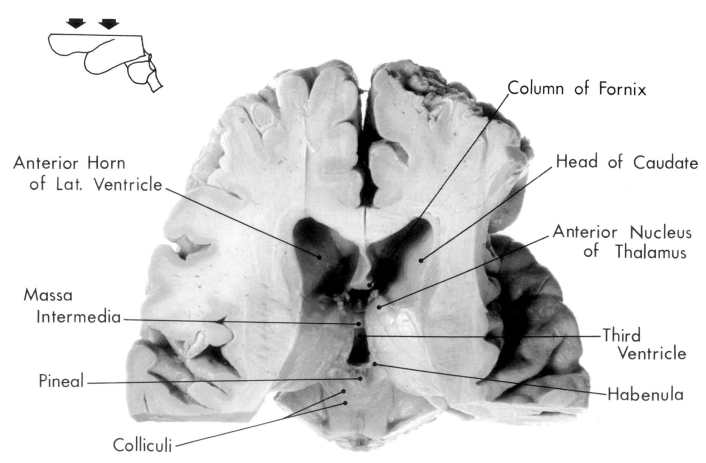

Anterior Horn
of Lat. Ventricle

Massa
Intermedia

Pineal

Colliculi

Column of Fornix

Head of Caudate

Anterior Nucleus
of Thalamus

Third
Ventricle

Habenula

3-9 Dissected view of the brain from the dorsal aspect, showing lateral and third ventricles, the dorsal surface of the diencephalon, the insula and transverse temporal gyri, and the colliculi. The majority of the fornix and the roof of the third ventricle have been removed. The small tufts of choroid plexus identify locations of the interventricular foramina. Note the massa intermedia traversing the third ventricle and other structures in addition to those labeled.

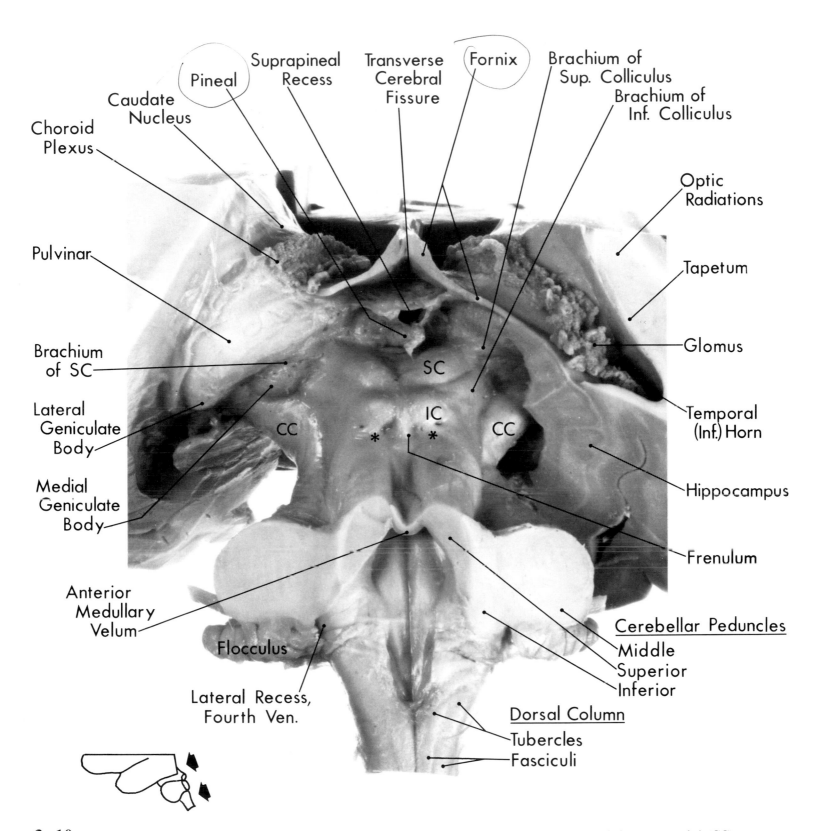

Choroid Plexus

Caudate Nucleus

Pineal

Suprapineal Recess

Transverse Cerebral Fissure

Fornix

Brachium of Sup. Colliculus

Brachium of Inf. Colliculus

Optic Radiations

Pulvinar

Tapetum

Brachium of SC

Glomus

SC

Lateral Geniculate Body

IC

CC

CC

Temporal (Inf.) Horn

Medial Geniculate Body

*   *

Hippocampus

Anterior Medullary Velum

Frenulum

Flocculus

Cerebellar Peduncles
Middle
Superior
Inferior

Lateral Recess, Fourth Ven.

Dorsal Column
Tubercles
Fasciculi

3–10 A dissected view showing caudal diencephalic structures, some telencephalic structures, and the interface of the mesencephalon with caudal parts of the thalamus. On the right side note the continuation between the fornix and hippocampus; on the left these structures have been removed to expose the underlying pulvinar. The superior (SC) and inferior (IC) colliculi and the crus cerebri (CC), as seen from the dorsal aspect, are indicated. The asterisks represent the exit points of the trochlear nerves. For further details of the dorsal brainstem see Figure 2-30 on page 32. Note structures in addition to those labeled.

Chapter 4

Meninges, Ventricles,
and Internal Morphology
of the Brain Dissections
of the Central Nervous System

Comparison of Cerebral versus Spinal Meninges

Cerebral	Spinal
Dura	Dura
adherent to inner table of skull	separated from vertebrae by epidural space
composed of 2 fused layers (periosteal and meningeal) which split to form sinuses	composed of one layer (spinal dura only; vertebrae have their own periosteum)
Arachnoid	Arachnoid
attached to dura in living condition (no subdural space)	attached to dura in living condition (no subdural space)
arachnoid villi (in superior sagittal sinus)	no arachnoid villi
arachnoid trabeculae	arachnoid trabeculae
subarachnoid space with several cisterns	subarachnoid space with one cistern
Pia	Pia
intimately adherent to surface of brain	intimately adherent to surface of cord
no pial specializations	specializations in the form of denticulate ligaments, filum terminale, and linea splendens
follows vessels as they pierce the cerebral cortex	follows vessels as they pierce the cord

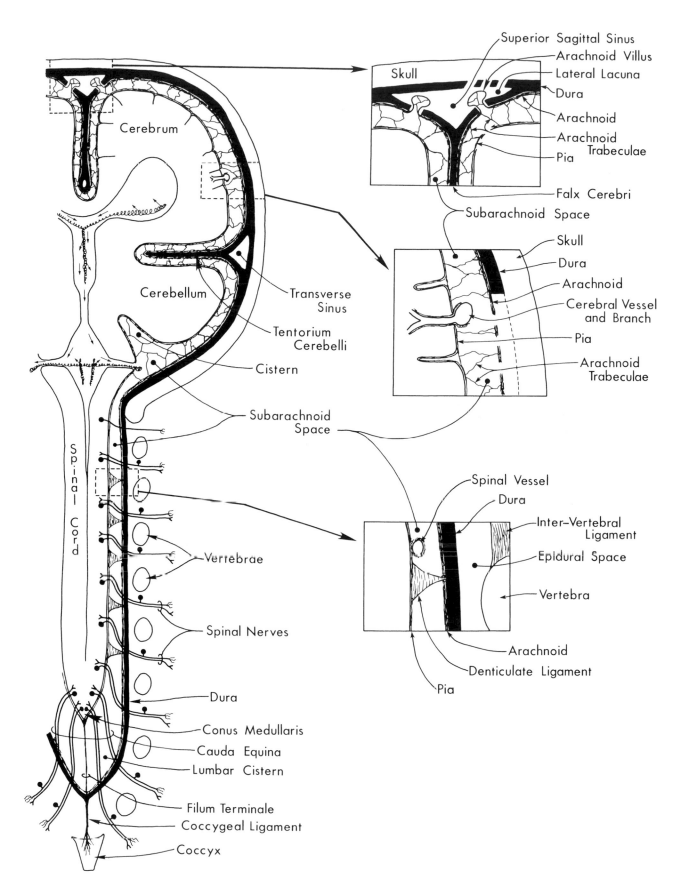

4–1   Semi-diagrammatic representation of the central nervous system and associated meninges. The detail drawings show the relationships of the meninges in the area of the superior sagittal sinus, on the lateral aspect of the cerebral hemisphere, and around the spinal cord. Cerebrospinal fluid is produced by the choroid plexi of lateral, third, and fourth ventricles. It circulates through the ventricular system (small arrows) and enters the subarachnoid space via the medial foramen of Magendie and the two lateral foramina of Luschka. In the living situation the arachnoid is attached to the inner surface of the dura. There is no *actual* or *potential* subdural space.

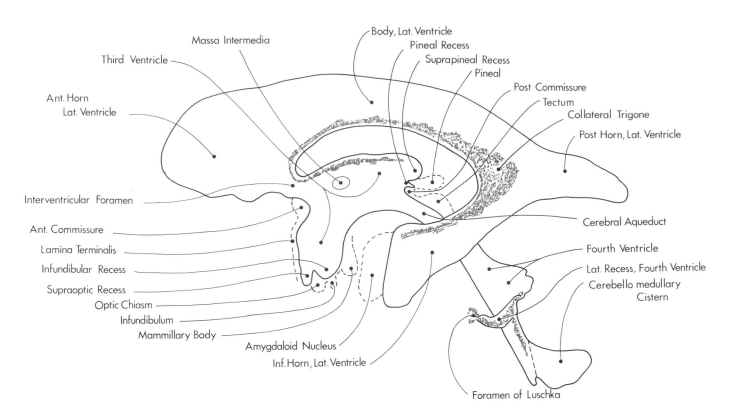

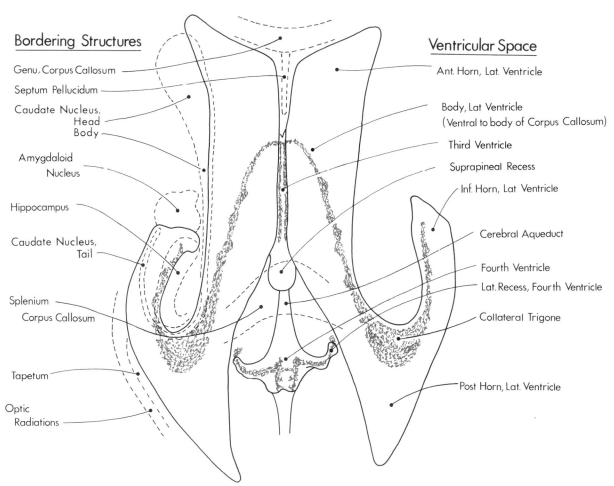

Bordering Structures

- Genu, Corpus Callosum
- Septum Pellucidum
- Caudate Nucleus, Head Body
- Amygdaloid Nucleus
- Hippocampus
- Caudate Nucleus, Tail
- Splenium Corpus Callosum
- Tapetum
- Optic Radiations

Ventricular Space

- Ant. Horn, Lat. Ventricle
- Body, Lat Ventricle (Ventral to body of Corpus Callosum)
- Third Ventricle
- Suprapineal Recess
- Inf. Horn, Lat Ventricle
- Cerebral Aqueduct
- Fourth Ventricle
- Lat. Recess, Fourth Ventricle
- Collateral Trigone
- Post Horn, Lat. Ventricle

4–2 Lateral (above) and dorsal (below) views of the ventricles and the choroid plexus (shown in red). The dashed lines show the approximate positions of some of the important structures that border on the ventricular space. Note the relationships between the choroid plexus and various parts of the ventricular system. The large expanded portion of the choroid plexus found in the area of the collateral trigone is the glomus (glomus choroideum).

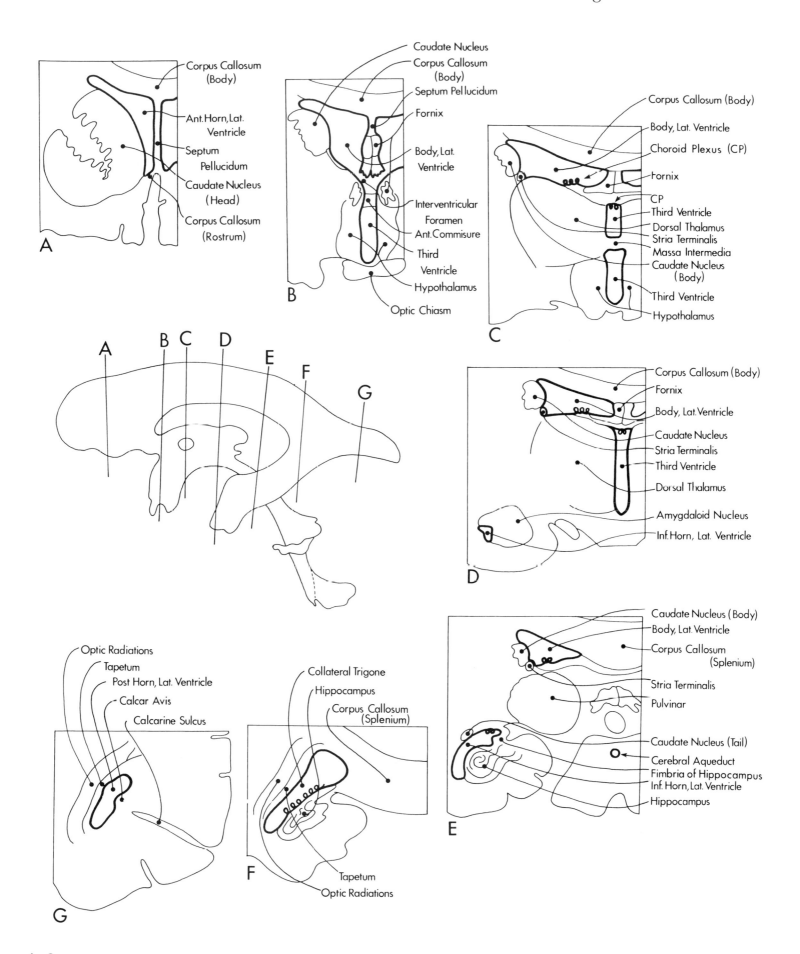

4–3 Lateral view of the ventricular system from rostral (A) to caudal (G) and corresponding semi-diagrammatic cross-sectional representations identifying specific structures that border on the ventricular space. In the cross-sections, the ventricle is outlined by a heavy line, and the majority of structures labeled have some direct relevance to the ventricular space at that particular level.

Figures:

4-13 4-12 4-11 4-10 4-9 4-8 4-7 4-6 4-5

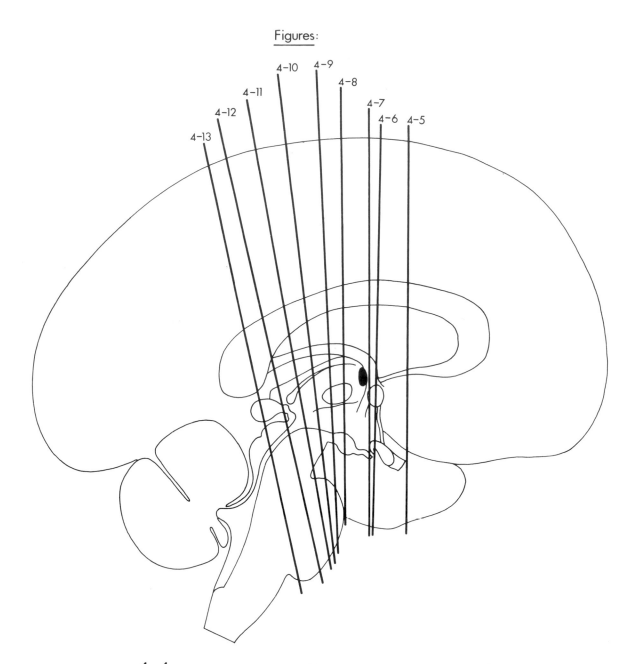

4–4 Mid-sagittal drawing of brain showing the planes of section for all coronal slices. The orientation of these slices is, in general, markedly similar to that seen in magnetic resonance imaging (MRI) and computerized tomography (CT) images when made in the coronal plane. Because a slice of brain has thickness and therefore dimension, the figure description for each coronal level specifies whether one is viewing the rostral or caudal surface of the slice. In addition, important landmarks that help to identify the level of the section appear in italics in the figure description.

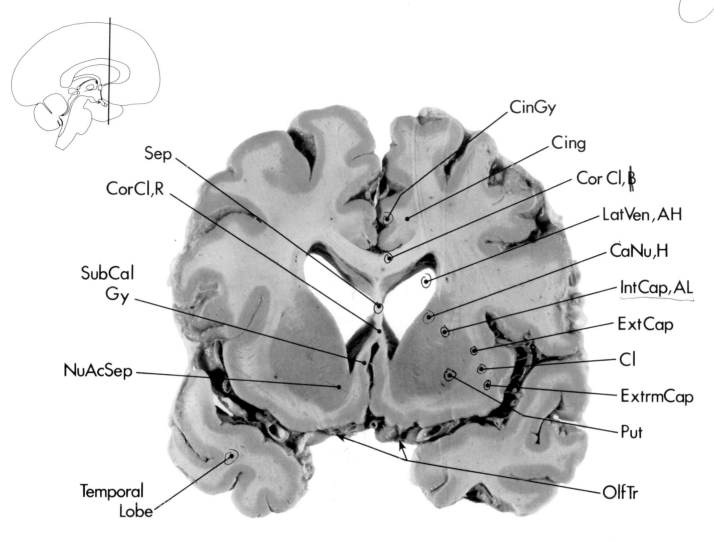

4–5 The caudal surface of a coronal section of brain through the *anterior limb of the internal capsule* and the *head of the caudate nucleus.*

Abbreviations

⌒CaNu,H	Caudate Nucleus, Head
Cing	Cingulum
CinGy	Cingulate Gyrus
⌒Cl	Claustrum
⌒CorCl,B	Corpus Callosum, Body
CorCl,R	Corpus Callosum, Rostrum
⌒ExtCap	External Capsule
⌒ExtrmCap	Extreme Capsule
⌒IntCap,AL	Internal Capsule, Anterior Limb
⌒LatVen,AH	Lateral Ventricle, Anterior Horn
NuAcSep	Nucleus Accumbens Septi
OlfTr	Olfactory Tract
⌒Put	Putamen
⌣Sep	Septum Pellucidum
SubCalGy	Subcallosal Gyrus

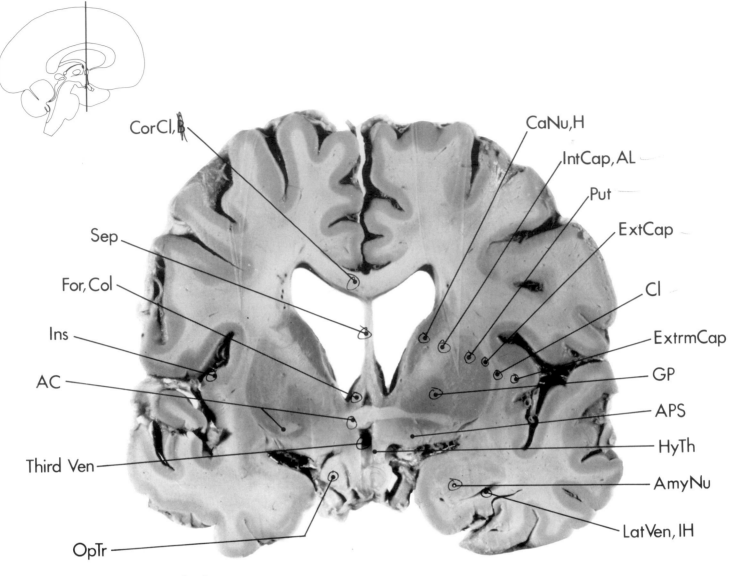

4–6 The caudal surface of a coronal section of brain through the level of the *anterior commissure*.

Abbreviations

AC	Anterior Commissure
AmyNu	Amygdaloid Nucleus (Complex)
APS	Anterior Perforated Substance
CaNu,H	Caudate Nucleus, Head
Cl	Claustrum
CorCl,B	Corpus Callosum, Body
ExtCap	External Capsule
ExtrmCap	Extreme Capsule
For,Col	Fornix, Column
GP	Globus Pallidus
HyTh	Hypothalamus
Ins	Insula
IntCap,AL	Internal Capsule, Anterior Limb Genu
LatVen,IH	Lateral Ventricle, Inferior Horn
OpTr	Optic Tract
Put	Putamen
Sep	Septum Pellucidum
Ven	Ventricle

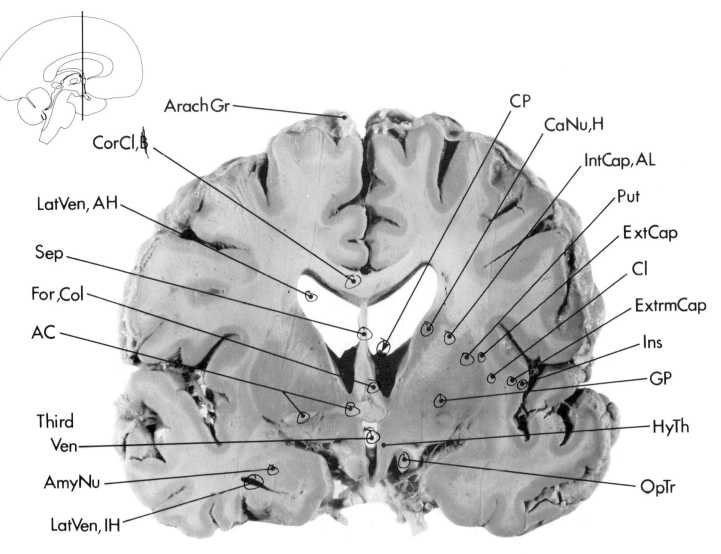

ArachGr

CP

CaNu,H

IntCap,AL

Put

ExtCap

Cl

ExtrmCap

Ins

GP

HyTh

OpTr

CorCl,B

LatVen,AH

Sep

For,Col

AC

Third
Ven

AmyNu

LatVen,IH

4–7 The rostral surface of a coronal section of brain through the level of the *anterior commissure* just rostral to the genu of internal capsule.

Abbreviations

AC	Anterior Commissure
AmyNu	Amygdaloid Nucleus (Complex)
ArachGr	Arachnoid Granulations
CaNu,H	Caudate Nucleus, Head
Cl	Claustrum
CorCl,B	Corpus Callosum, Body
CP	Choroid Plexus
ExtCap	External Capsule
ExtrmCap	Extreme Capsule
For,Col	Fornix, Column
GP	Globus Pallidus
HyTh	Hypothalamus
Ins	Insula
IntCap,AL	Internal Capsule, ~~Anterior Limb~~ Genu .
LatVen,AH	Lateral Ventricle, Anterior Horn
LatVen,IH	Lateral Ventricle, Inferior Horn
OpTr	Optic Tract
Put	Putamen
Sep	Septum Pellucidum
Ven	Ventricle

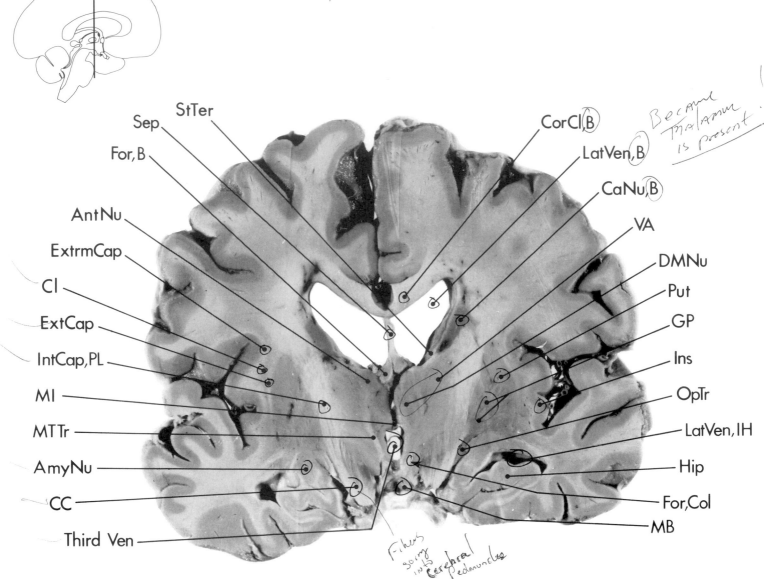

Sep

StTer

For,B

AntNu

ExtrmCap

Cl

ExtCap

IntCap,PL

MI

MTTr

AmyNu

CC

Third Ven

CorCl,B

LatVen,B

Become Thalamus is present

CaNu,B

VA

DMNu

Put

GP

Ins

OpTr

LatVen,IH

Hip

For,Col

MB

Fibers going into Cerebral peduncles

4–8 The caudal surface of a section of brain through the *anterior nucleus of the thalamus, mamillothalamic tract,* and the rostral portion of the *crus cerebri.*

Abbreviations

AmyNu	Amygdaloid Nucleus (Complex)	**Ins**	Insula
AntNu	Anterior Nucleus of Thalamus	**IntCap,PL**	Internal Capsule, Posterior Limb
CaNu,B	Caudate Nucleus, Body	**LatVen,B**	Lateral Ventricle, Body
CC	Crus Cerebri	**LatVen,IH**	Lateral Ventricle, Inferior Horn
Cl	Claustrum	**MB**	Mammillary Body
CorCl,B	Corpus Callosum, Body	**MI**	Massa Intermedia
DMNu	Dorsomedial Nucleus of Thalamus	**MTTr**	Mammillothalamic Tract
ExtCap	External Capsule	**OpTr**	Optic Tract
ExtrmCap	Extreme Capsule	**Put**	Putamen
For,B	Fornix, Body	**Sep**	Septum Pellucidum
For,Col	Fornix, Column	**StTer**	Stria Terminalis
GP	Globus Pallidus	**VA**	Ventral Anterior Nucleus of Thalamus
Hip	Hippocampal Formation	**Ven**	Ventricle

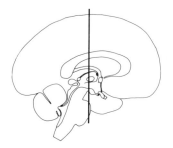

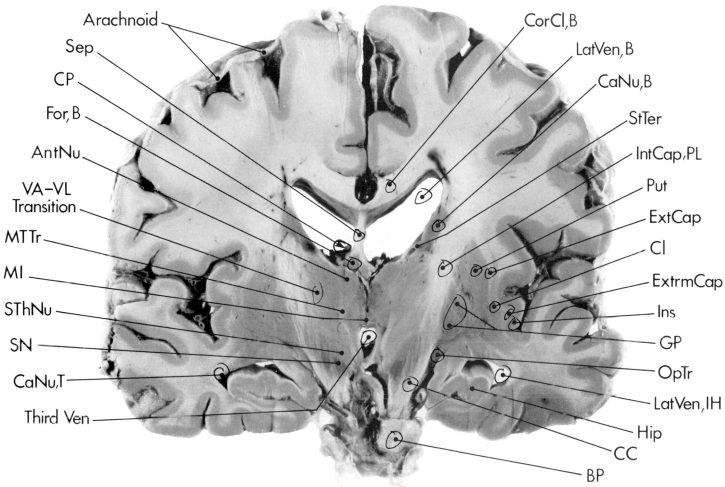

Arachnoid

Sep

CP

For, B

AntNu

VA–VL
Transition

MTTr

MI

SThNu

SN

CaNu,T

Third Ven

CorCl,B

LatVen,B

CaNu,B

StTer

IntCap,PL

Put

ExtCap

Cl

ExtrmCap

Ins

GP

OpTr

LatVen,IH

Hip

CC

BP

4–9 The rostral surface of a coronal section of brain through caudal parts of the *anterior nucleus*, the *massa intermedia*, and the *subthalamic nucleus*.

Abbreviations

AntNu	Anterior Nucleus of Thalamus	**LatVen,B**	Lateral Ventricle, Body
BP	Basilar Pons	**LatVen,IH**	Lateral Ventricle, Inferior Horn
CaNu,B	Caudate Nucleus, Body	**MI**	Massa Intermedia
CaNu,T	Caudate Nucleus, Tail	**MTTr**	Mammillothalamic Tract
CC	Crus Cerebri	**OpTr**	Optic Tract
Cl	Claustrum	**Put**	Putamen
CorCl,B	Corpus Callosum, Body	**Sep**	Septum Pellucidum
CP	Choroid Plexus	**SN**	Substantia Nigra
ExtCap	External Capsule	**SThNu**	Subthalamic Nucleus
ExtrmCap	Extreme Capsule	**StTer**	Stria Terminalis
For,B	Fornix, Body	**VA**	Ventral Anterior Nucleus of Thalamus
GP	Globus Pallidus		
Hip	Hippocampal Formation	**Ven**	Ventricle
Ins	Insula	**VL**	Ventral Lateral Nucleus of Thalamus
IntCap,PL	Internal Capsule, Posterior Limb		

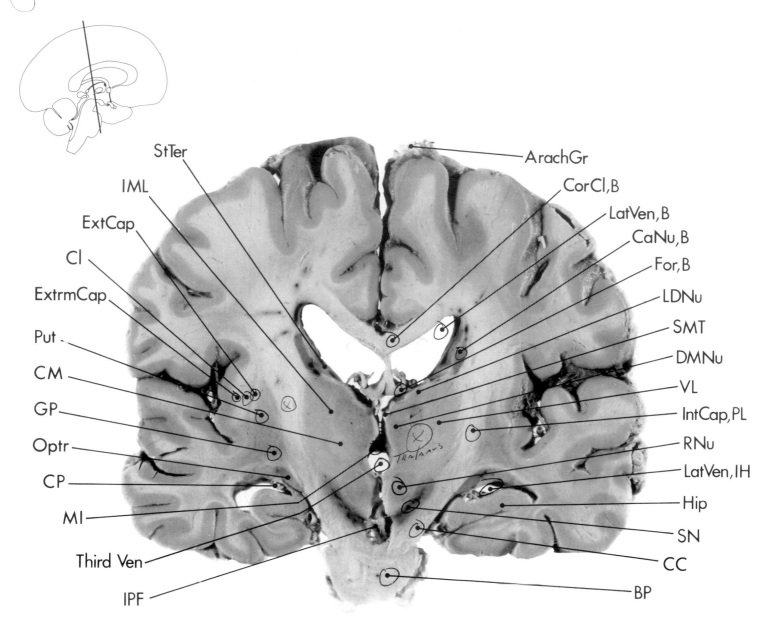

StTer

IML

ExtCap

Cl

ExtrmCap

Put

CM

GP

Optr

CP

MI

Third Ven

IPF

ArachGr

CorCl,B

LatVen,B

CaNu,B

For,B

LDNu

SMT

DMNu

VL

IntCap,PL

RNu

LatVen,IH

Hip

SN

CC

BP

4–10 The caudal surface of a coronal section of brain through middle levels of dorsal thalamus and through rostral midbrain (*red nucleus*) and rostral portions of *basilar pons*.

Abbreviations

ArachGr	Arachnoid Granulations	**IntCap,PL**	Internal Capsule, Posterior Limb
BP	Basilar Pons	**IPF**	Interpeduncular Fossa
CaNu,B	Caudate Nucleus, Body	**LatVen,B**	Lateral Ventricle, Body
CC	Crus Cerebri	**LatVen,IH**	Lateral Ventricle, Inferior Horn
Cl	Claustrum	**LDNu**	Lateral Dorsal Nucleus
CM	Centromedian Nucleus of Thalamus	**MI**	Massa Intermedia
CorCl,B	Corpus Callosum, Body	**OpTr**	Optic Tract
CP	Choroid Plexus	**Put**	Putamen
DMNu	Dorsomedial Nucleus of Thalamus	**RNu**	Red Nucleus
ExtCap	External Capsule	**SMT**	Stria Medullaris Thalami
ExtrmCap	Extreme Capsule	**SN**	Substantia Nigra
For,B	Fornix, Body	**StTer**	Stria Terminalis
GP	Globus Pallidus	**Ven**	Ventricle
Hip	Hippocampal Formation	**VL**	Ventral Lateral Nucleus of Thalamus
IML	Internal Medullary Lamina		

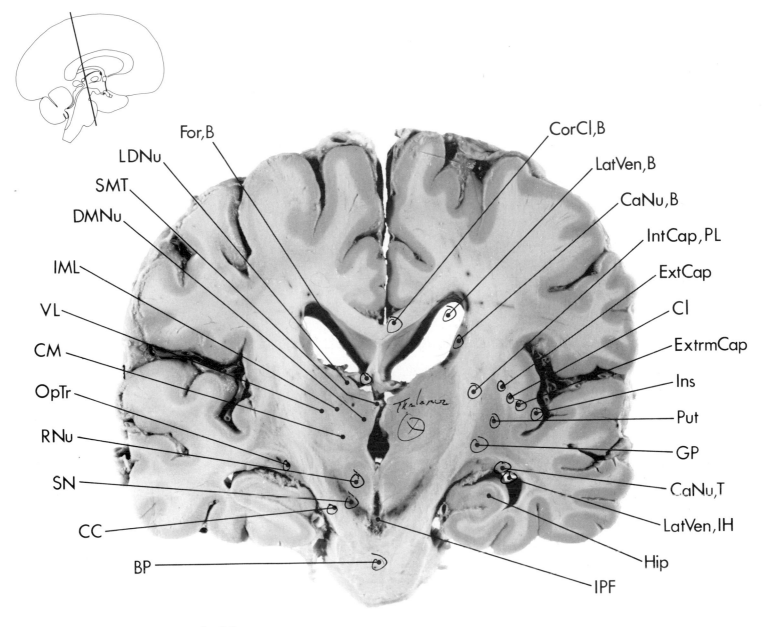

For,B
LDNu
SMT
DMNu
IML
VL
CM
OpTr
RNu
SN
CC
BP

CorCl,B
LatVen,B
CaNu,B
IntCap,PL
ExtCap
Cl
ExtrmCap
Ins
Put
GP
CaNu,T
LatVen,IH
Hip
IPF

Thalamus

4–11 The rostral surface of a coronal section of brain at a mid to caudal thalamic level and through rostral midbrain (*red nucleus*) and rostral portions of *basilar pons*.

Abbreviations

BP	Basilar Pons		**IML**	Internal Medullary Lamina
CaNu,B	Caudate Nucleus, Body		**Ins**	Insula
CaNu,T	Caudate Nucleus, Tail		**IntCap,PL**	Internal Capsule, Posterior Limb
CC	Crus Cerebri		**IPF**	Interpeduncular Fossa
Cl	Claustrum		**LatVen,B**	Lateral Ventricle, Body
CM	Centromedian Nucleus of Thalamus		**LatVen,IH**	Lateral Ventricle, Inferior Horn
CorCl,B	Corpus Callosum, Body		**LDNu**	Lateral Dorsal Nucleus of Thalamus
DMNu	Dorsomedial Nucleus of Thalamus		**OpTr**	Optic Tract
ExtCap	External Capsule		**Put**	Putamen
ExtrmCap	Extreme Capsule		**RNu**	Red Nucleus
For,B	Fornix, Body		**SMT**	Stria Medullaris Thalami
GP	Globus Pallidus		**SN**	Substantia Nigra
Hip	Hippocampal Formation		**VL**	Ventral Lateral Nucleus of Thalamus

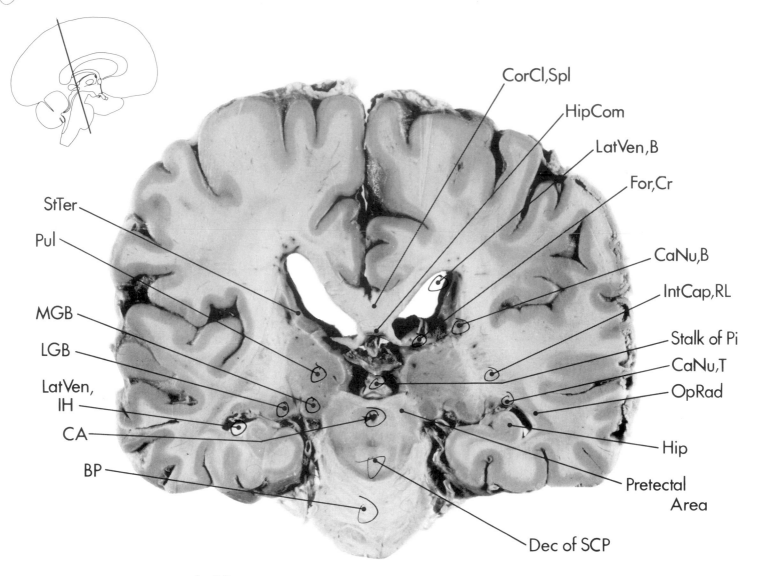

StTer

Pul

MGB

LGB

LatVen,
IH

CA

BP

CorCl,Spl

HipCom

LatVen,B

For,Cr

CaNu,B

IntCap,RL

Stalk of Pi

CaNu,T

OpRad

Hip

Pretectal
Area

Dec of SCP

4–12   The caudal surface of a coronal section of brain through the *pulvinar nucleus* of thalamus, *geniculate bodies, pretectal area, decussation of the superior cerebellar peduncle,* and middle portions of *basilar pons.*

Abbreviations

BP	Basilar Pons
CA	Cerebral Aqueduct
CaNu,B	Caudate Nucleus, Body
CaNu,T	Caudate Nucleus, Tail
CorCl,Spl	Corpus Callosum, Splenium
Dec of SCP	Decussation of Superior Cerebellar Peduncle
For,Cr	Fornix, Crus
Hip	Hippocampal Formation
HipCom	Hippocampal Commissure
IntCap,RL	Internal Capsule, Retrolenticular Limb
LatVen,B	Lateral Ventricle, Body
LatVen,IH	Lateral Ventricle, Inferior Horn
LGB	Lateral Geniculate Body (Nucleus)
MGB	Medial Geniculate Body (Nucleus)
OpRad	Optic Radiations
Pi	Pineal
Pul	Pulvinar
StTer	Stria Terminalis

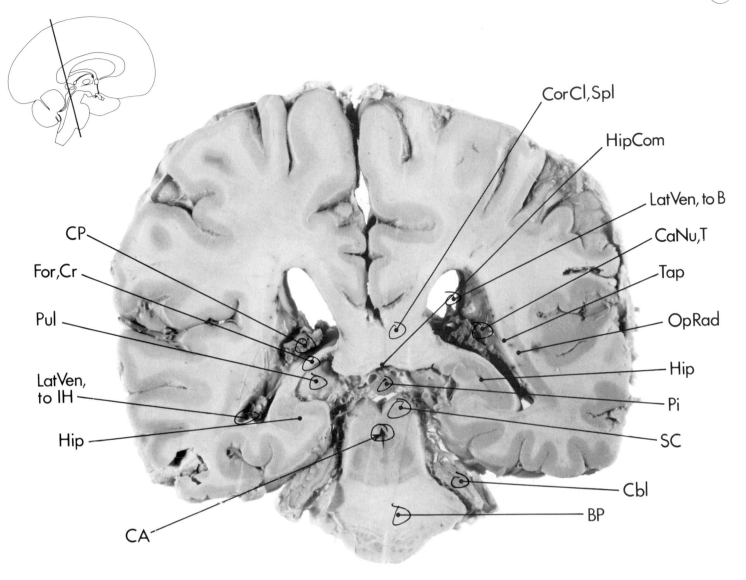

4–13 The caudal surface of a coronal section of brain through the *splenium of corpus callosum*, the *superior colliculus*, and the junction of the *crus of fornix* with the *hippocampal formation*. The plane of section is also through the collateral trigone of the lateral ventricles.

Abbreviations

BP	Basilar Pons
CA	Cerebral Aqueduct
CaNu,T	Caudate Nucleus, Tail
Cbl	Cerebellum
CorCl,Spl	Corpus Callosum, Splenium
CP	Choroid Plexus
For,Cr	Fornix, Crus
Hip	Hippocampal Formation
HipCom	Hippocampal Commissure
LatVen,toB	Lateral Ventricle, towards Body
LatVen,toIH	Lateral Ventricle, towards Inferior Horn
OpRad	Optic Radiations
Pi	Pineal
Pul	Pulvinar
SC	Superior Colliculus
Tap	Tapetum

Figures:

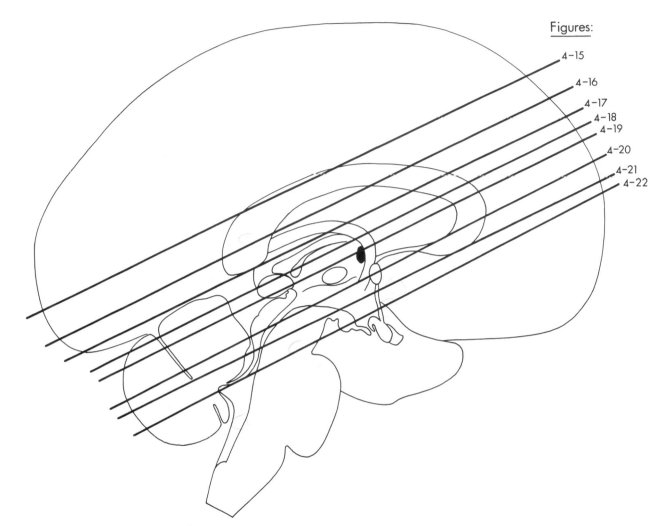

4-15
4-16
4-17
4-18
4-19
4-20
4-21
4-22

4–14 Mid-sagittal drawing of brain showing the planes of section for all axial (horizontal) slices. Technically these brain slices are not truly axial (horizontal), but are actually somewhat oblique (25^0-30^0 off the horizontal) so as to be similar to, and correlate with, planes through the brain as visualized in CT and MRI scans. While anatomists commonly refer to sections in this general plane as "horizontal," clinicians usually describe this as the axial plane. Correlations between these slices and CT and MRI scans are shown in Chapter 8. Because a slice of brain has thickness and therefore dimension, the figure description for each axial (horizontal) level specifies whether one is viewing the dorsal or the ventral surface of the slice. In addition, important landmarks that help to identify the level of the section appear in italics in the figure description.

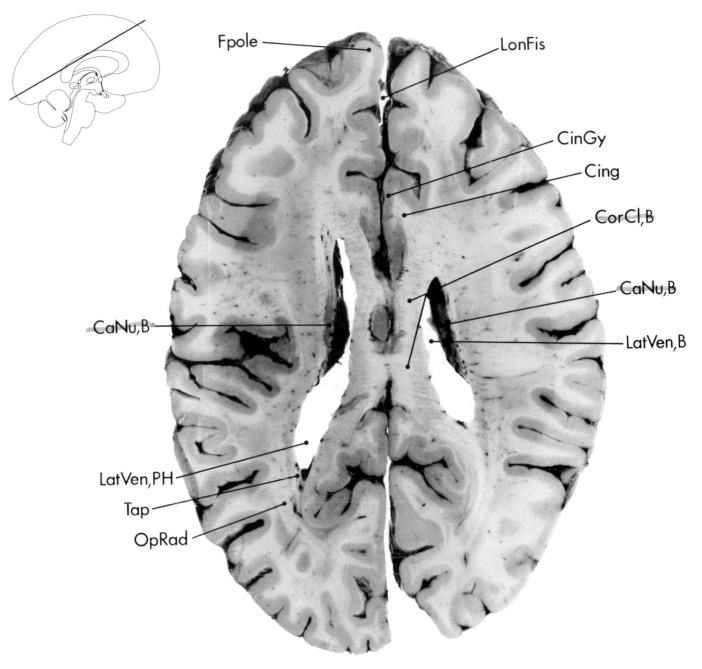

Fpole — LonFis — CinGy — Cing — CorCl,B — CaNu,B — LatVen,B — CaNu,B — LatVen,PH — Tap — OpRad

4–15 Dorsal surface of an axial (horizontal) section of brain through dorsal portions of *corpus callosum*. The plane of section just touches the upper portion of the *body of caudate nucleus*.

Abbreviations

CaNu,B	Caudate Nucleus, Body
Cing	Cingulum
CinGy	Cingulate Gyrus
CorCl,B	Corpus Callosum, Body
Fpole	Frontal Pole
LatVen,B	Lateral Ventricle, Body
LatVen,PH	Lateral Ventricle, Posterior Horn
LonFis	Longitudinal Fissure
OpRad	Optic Radiations
Tap	Tapetum

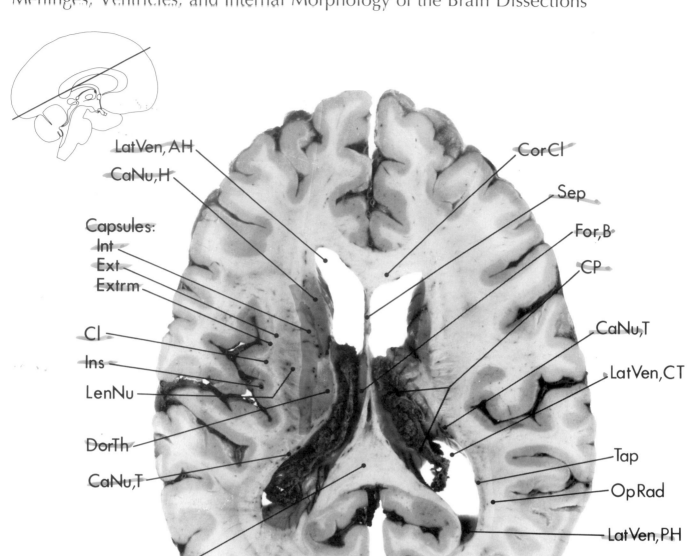

LatVen,AH
CaNu,H
Capsules:
Int
Ext
Extrm
Cl
Ins
LenNu
DorTh
CaNu,T
CorCl,Spl

CorCl
Sep
For,B
CP
CaNu,T
LatVen,CT
Tap
OpRad
LatVen,PH

4–16 Dorsal surface of an axial (horizontal) section of brain through the *splenium of corpus callosum* and dorsal portions of the *head of caudate nucleus*. This plane is just above the *body of fornix* and includes only a small portion of *dorsal thalamus*.

Abbreviations

CaNu,H	Caudate Nucleus, Head	**Ins**	Insula
CaNu,T	Caudate Nucleus, Tail	**IntCap**	Internal Capsule
Cl	Claustrum	**LatVen,AH**	Lateral Ventricle, Anterior Horn
CorCl	Corpus Callosum	**LatVen,CT**	Lateral Ventricle, Collateral Trigone
CorCl,Spl	Corpus Callosum, Splenium	**LatVen,PH**	Lateral Ventricle, Posterior Horn
CP	Choroid Plexus	**LenNu**	Lenticular Nucleus
DorTh	Dorsal Thalamus	**OpRad**	Optic Radiations
ExtCap	External Capsule	**Sep**	Septum Pellucidum
ExtrmCap	Extreme Capsule	**Tap**	Tapetum
For,B	Fornix, Body		

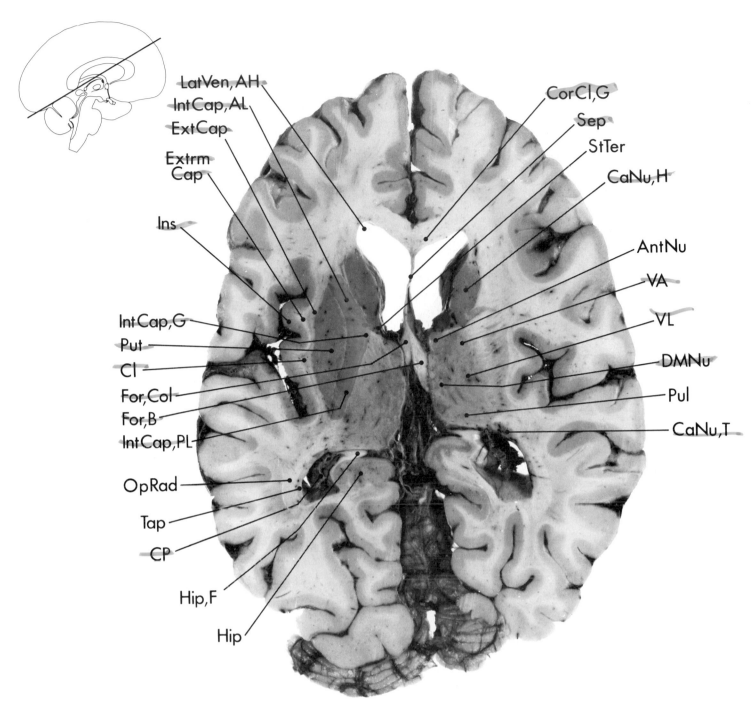

4–17   Dorsal surface of an axial (horizontal) section of brain through the *genu of corpus callosum, head of caudate nucleus,* and dorsal portions of the *pulvinar.* This section is just dorsal to the pineal and roof of the third ventricle, yet passes ventral to the splenium of corpus callosum.

Abbreviations

AntNu	Anterior Nucleus of Thalamus		**Ins**	Insula
CaNu,H	Caudate Nucleus, Head		**IntCap,AL**	Internal Capsule, Anterior Limb
CaNu,T	Caudate Nucleus, Tail		**IntCap,G**	Internal Capsule, Genu
Cl	Claustrum		**IntCap,PL**	Internal Capsule, Posterior Limb
CorCl,G	Corpus Callosum, Genu		**LatVen,AH**	Lateral Ventricle, Anterior Horn
CP	Choroid Plexus		**OpRad**	Optic Radiations
DMNu	Dorsomedial Nucleus of Thalamus		**Pul**	Pulvinar
ExtCap	External Capsule		**Put**	Putamen
ExtrmCap	Extreme Capsule		**Sep**	Septum Pellucidum
For,B	Fornix, Body		**StTer**	Stria Terminalis
For,Col	Fornix, Column		**Tap**	Tapetum
Hip	Hippocampal Formation		**VA**	Ventral Anterior Nucleus of Thalamus
Hip,F	Hippocampus, Fimbria of		**VL**	Ventral Lateral Nucleus of Thalamus

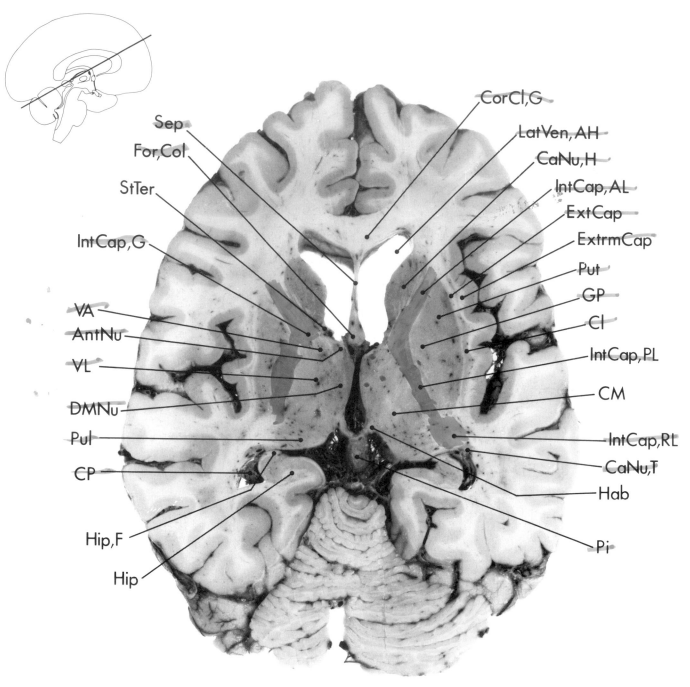

4–18   Ventral surface of an axial (horizontal) section of brain through the *column of fornix, anterior thalamic nucleus, habenula,* and dorsal aspects of the *pineal.* At this plane the major nuclei of the dorsal thalamus are especially obvious. The dark midline area is the bottom surface of the roof of the third ventricle.

Abbreviations

AntNu	Anterior Nucleus of Thalamus
CaNu,H	Caudate Nucleus, Head
CaNu,T	Caudate Nucleus, Tail
Cl	Claustrum
CM	Centromedian Nucleus of Thalamus
CorCl,G	Corpus Callosum, Genu
CP	Choroid Plexus
DMNu	Dorsomedial Nucleus of Thalamus
ExtCap	External Capsule
ExtrmCap	Extreme Capsule
For,Col	Fornix, Column
GP	Globus Pallidus
Hab	Habenula
Hip	Hippocampal Formation
Hip,F	Hippocampus, Fimbria of
IntCap,AL	Internal Capsule, Anterior Limb
IntCap,G	Internal Capsule, Genu
IntCap,PL	Internal Capsule, Posterior Limb
IntCap,RL	Internal Capsule, Retrolenticular Limb
LatVen,AH	Lateral Ventricle, Anterior Horn
Pi	Pineal
Pul	Pulvinar
Put	Putamen
Sep	Septum Pellucidum
StTer	Stria Terminalis
VA	Ventral Anterior Nucleus of Thalamus
VL	Ventral Lateral Nucleus of Thalamus

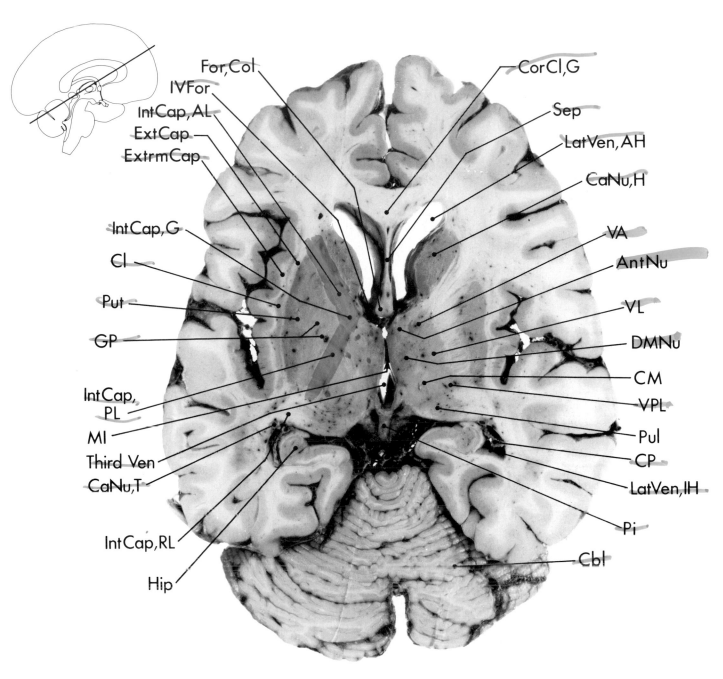

4–19 Dorsal surface of an axial (horizontal) section of brain through the *interventricular foramina*, third ventricle just dorsal to the *massa intermedia*, and ventral portions of the *pulvinar*.

on pg 61
CaNU, Body - Superior to Thal.

Abbreviations

AntNu	Anterior Nucleus of Thalamus	**IntCap,G**	Internal Capsule, Genu
CaNu,H	Caudate Nucleus, Head - Ant. to Thal.	**IntCap,PL**	Internal Capsule, Posterior Limb
CaNu,T	Caudate Nucleus, Tail ~ Post - Inf to Thalamu.	**IntCap,RL**	Internal Capsule, Retrolenticular Limb
Cbl	Cerebellum	**IVFor**	Interventricular Foramen
Cl	Claustrum	**LatVen,AH**	Lateral Ventricle, Anterior Horn
CM	Centromedian Nucleus of Thalamus	**LatVen,IH**	Lateral Ventricle, Inferior Horn
CorCl,G	Corpus Callosum, Genu	**MI**	Massa Intermedia
CP	Choroid Plexus	**Pi**	Pineal
DMNu	Dorsomedial Nucleus of Thalamus	**Pul**	Pulvinar
ExtCap	External Capsule	**Put**	Putamen
ExtrmCap	Extreme Capsule	**Sep**	Septum Pellucidum
For,Col	Fornix, Column	**VA**	Ventral Anterior Nucleus of Thalamus
GP	Globus Pallidus	**Ven**	Ventricle
Hip	Hippocampal Formation	**VL**	Ventral Lateral Nucleus of Thalamus
IntCap,AL	Internal Capsule, Anterior Limb	**VPL**	Ventral Posterolateral Nucleus of Thalamus

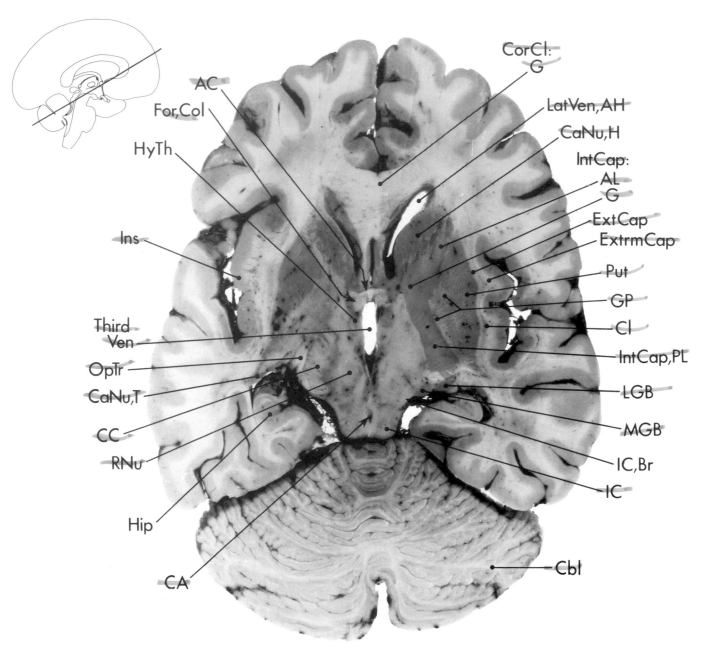

4–20 Dorsal surface of an axial (horizontal) section of brain through the *anterior commissure, column of fornix, red nucleus, inferior colliculus,* and *geniculate bodies.* With the brainstem *in situ,* this plane of section is actually somewhat oblique through the midbrain.

Abbreviations

AC	Anterior Commissure		**IC,Br**	Inferior Colliculus, Brachium
CA	Cerebral Aqueduct		**Ins**	Insula
CaNu,H	Caudate Nucleus, Head		**IntCap**	Internal Capsule
CaNu,T	Caudate Nucleus, Tail		**AL**	Anterior Limb
Cbl	Cerebellum		**G**	Genu
CC	Crus Cerebri		**IntCap,PL**	Internal Capsule, Posterior Limb
CI	Claustrum		**LatVen,AH**	Lateral Ventricle, Anterior Horn
CorCl,G	Corpus Callosum, Genu		**LGB**	Lateral Geniculate Body (Nucleus)
ExtCap	External Capsule		**MGB**	Medial Geniculate Body (Nucleus)
ExtrmCap	Extreme Capsule			
For,Col	Fornix, Column		**OpTr**	Optic Tract
GP	Globus Pallidus		**Put**	Putamen
Hip	Hippocampal Formation		**RNu**	Red Nucleus
HyTh	Hypothalamus		**Ven**	Ventricle
IC	Inferior Colliculus			

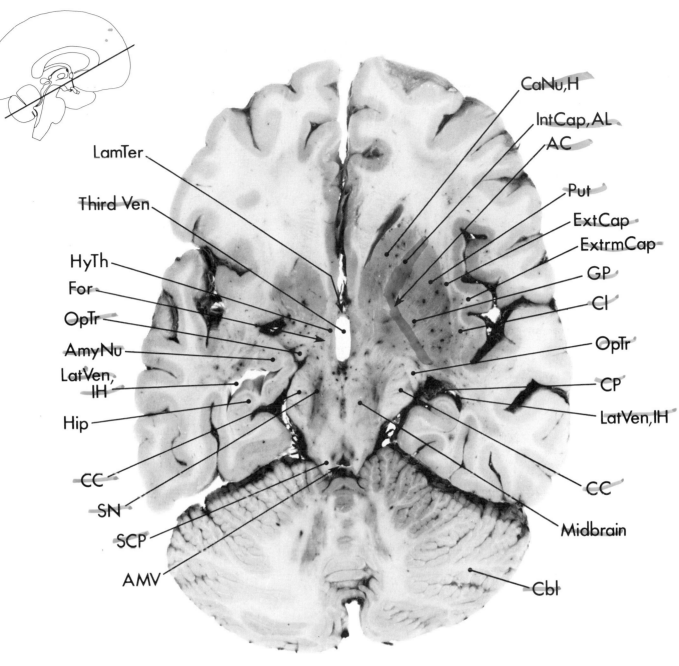

4–21 Dorsal surface of an axial (horizontal) section of brain through the basal portion of the forebrain and extending obliquely through the midbrain.

Abbreviations

AC	Anterior Commissure
AMV	Anterior Medullary Velum
AmyNu	Amygdaloid Nucleus (Complex)
CaNu,H	Caudate Nucleus, Head
Cbl	Cerebellum
CC	Crus Cerebri
CI	Claustrum
CP	Choroid Plexus
ExtCap	External Capsule
ExtrmCap	Extreme Capsule
For	Fornix
GP	Globus Pallidus

Hip	Hippocampal Formation
HyTh	Hypothalamus
IntCap,AL	Internal Capsule, Anterior Limb
LamTcr	Lamina Terminalis
LatVen,IH	Lateral Ventricle, Inferior Horn
OpTr	Optic Tract
Put	Putamen
SCP	Superior Cerebellar Peduncle (Brachium Conjunctivum)
SN	Substantia Nigra
Ven	Ventricle

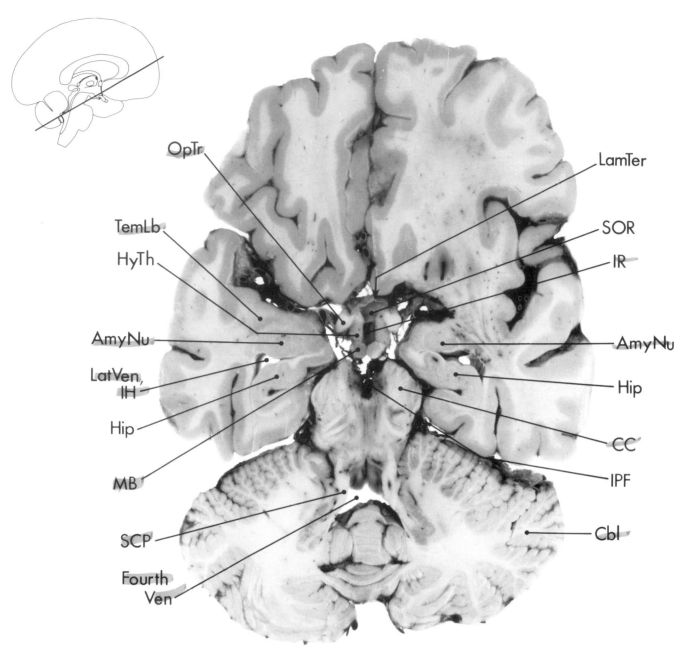

OpTr
TemLb
HyTh
AmyNu
LatVen, IH
Hip
MB
SCP
Fourth Ven
LamTer
SOR
IR
AmyNu
Hip
CC
IPF
Cbl

4–22   Dorsal surface of an axial (horizontal) section of brain through ventral portions of the *hypothalamus* and extending obliquely through the midbrain into the *superior cerebellar peduncle*. Note the characteristic appearance of the third ventricle and immediately adjacent hypothalamic structures.

Abbreviations

AmyNu	Amygdaloid Nucleus (Complex)	**LamTer**	Lamina Terminalis
Cbl	Cerebellum	**OpTr**	Optic Tract
CC	Crus Cerebri	**MB**	Mammillary Body
Hip	Hippocampal Formation	**SCP**	Superior Cerebellar Peduncle (Brachium Conjunctivum)
HyTh	Hypothalamus		
IPF	Interpeduncular Fossa	**SOR**	Supraoptic Recess of Third Ventricle
IR	Infundibular Recess of Third Ventricle	**TemLb**	Temporal Lobe
LatVen,IH	Lateral Ventricle, Inferior Horn	**Ven**	Ventricle

Chapter 5

Internal Morphology
of the Spinal Cord and Brain
in Stained Sections

5-1   Transverse section of spinal cord showing the characteristics of a sacral level. Gray matter occupies most of the cross-section; its H-shaped appearance is not obvious at sacral-coccygeal levels. The white matter is a comparatively thin mantle.

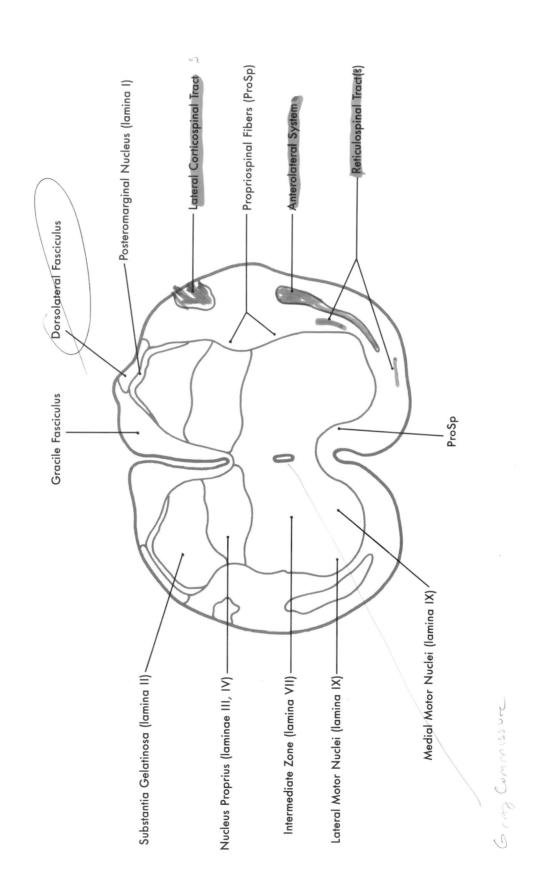

Dorsolateral Fasciculus

Posteromarginal Nucleus (lamina I)

Lateral Corticospinal Tract

Propriospinal Fibers (ProSp)

Anterolateral System

Reticulospinal Tract(s)

Gracile Fasciculus

ProSp

Substantia Gelatinosa (lamina II)

Nucleus Proprius (laminae III, IV)

Intermediate Zone (lamina VII)

Lateral Motor Nuclei (lamina IX)

Medial Motor Nuclei (lamina IX)

Gray Commissure

Gray Matter Shaped like an
'H'

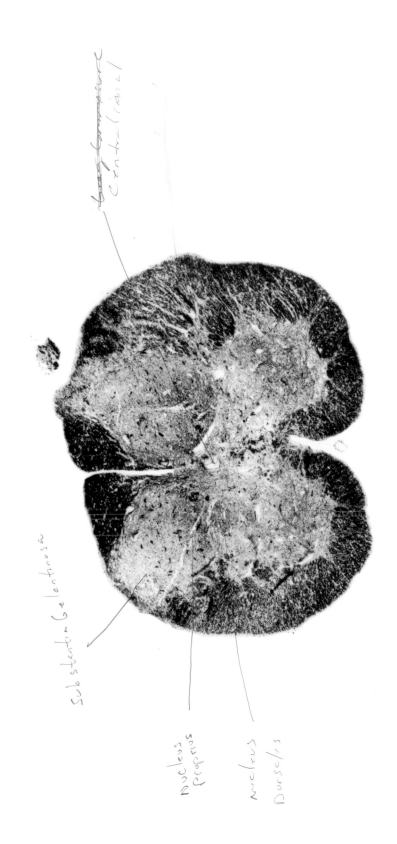

Blood vessel
Central canal

Substantia Gelatinosa

Nucleus Proprius

Nucleus Dorsalis

Little Gray Matter to white mather.

5-2 Transverse section of spinal cord showing its characteristic appearance at lumbar levels (L4). Dorsal and ventral horns are large in relation to a modest amount of white matter. Fibers of the medial division of the dorsal root directly enter the gracile fasciculus.

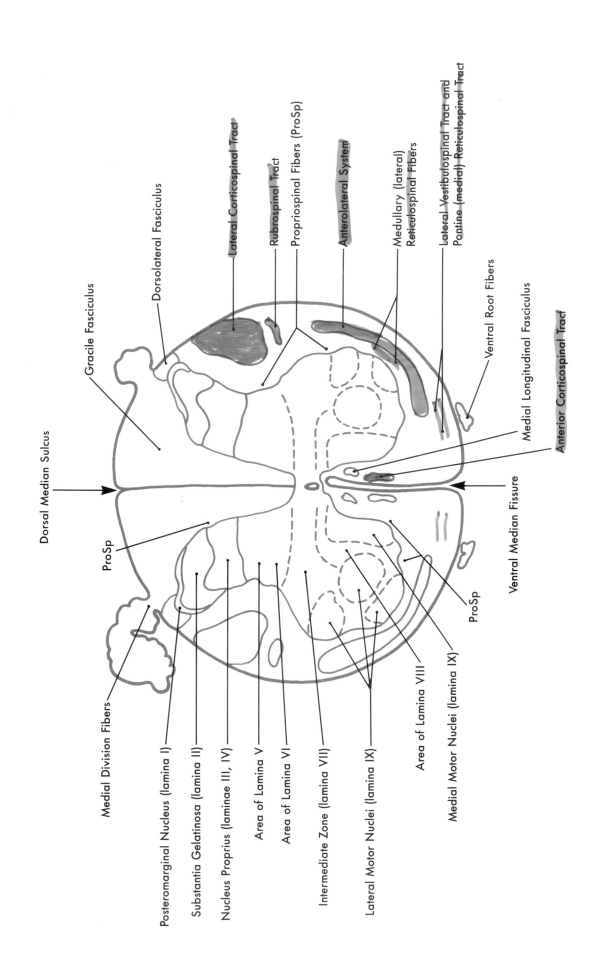

Lateral Corticospinal Tract

Rubrospinal Tract

Propriospinal Fibers (ProSp)

Anterolateral System

Medullary (lateral) Reticulospinal Fibers

Lateral Vestibulospinal Tract and Pontine (medial) Reticulospinal Tract

Ventral Root Fibers

Medial Longitudinal Fasciculus

Anterior Corticospinal Tract

Dorsolateral Fasciculus

Gracile Fasciculus

Dorsal Median Sulcus

ProSp

Ventral Median Fissure

ProSp

Medial Division Fibers

Posteromarginal Nucleus (lamina I)

Substantia Gelatinosa (lamina II)

Nucleus Proprius (laminae III, IV)

Area of Lamina V

Area of Lamina VI

Intermediate Zone (lamina VII)

Lateral Motor Nuclei (lamina IX)

Area of Lamina VIII

Medial Motor Nuclei (lamina IX)

Grey matter > white matter.

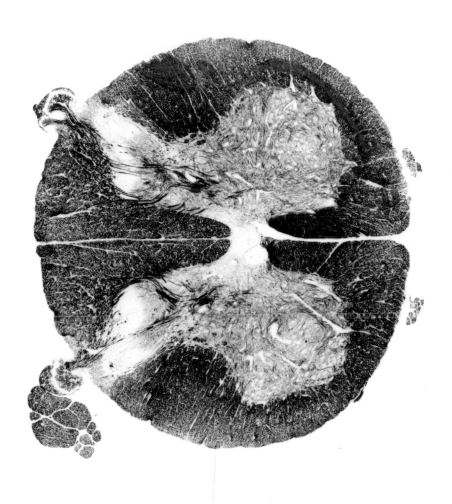

5–3 Transverse section of spinal cord showing its characteristic appearance at thoracic levels (T4). The white matter appears large in relation to the rather diminutive amount of gray matter. Dorsal and ventral horns are small especially when compared to low cervical and to lumbar levels. The overall shape of the cord is round.

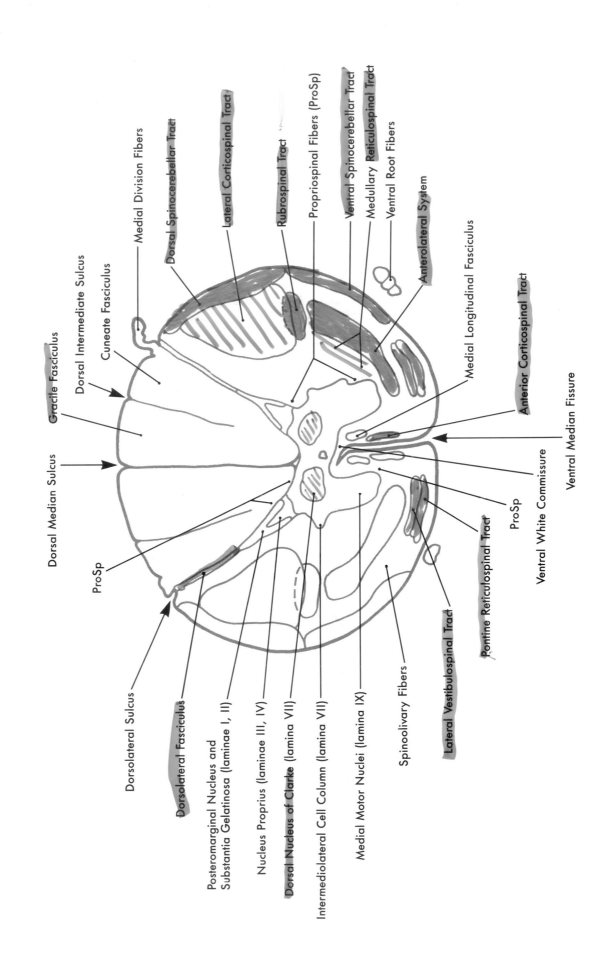

I forgot
Thin Dorsal Root

Dorsal nucleus
clarke column.

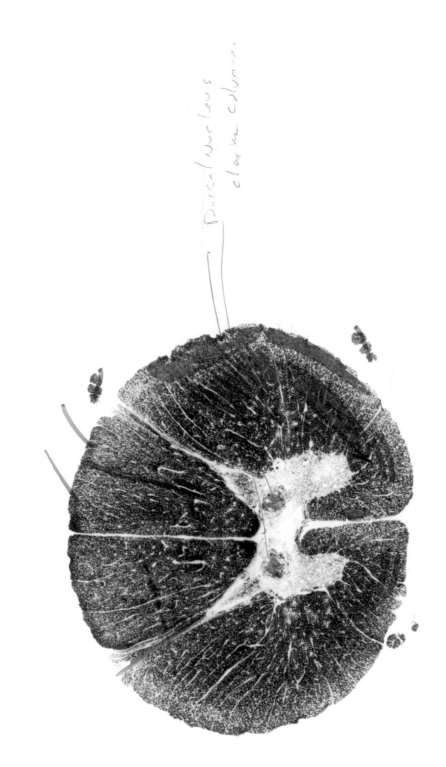

5–4   Transverse section of spinal cord showing its characteristic appearance at lower cervical levels (C7). The ventral horn is large and there is, proportionally and absolutely, a large amount of white matter. The overall shape of the cord is oval.

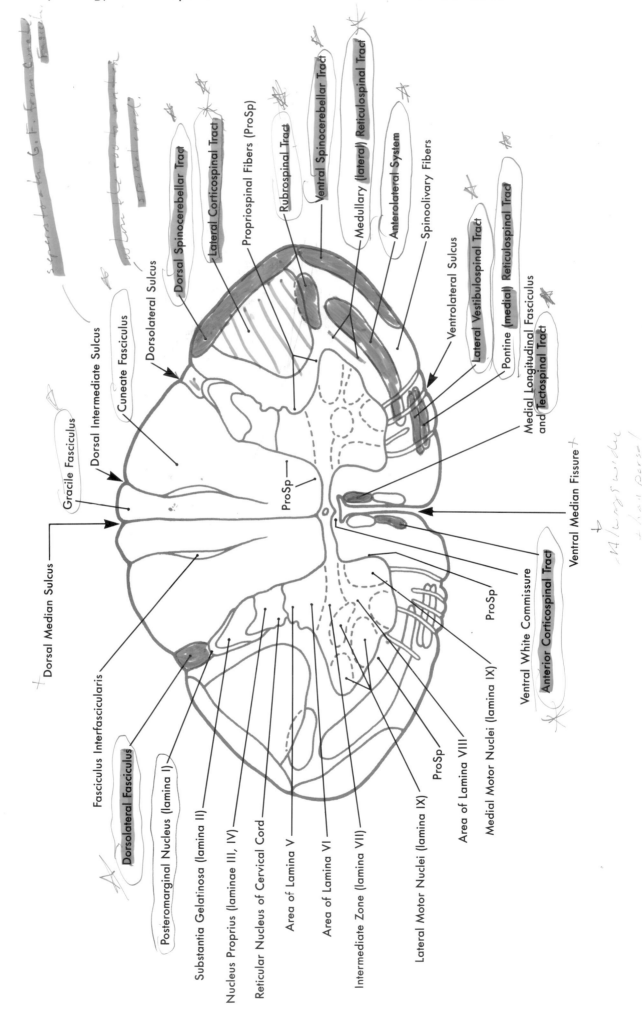

Dorsal Spinocerebellar Tract

Lateral Corticospinal Tract

Propriospinal Fibers (ProSp)

Rubrospinal Tract

Ventral Spinocerebellar Tract

Medullary (lateral) Reticulospinal Tract

Anterolateral System

Spinoolivary Fibers

Ventrolateral Sulcus

Lateral Vestibulospinal Tract

Pontine (medial) Reticulospinal Tract

Medial Longitudinal Fasciculus and Tectospinal Tract

Ventral Median Fissure

Dorsolateral Sulcus

Cuneate Fasciculus

Dorsal Intermediate Sulcus

Gracile Fasciculus

ProSp

Dorsal Median Sulcus

Fasciculus Interfascicularis

Dorsolateral Fasciculus

Posteromarginal Nucleus (lamina I)

Substantia Gelatinosa (lamina II)

Nucleus Proprius (laminae III, IV)

Reticular Nucleus of Cervical Cord

Area of Lamina V

Area of Lamina VI

Intermediate Zone (lamina VII)

Lateral Motor Nuclei (lamina IX)

ProSp

Area of Lamina VIII

Medial Motor Nuclei (lamina IX)

Ventral White Commissure

Anterior Corticospinal Tract

ProSp

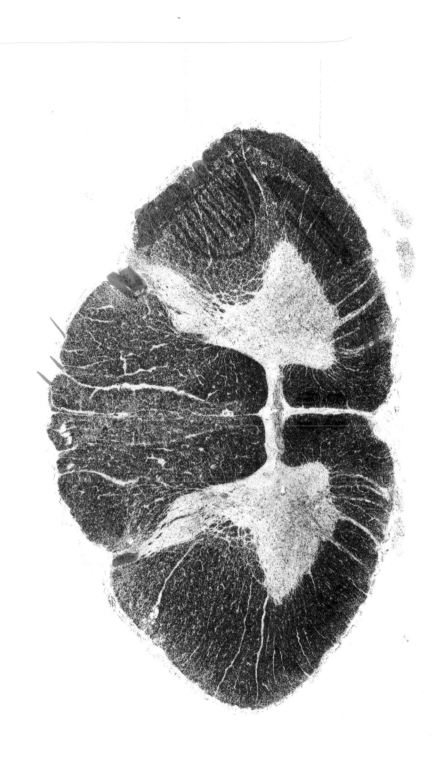

Ident to:

Oval shaped

5-5 Transverse section of spinal cord at the C1 level. Lateral corticospinal fibers are now located medially toward the pyramidal decussation (see also Fig. 5-8 on page 84). At this level, fibers of the spinal trigeminal tract interdigitate with those of the dorsolateral fasciculus.

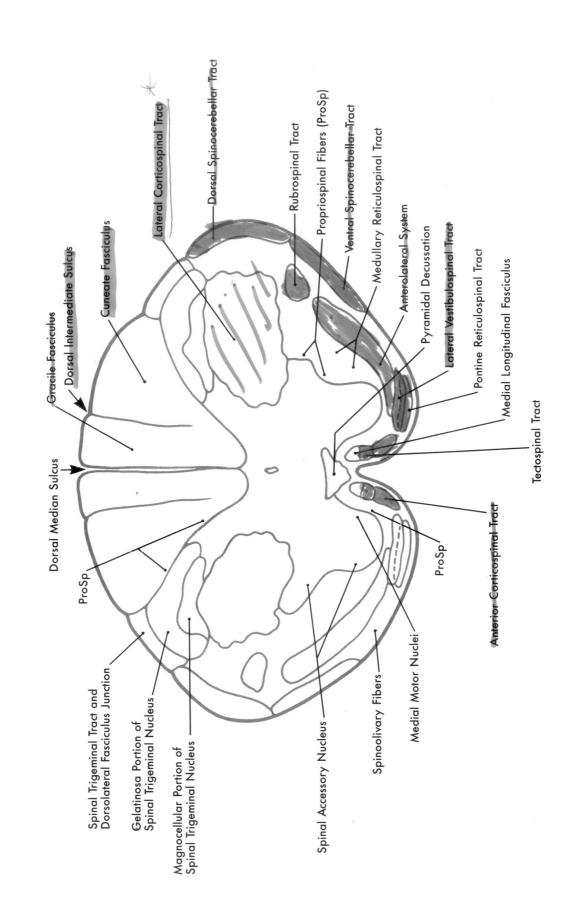

Gracile Fasciculus

Dorsal Intermediate Sulcus

Cuneate Fasciculus

Lateral Corticospinal Tract

Dorsal Spinocerebellar Tract

Rubrospinal Tract

Propriospinal Fibers (ProSp)

Ventral Spinocerebellar Tract

Medullary Reticulospinal Tract

Anterolateral System

Pyramidal Decussation

Lateral Vestibulospinal Tract

Pontine Reticulospinal Tract

Medial Longitudinal Fasciculus

Tectospinal Tract

Anterior Corticospinal Tract

Dorsal Median Sulcus

ProSp

Spinal Trigeminal Tract and Dorsolateral Fasciculus Junction

Gelatinosa Portion of Spinal Trigeminal Nucleus

Magnocellular Portion of Spinal Trigeminal Nucleus

Spinal Accessory Nucleus

Spinoolivary Fibers

Medial Motor Nuclei

ProSp

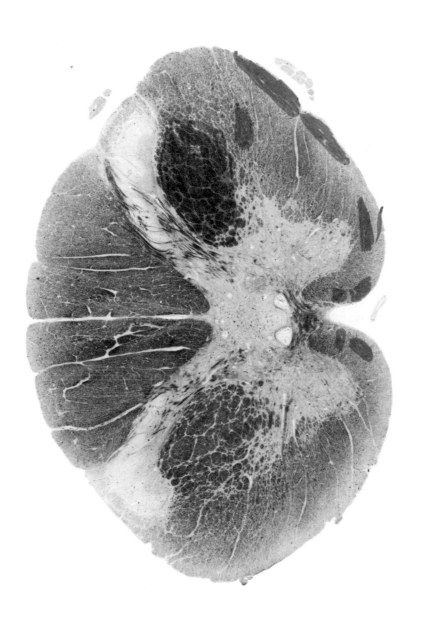

5-6   Semi-diagrammatic representation of internal blood supply to the spinal cord. This is an actual tracing of a C4 level, with the positions of principal tracts superimposed on the left and the general pattern of blood vessels superimposed on the right.

Abbreviations

A	representation of Arm areas
ACSp	Anterior Corticospinal Tract
ALS	Anterolateral System
DH	Dorsal Horn
DSCT	Dorsal Spinocerebellar Tract
FCu	Cuneate Fasciculus
FGr	Gracile Fasciculus
IZ	Intermediate Zone
L	representation of Leg areas
LCSp	Lateral Corticospinal Tract
MLF	Medial Longitudinal Fasciculus
N	representation of Neck areas
ProSp	Propriospinal Fibers
RetSp	Reticulospinal Tract
RuSp	Rubrospinal Tract
S	representation of Sacral areas
T	representation of Trunk areas
VesSp	Vestibulospinal Tract
VH	Ventral Horn
VSCT	Ventral Spinocerebellar Tract

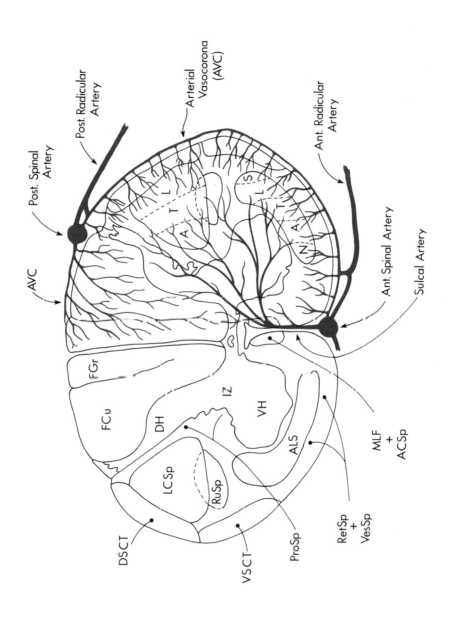

5–7 All of the brainstem sections used in Figures 5-9 through 5-13 (medulla), 5-17 through 5-20 (pons), and 5-22 through 5-25 (midbrain) are from an individual who had an infarct (green in drawing) in the posterior limb of the internal capsule. This lesion damaged corticospinal fibers (red in drawing), producing a contralateral hemiplegia of the arm and leg, and damaged sensory radiations that travel from thalamic nuclei to the somatosensory cortex.

Although the patient survived the initial episode, corticospinal fibers (red) distal to the lesion (green) underwent degenerative changes and largely disappeared. This Wallerian (anterograde) degeneration takes place because the capsular infarct effectively separates the descending corticospinal fibers from their cell bodies in the cerebral cortex. Consequently, the location of corticospinal fibers in the middle third of the crus cerebri of the midbrain, in the basilar pons, and in the pyramid of the medulla is characterized by the obvious lack of myelinated axons in these structures when compared to the opposite side. In the brainstem, these degenerated fibers are ipsilateral to their cells of origin but are contralateral to their former destination in the spinal cord; hence the contralateral motor deficit.

These photographs give the user the unique opportunity of seeing where corticospinal fibers are located at all levels of the brainstem. Also, one is constantly reminded of (1) the relationship of corticospinal fibers to other structures, (2) the deficits one can expect to see at representative levels due to this lesion, and (3) the general appearance of degenerated fibers in the human central nervous system (CNS). These images can be adapted to a wide range of instructional formats.

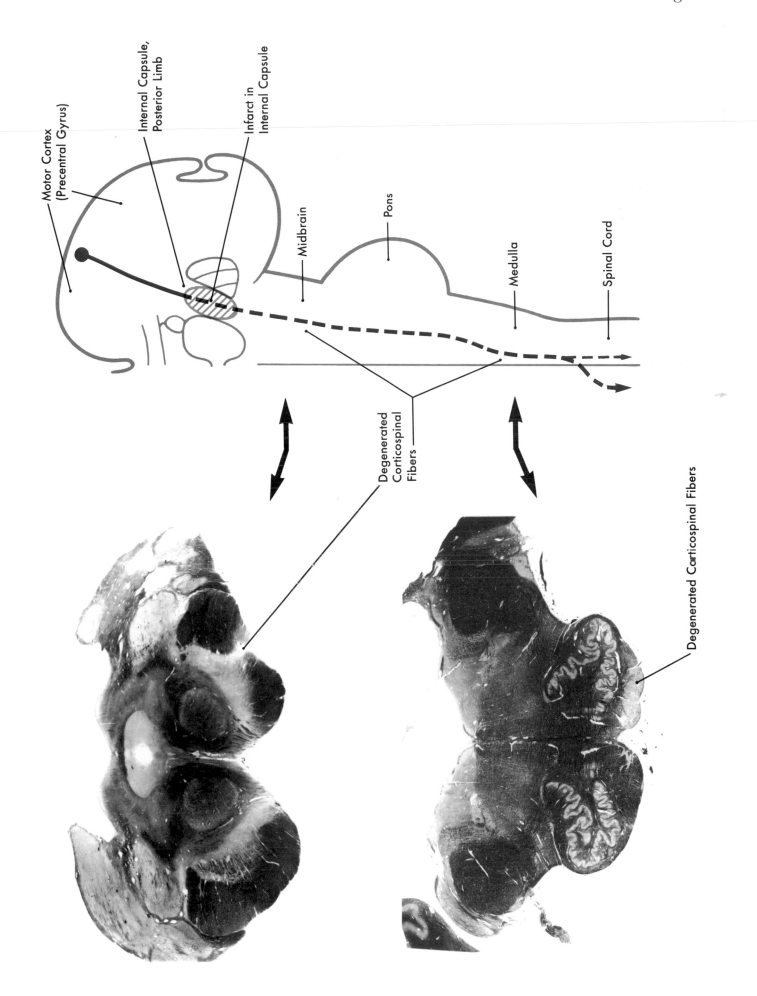

Motor Cortex (Precentral Gyrus)

Internal Capsule, Posterior Limb

Infarct in Internal Capsule

Midbrain

Pons

Medulla

Spinal Cord

Degenerated Corticospinal Fibers

Degenerated Corticospinal Fibers

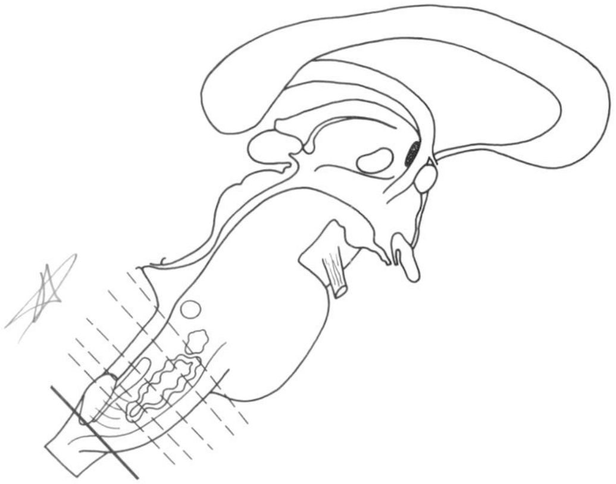

5-8   Transverse section of medulla through the *pyramidal decussation* (motor decussation, crossing of corticospinal fibers). This is the level of the spinal cord-medulla transition.

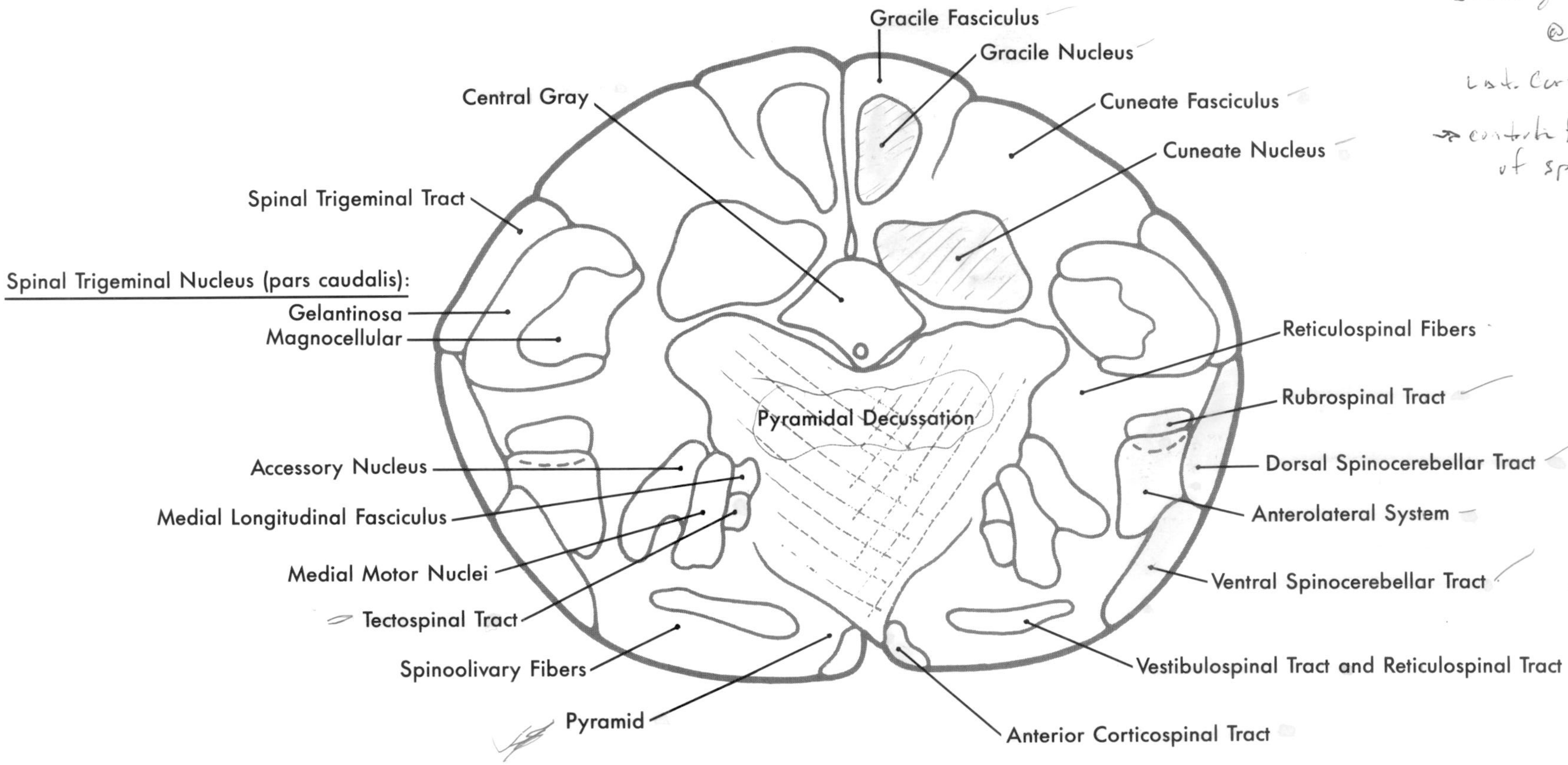

Gracile Fasciculus
Gracile Nucleus
Cuneate Fasciculus
Cuneate Nucleus
Central Gray
Spinal Trigeminal Tract
Spinal Trigeminal Nucleus (pars caudalis):
Gelantinosa
Magnocellular
Accessory Nucleus
Medial Longitudinal Fasciculus
Medial Motor Nuclei
Tectospinal Tract
Spinoolivary Fibers
Pyramid
Pyramidal Decussation

Reticulospinal Fibers
Rubrospinal Tract
Dorsal Spinocerebellar Tract
Anterolateral System
Ventral Spinocerebellar Tract
Vestibulospinal Tract and Reticulospinal Tract
Anterior Corticospinal Tract

Handwritten annotations:
Crossy Spinal Tract @ Decussation
Lat. Corticol Spinal Tract
gentsh fine movement of spinal Tract.

Spinal medulla ts. Transverse

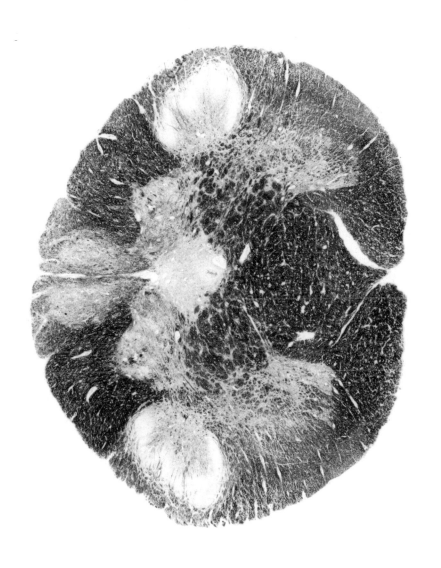

5-9 Transverse section of medulla through the _dorsal column nuclei_, caudal portions of the _hypoglossal nucleus_, caudal end of the _principal (inferior) olivary nucleus_, and middle portions of the _sensory decussation_.

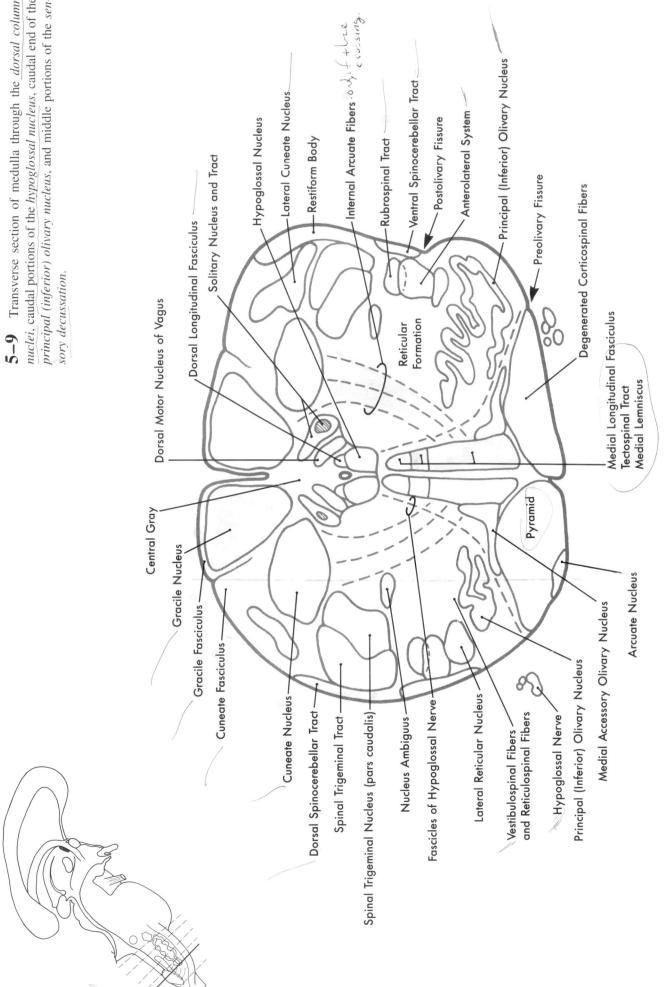

Dorsal Longitudinal Fasciculus

Solitary Nucleus and Tract

Hypoglossal Nucleus

Lateral Cuneate Nucleus

Restiform Body

Internal Arcuate Fibers and if the crossing.

Rubrospinal Tract

Ventral Spinocerebellar Tract

Postolivary Fissure

Anterolateral System

Principal (Inferior) Olivary Nucleus

Preolivary Fissure

Degenerated Corticospinal Fibers

Medial Longitudinal Fasciculus
Tectospinal Tract
Medial Lemniscus

Reticular Formation

Pyramid

Dorsal Motor Nucleus of Vagus

Central Gray

Gracile Nucleus

Gracile Fasciculus

Cuneate Fasciculus

Cuneate Nucleus

Dorsal Spinocerebellar Tract

Spinal Trigeminal Tract

Spinal Trigeminal Nucleus (pars caudalis)

Nucleus Ambiguus

Fascicles of Hypoglossal Nerve

Lateral Reticular Nucleus

Vestibulospinal Fibers
and Reticulospinal Fibers

Hypoglossal Nerve

Principal (Inferior) Olivary Nucleus

Medial Accessory Olivary Nucleus

Arcuate Nucleus

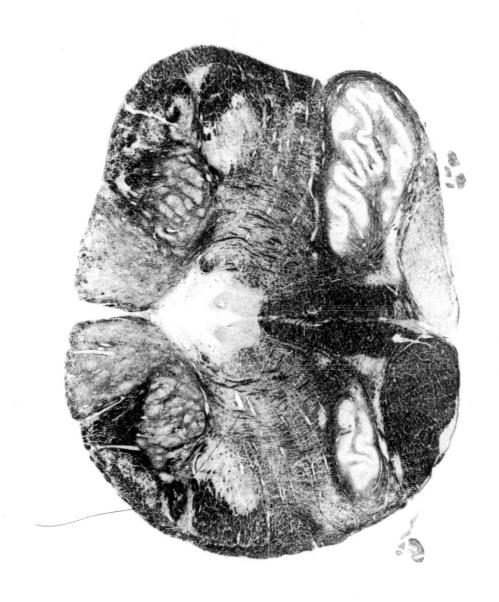

5–10 Transverse section of medulla through rostral portions of the sensory decussation (*internal arcuate fibers*), *obex*, and *caudal thirds of the hypoglossal and principal (inferior) olivary nuclei.*

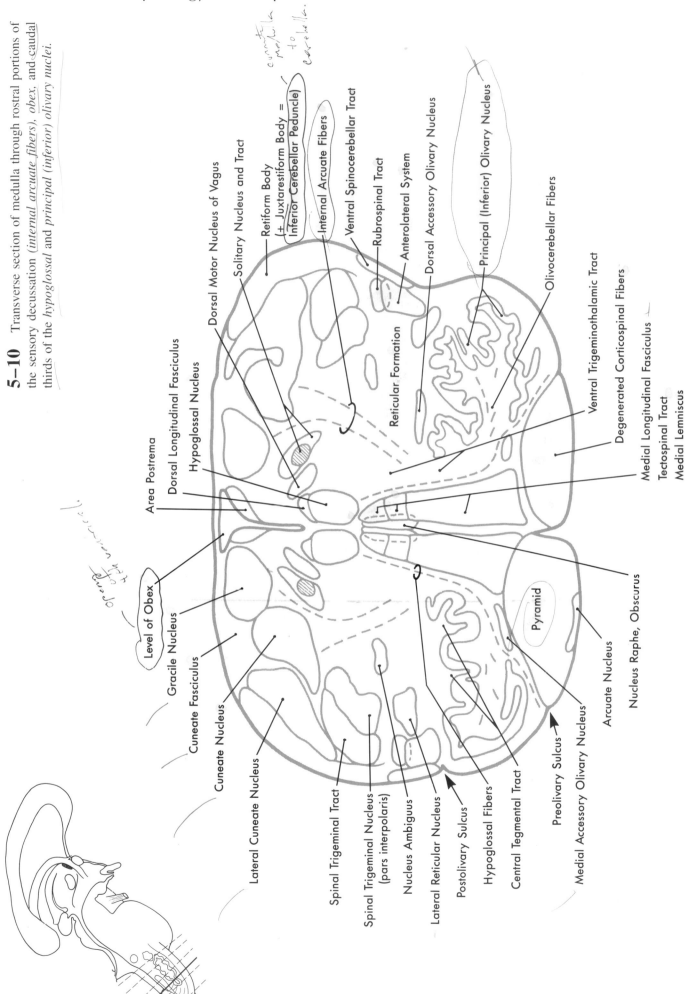

Dorsal Motor Nucleus of Vagus

Solitary Nucleus and Tract

Retiform Body
(+ Juxtarestiform Body =
Inferior Cerebellar Peduncle)

current medulla to cerebella.

Internal Arcuate Fibers

Ventral Spinocerebellar Tract

Rubrospinal Tract

Anterolateral System

Dorsal Accessory Olivary Nucleus

Principal (Inferior) Olivary Nucleus

Olivocerebellar Fibers

Reticular Formation

Ventral Trigeminothalamic Tract

Degenerated Corticospinal Fibers

Medial Longitudinal Fasciculus

Tectospinal Tract

Medial Lemniscus

Area Postrema

Dorsal Longitudinal Fasciculus

Hypoglossal Nucleus

Level of Obex

Gracile Nucleus

Cuneate Fasciculus

Cuneate Nucleus

Lateral Cuneate Nucleus

Spinal Trigeminal Tract

Spinal Trigeminal Nucleus
(pars interpolaris)

Nucleus Ambiguus

Lateral Reticular Nucleus

Postolivary Sulcus

Hypoglossal Fibers

Central Tegmental Tract

Medial Accessory Olivary Nucleus

Preolivary Sulcus

Arcuate Nucleus

Nucleus Raphe, Obscurus

Pyramid

obex ? [handwritten]

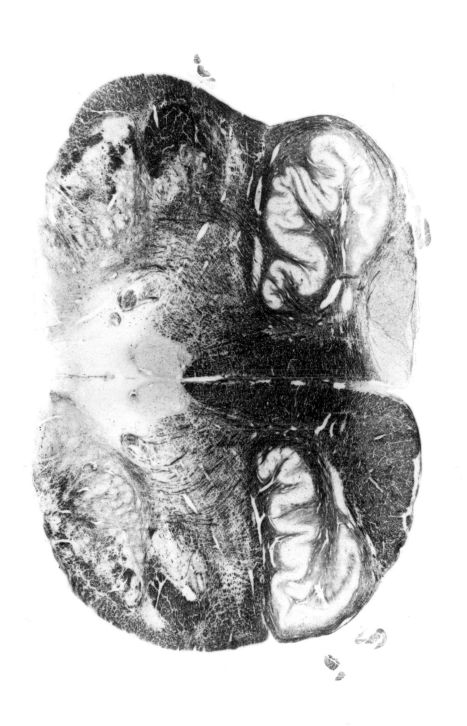

5–11 Transverse section of medulla through rostral portions of the *hypoglossal nucleus* and the middle portions of the *principal (inferior) olivary nucleus.*

Dorsal Longitudinal Fasciculus

Hypoglossal Nucleus

Sulcus Limitans

Solitary Nucleus and Tract

Spinal Trigeminal Tract

Spinal Trigeminal Nucleus (pars interpolaris)

Ventral Spinocerebellar Tract

Rubrospinal Tract

Anterolateral System

Central Tegmental Tract

Olivocerebellar Fibers

Ventral Trigeminothalamic Tract

Degenerated Corticospinal Fibers

Reticular Formation

Medial Longitudinal Fasciculus
Tectospinal Tract
Medial Lemniscus

Nucleus Raphe, Obscurus

Dorsal Motor Nucleus of the Vagus

Medial Vestibular Nucleus

Spinal (Inferior) Vestibular Nucleus

Lateral Cuneate Nucleus

Restiform Body
(+ Juxtarestiform Body =
Inferior Cerebellar Peduncle)

Nucleus Ambiguus

Vagus Nerve

Lateral Reticular Nucleus

Dorsal Accessory
Olivary Nucleus

Principal (Inferior)
Olivary Nucleus

Hypoglossal Nerve

Medial Accessory Olivary Nucleus

Arcuate Nucleus

Nucleus Raphe, Pallidus

Pyramid

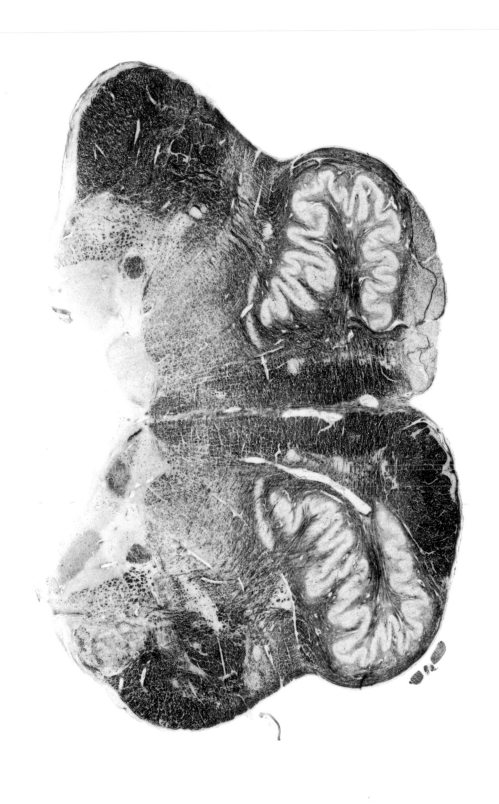

5-12 Transverse section of medulla through the *dorsal* and *ventral cochlear nuclei* and *root of the glossopharyngeal nerve.* This corresponds to approximately the rostral third to fourth of the *principal (inferior) olivary nucleus.*

Ventral Cochlear Nucleus

Dorsal Cochlear Nucleus

Pontobulbar Nucleus

Spinal Trigeminal Nucleus (pars oralis)

Spinal Trigeminal Tract

Nucleus Ambiguus

Rubrospinal Tract

Anterolateral System

Central Tegmental Tract

Olivocerebellar Fibers

Degenerated Corticospinal Fibers

Ventral Trigeminothalamic Tract

Nucleus Raphe, Pallidus

Spinal (or Inferior) Vestibular Nucleus

Stria Medullares of Fourth Ventricle

Medial Vestibular Nucleus

Nucleus Prepositus

Dorsal Longitudinal Fasciculus

Reticular Formation

Nucleus Raphe, Obscurus

Inferior Salivatory Nucleus

Solitary Nucleus

Solitary Tract

Restiform Body

Cerebellum

Dorsal Cochlear Nucleus

Ventral Cochlear Nucleus

Cochlear Nerve

Glossopharyngeal Nerve

Ventral Spinocerebellar Tract

Reticulospinal Fibers

Dorsal Accessory Olivary Nucleus

Principal (Inferior) Olivary Nucleus

Medial Accessory Olivary Nucleus

Arcuate Nucleus

Pyramid

Medial Longitudinal Fasciculus

Tectospinal Tract

Medial Lemniscus

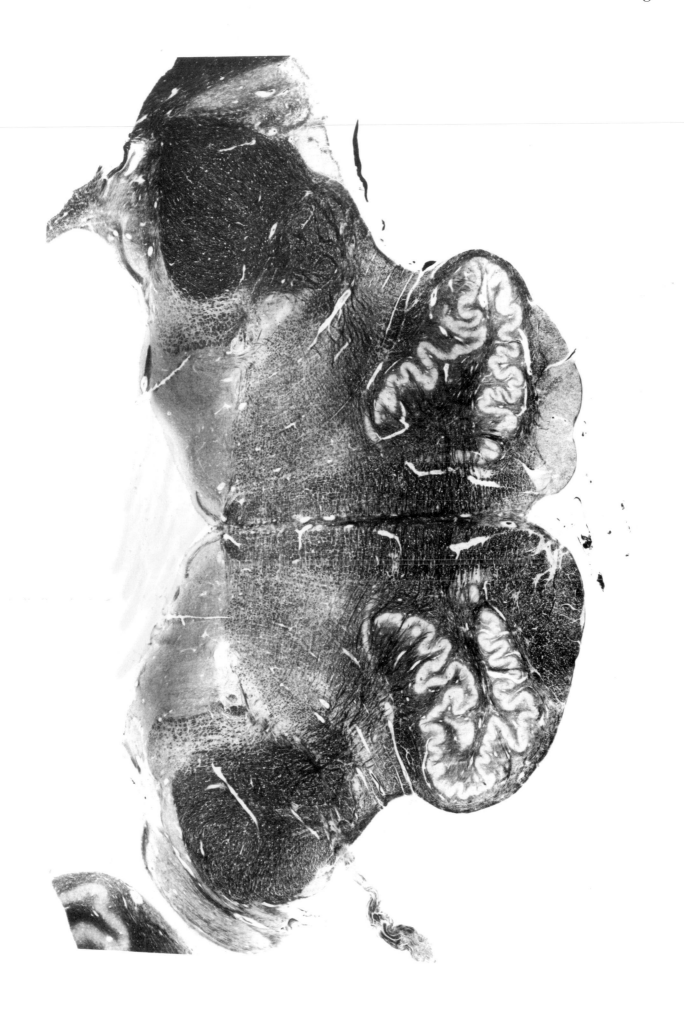

5–13   Transverse section of medulla-pons junction through the rostral pole of the *principal (inferior) olivary nucleus* and the *facial nucleus*. This plane is just caudal to the abducens nucleus. Pontine nuclei at this level may also be called arcuate nuclei.

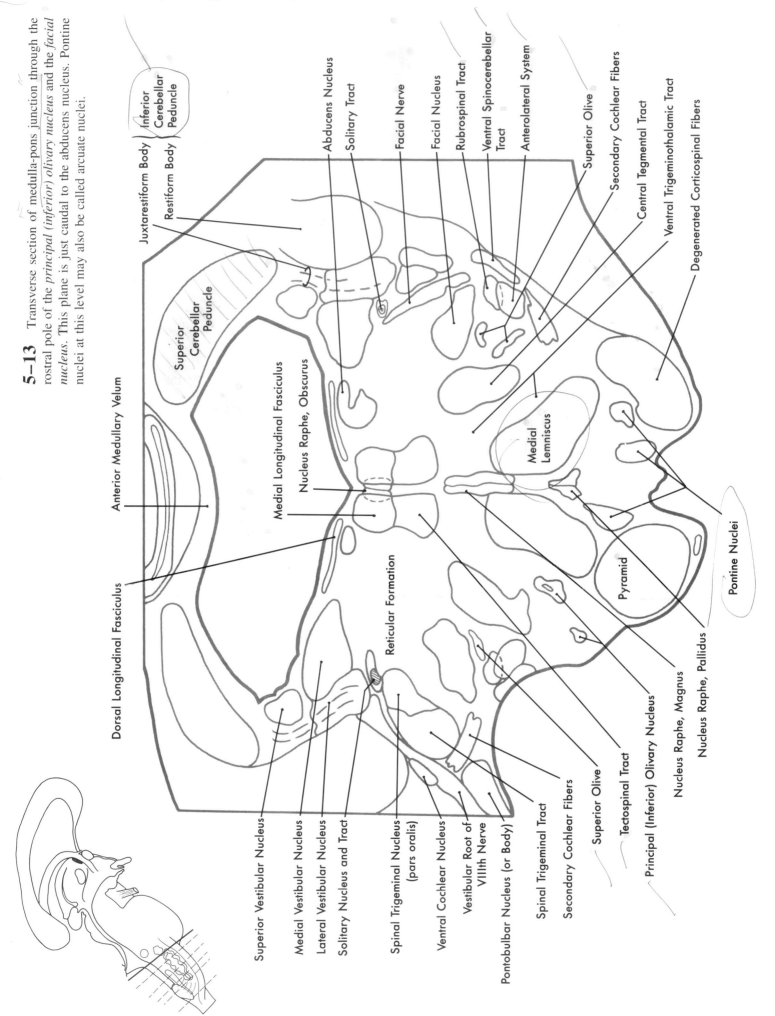

Inferior Cerebellar Peduncle

Restiform Body

Juxtarestiform Body

Abducens Nucleus

Solitary Tract

Facial Nerve

Facial Nucleus

Rubrospinal Tract

Ventral Spinocerebellar Tract

Anterolateral System

Superior Olive

Secondary Cochlear Fibers

Central Tegmental Tract

Ventral Trigeminothalamic Tract

Degenerated Corticospinal Fibers

Superior Cerebellar Peduncle

Anterior Medullary Velum

Medial Longitudinal Fasciculus

Nucleus Raphe, Obscurus

Medial Lemniscus

Dorsal Longitudinal Fasciculus

Reticular Formation

Pyramid

Pontine Nuclei

Superior Vestibular Nucleus

Medial Vestibular Nucleus

Lateral Vestibular Nucleus

Solitary Nucleus and Tract

Spinal Trigeminal Nucleus (pars oralis)

Ventral Cochlear Nucleus

Vestibular Root of VIIIth Nerve

Pontobulbar Nucleus (or Body)

Spinal Trigeminal Tract

Secondary Cochlear Fibers

Superior Olive

Tectospinal Tract

Principal (Inferior) Olivary Nucleus

Nucleus Raphe, Magnus

Nucleus Raphe, Pallidus

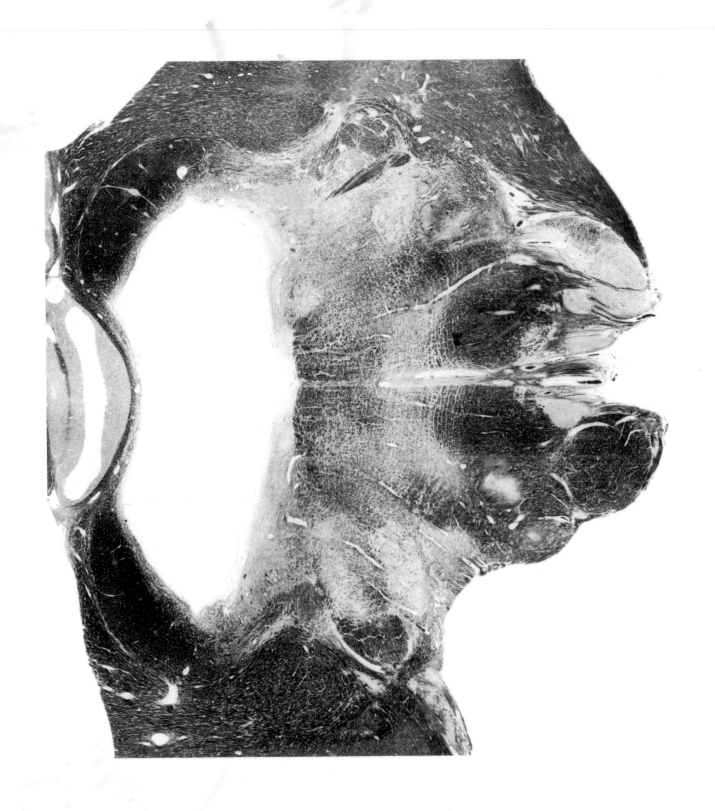

5–14 Semi-diagrammatic representation of the internal distribution of arteries in the medulla oblongata. Selected main structures are labeled on the left side of each section and the general pattern of arterial distribution overlies these structures on the right.

Abbreviations

ALS	Anterolateral System
CSp	Corticospinal Fibers
DVagNu	Dorsal Motor Nucleus of Vagus
DCNu	Dorsal Cochlear Nucleus
DSCT	Dorsal Spinocerebellar Tract
FCu	Cuneate Fasciculus
FGr	Gracile Fasciculus
HyNr	Hypoglossal Nerve
HyNu	Hypoglossal Nucleus
IAF	Internal Arcuate Fibers
LCSp	Lateral Corticospinal Tract
ML	Medial Lemniscus
MLF	Medial Longitudinal Fasciculus
NuAm	Nucleus Ambiguus
NuCu	Cuneate Nucleus
NuGr	Gracile Nucleus
NuPp	Nucleus Prepositus
Py	Pyramid
PyDec	Pyramidal Decussation
RB	Restiform Body (+ Juxtarestiform Body = Inferior Cerebellar Peduncle)
RetF	Reticular Formation
RuSp	Rubrospinal Tract
SolNu	Solitary Nucleus
SpTTr & Nu	Spinal Trigeminal Tract and Nucleus
TecSp	Tectospinal Tract
Ven	Ventricle
VesNu	Vestibular Nuclei
VSCT	Ventral Spinocerebellar Tract

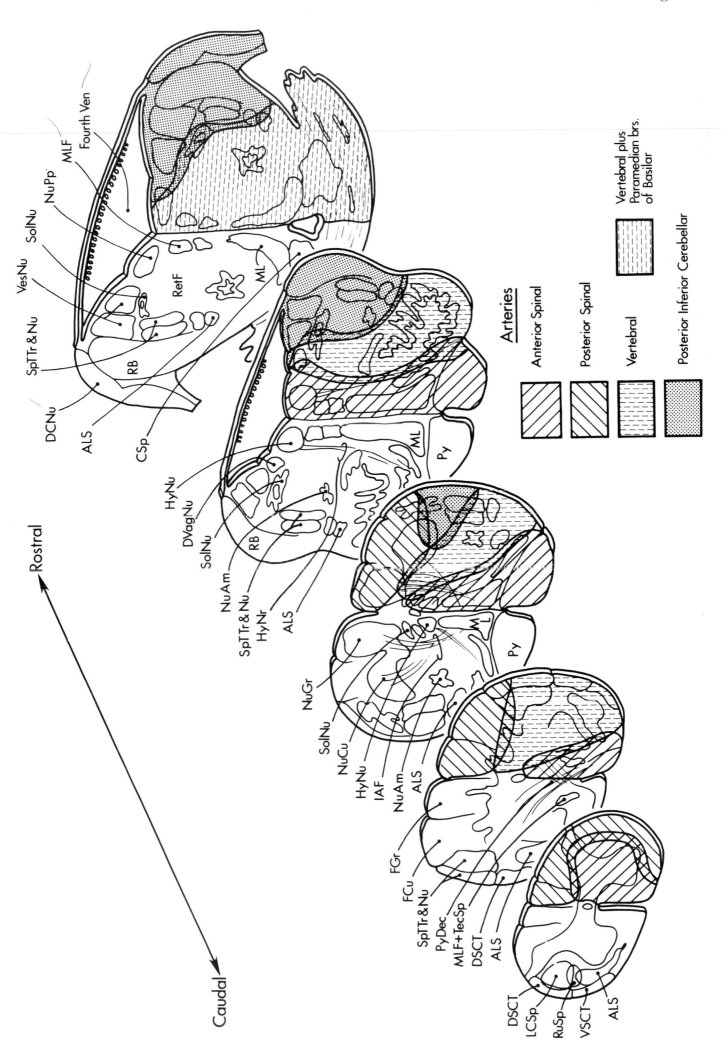

Rostral

Caudal

Fourth Ven
MLF
NuPp
SolNu
VesNu
SpTr &Nu
DCNu
ALS
CSp
RetF
ML
RB

HyNu
DVagNu
SolNu
RB
NuAm
SpTTr &Nu
HyNr
ALS
ML
Py

NuGr
SolNu
NuCu
HyNu
IAF
NuAm
ALS
ML
Py

FGr
FCu
SpTr &Nu
PyDec
MLF+TecSp
DSCT
ALS

DSCT
LCSp
RuSp
VSCT
ALS

Arteries

Anterior Spinal

Posterior Spinal

Vertebral

Posterior Inferior Cerebellar

Vertebral plus
Paramedian brs.
of Basilar

5-15 Transverse section through the dorsal aspects of medulla at the level of the *cochlear nuclei* and the *cerebellar nuclei*. The plane corresponds to about the middle of the *dentate nucleus* and caudal portions of the *globosus* and *emboliform nuclei*. For additional details of the medulla at this level see Figure 5-12 on page 92.

Dentate Nucleus, DNu
(Lateral Cerebellar Nucleus)

Globose Nucleus, GNu
(Posterior Interposed Cerebellar Nucleus)

Ventral Paraflocculus
(Tonsil)

Dorsal Cochlear Nucleus

Lateral Recess of
Fourth Ventricle

Restiform Body

Solitary Nucleus and Tract

Spinal (or Inferior)
Vestibular Nucleus

Medial Vestibular Nucleus

Fastigial Nucleus, FNu
(Medial Cerebellar Nucleus)

Uvula

Nodulus

Nucleus Prepositus

Medial Longitudinal Fasciculus

Tectospinal Tract

Spinal Trigeminal Tract

Spinal Trigeminal Nucleus (pars oralis)

Ventral Cochlear Nucleus

Choroid Plexus

Tela Choroidea

Hilus of Dentate Nucleus

Inferior (or Posterior)
Medullary Velum

Emboliform Nucleus
(Anterior Interposed
Cerebellar Nucleus)

DNu

GNu

FNu

DNu

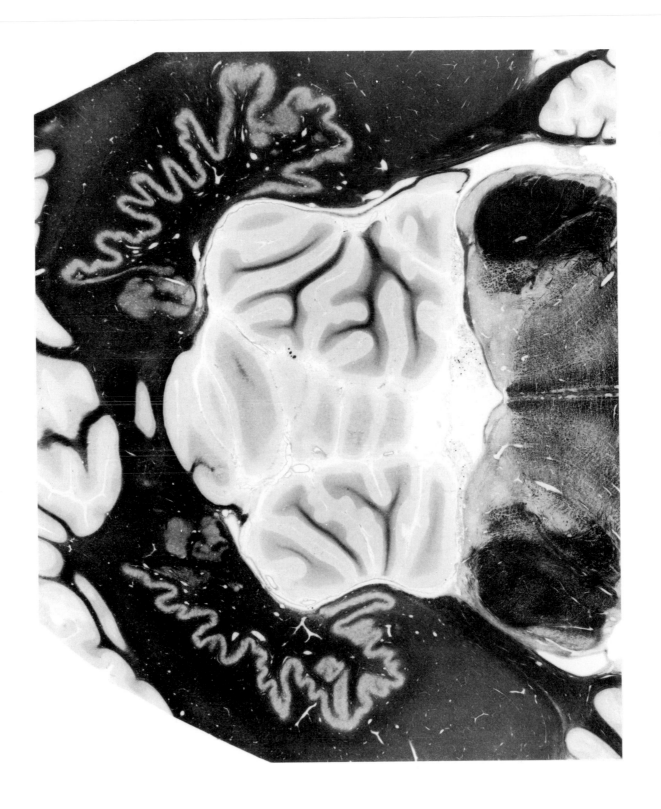

5–16   Transverse section through dorsal portions of pons at the level of the *abducens nucleus* (and *facial colliculus*) and through rostral portions of the *cerebellar nuclei*. For additional details of the pons at this level see Figure 5-17 on page 102.

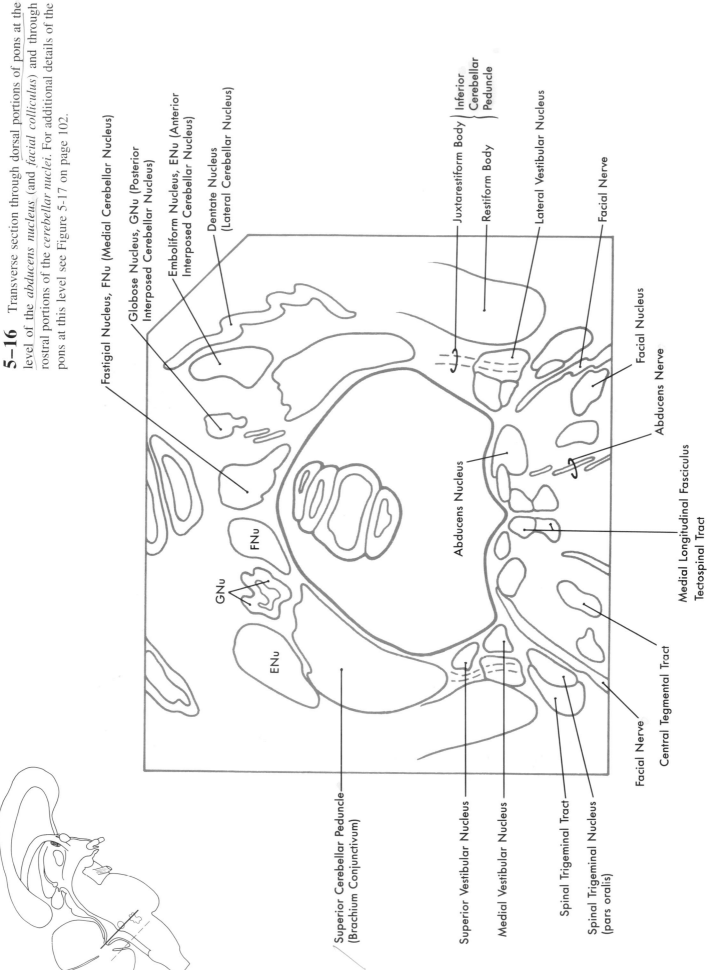

Fastigial Nucleus, FNu (Medial Cerebellar Nucleus)

Globose Nucleus, GNu (Posterior Interposed Cerebellar Nucleus)

Emboliform Nucleus, ENu (Anterior Interposed Cerebellar Nucleus)

Dentate Nucleus (Lateral Cerebellar Nucleus)

Juxtarestiform Body ⎫ Inferior
Restiform Body ⎭ Cerebellar Peduncle

Lateral Vestibular Nucleus

Facial Nerve

Facial Nucleus

Abducens Nerve

Abducens Nucleus

Medial Longitudinal Fasciculus

Tectospinal Tract

Facial Nerve

Central Tegmental Tract

Superior Cerebellar Peduncle (Brachium Conjunctivum)

Superior Vestibular Nucleus

Medial Vestibular Nucleus

Spinal Trigeminal Tract

Spinal Trigeminal Nucleus (pars oralis)

GNu

FNu

ENu

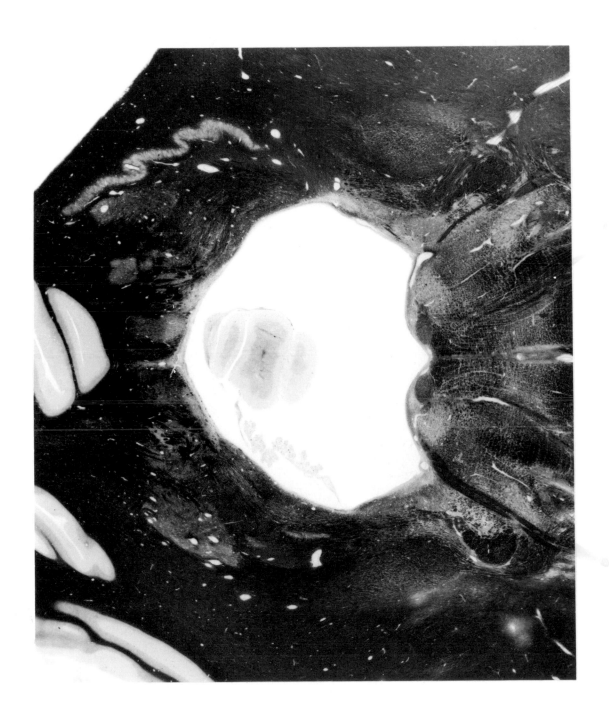

5-17   Transverse section of caudal pons through the *facial nucleus*, *abducens nucleus* (and facial colliculus), and the intramedullary course of fibers of *facial* and *abducens nerves*.

Superior Vestibular Nucleus
Restiform Body
Facial Nerve, Internal Genu
Mesencephalic Tract and Nucleus
Superior Salivatory Nucleus, SSNu
Principal Sensory Nucleus
Trigeminal Motor Nucleus
Trigeminal Nerve
Ventral Spinocerebellar Tract
Rubrospinal Tract
Anterolateral System
Central Tegmental Tract
Trapezoid Body and Nuclei
Pontocerebellar Fibers
Pontine Nuclei
Degenerated Corticospinal Fibers

Superior Cerebellar Peduncle
Reticular Formation
Medial Lemniscus
Medial Longitudinal Fasciculus
Tectospinal Tract

Anterior Medullary Velum

SSNu

Dorsal Longitudinal Fasciculus

Ventral Trigeminothalamic Tract
Nucleus Raphe, Magnus
Corticospinal Fibers
Pontine Nuclei
Abducens Nerve
Superior Olive
Lateral Lemniscus
Abducens Nucleus
Facial Nucleus
Facial Nerve
Spinal Trigeminal Nucleus (pars oralis)
Solitary Nucleus and Tract
Spinal Trigeminal Tract
Lateral Vestibular Nucleus
Medial Vestibular Nucleus
Juxtarestiform Body
Superior Vestibular Nucleus

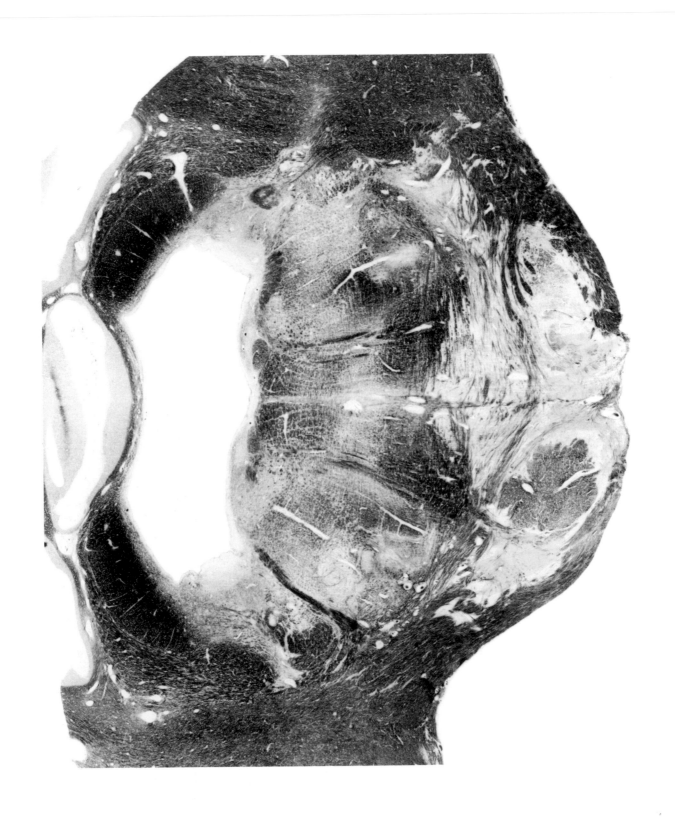

5-18 Transverse section of pons through the rostral pole of the *facial nucleus and the internal genu of the facial nerve.*

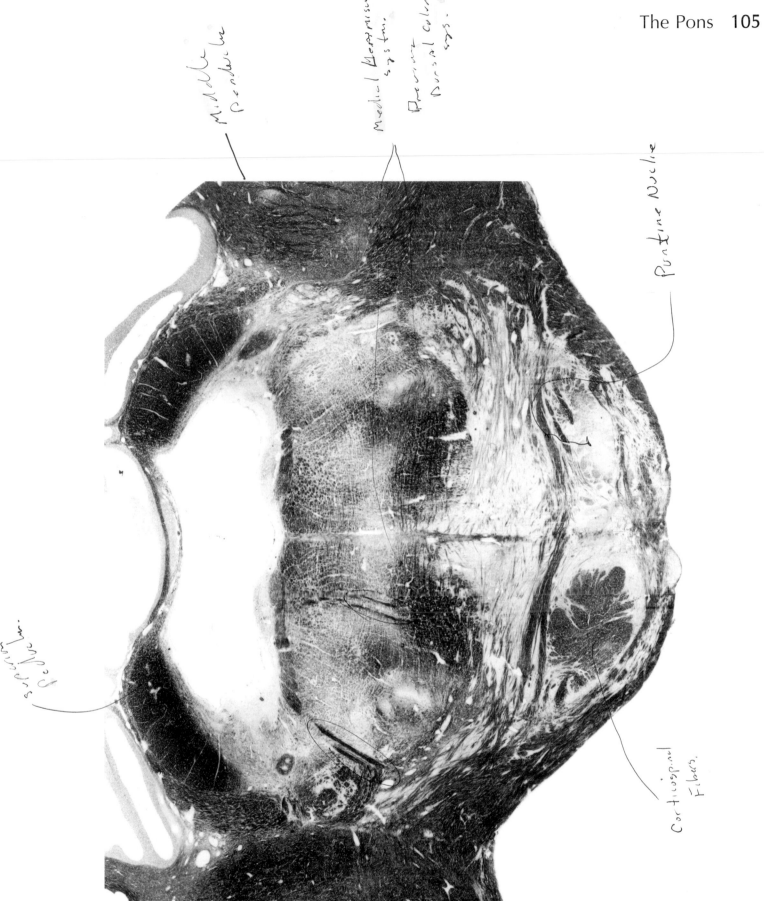

Middle Peduncle

Medial Lemniscus system.

Present Dorsal Colm sys.

Pontine Nuclei

Pontine Nuclei

Corticospinal Fibers.

Cerebellum.

5-19 Transverse section of pons through the chief sensory nucleus and motor nucleus of the trigeminal nerve.

Mesencephalic Tract

Superior Cerebellar Peduncle (Brachium Conjunctivum)

Ventral Spinocerebellar Tract (VSCT)

Locus Ceruleus

Trigeminal Motor Nucleus

Lateral Lemniscus

Middle Cerebellar Peduncle (Brachium Pontis)

VSCT

Anterolateral System

Rubrospinal Tract

Central Tegmental Tract

Ventral Trigeminothalamic Tract

Pontocerebellar Fibers

Degenerated Corticospinal Fibers

Central Gray (Periventricular Gray)

Mesencephalic Nucleus

Anterior Medullary Velum

Medial Longitudinal Fasciculus

Dorsal Longitudinal Fasciculus

Tectospinal Tract

Reticular Formation

Pontine Nuclei

Pontine Nuclei

Chief Sensory Nucleus

Trigeminal Motor Nucleus

Trigeminal Nerve

Lateral Lemniscus

Superior Olive

Lateral Lemniscus, Nucleus

Medial Lemniscus

Reticulotegmental Nucleus

Nucleus Raphe, Pontis

Corticospinal Fibers

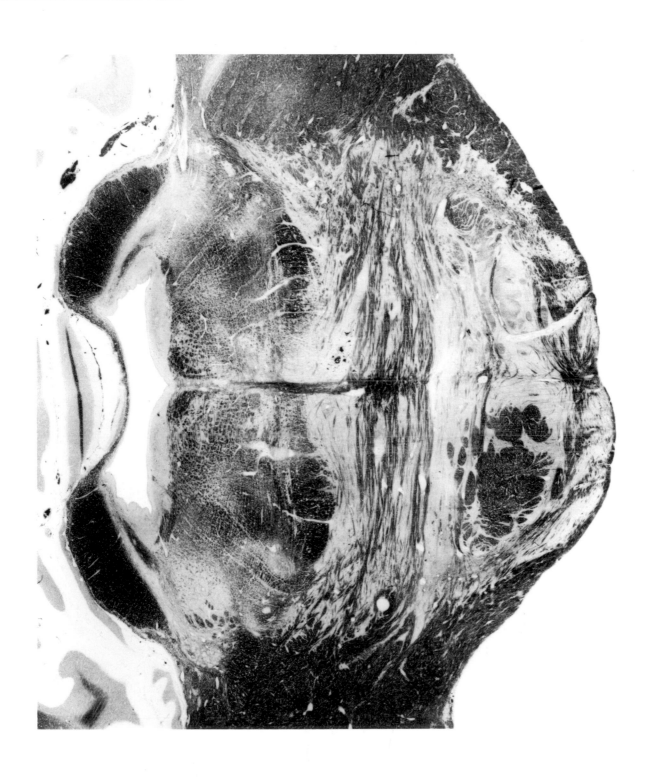

5–20 Transverse section of rostral pons through the *exit of the trochlear nerve* and rostral portions of the exit of the *trigeminal nerve.*

Frenulum

Cerebral Aqueduct

Central Gray (Periaqueductal Gray)

Trochlear Nerve, Exit

Dorsal Trigeminothalamic Tract

Superior Cerebellar Peduncle (Brachium Conjunctivum)

Central Tegmental Tract

Nucleus Centralis, Superior

Anterolateral System

Medial Lemniscus

Middle Cerebellar Peduncle (Brachium Pontis)

Trigeminal Nerve

Basilar Pons

Corticospinal Fibers

Nucleus Raphe, Dorsalis

Locus Ceruleus

Mesencephalic Nucleus and Tract

Medial Longitudinal Fasciculus

Reticular Formation

Lateral Lemniscus and Nuclei of Lateral Lemniscus

Tectospinal Tract

Ventral Trigeminothalamic Tract

Rubrospinal Tract

Pontine Nuclei

Pontocerebellar Fibers

Degenerated Corticospinal Fibers

Medial TP via ferrure.

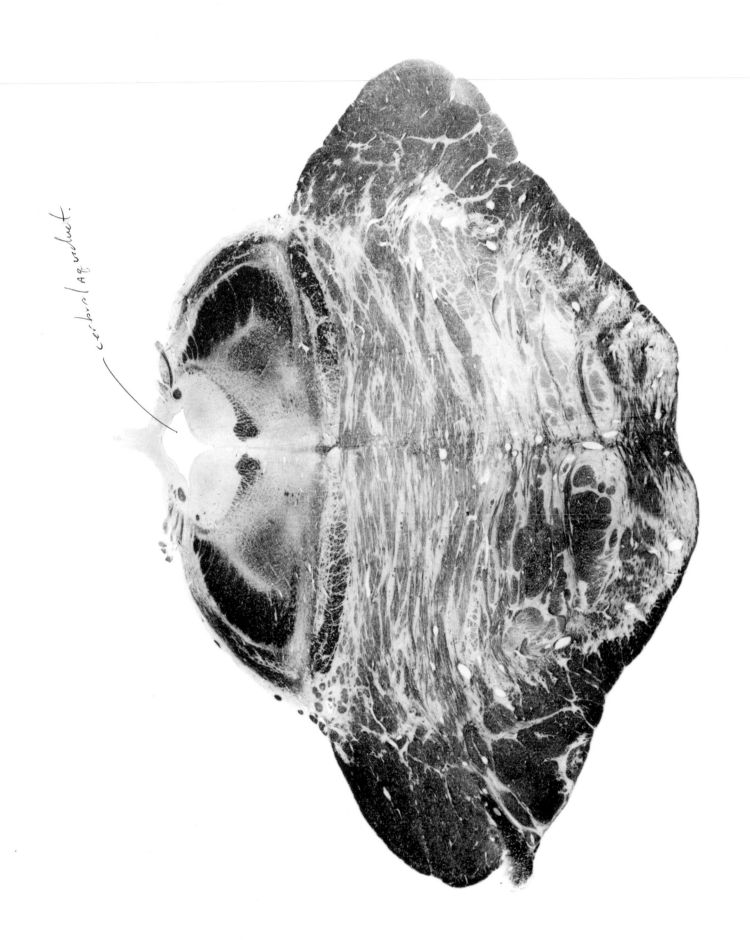

cerebral aqueduct.

5-21 Semi-diagrammatic representation of the internal distribution of arteries in the pons. Selected main structures are labeled on the left side of each section; the general pattern of arterial distribution overlies these structures on the right.

Abbreviations

AbdNr	Abducens Nerve
AbdNu	Abducens Nucleus
ALS	Anterolateral System
AMV	Anterior Medullary Velum
BP	Basilar Pons
CSp	Corticospinal Fibers
CTT	Central Tegmental Tract
FacNr	Facial Nerve
FacNu	Facial Nucleus
LL	Lateral Lemniscus
MCP	Middle Cerebellar Peduncle (Brachium Pontis)
MesNu	Mesencephalic Nucleus
ML	Medial Lemniscus
MLF	Medial Longitudinal Fasciculus
PonNu	Pontine Nuclei
RB	Restiform Body (+ Juxtarestiform Body = Inferior Cerebellar Peduncle)
RetF	Reticular Formation
SCP	Superior Cerebellar Peduncle (Brachium Conjunctivum)
SpTNu	Spinal Trigeminal Nucleus
SpTTr	Spinal Trigeminal Tract
TrapB	Trapezoid Body
TriNr	Trigeminal Nerve
Trigeminal Nu	Trigeminal Nuclei
CS	Chief Sensory
Mes	Mesencephalic
Mo	Motor
TroNr	Trochlear Nerve
VesNu	Vestibular Nuclei
VSCT	Ventral Spinocerebellar Tract

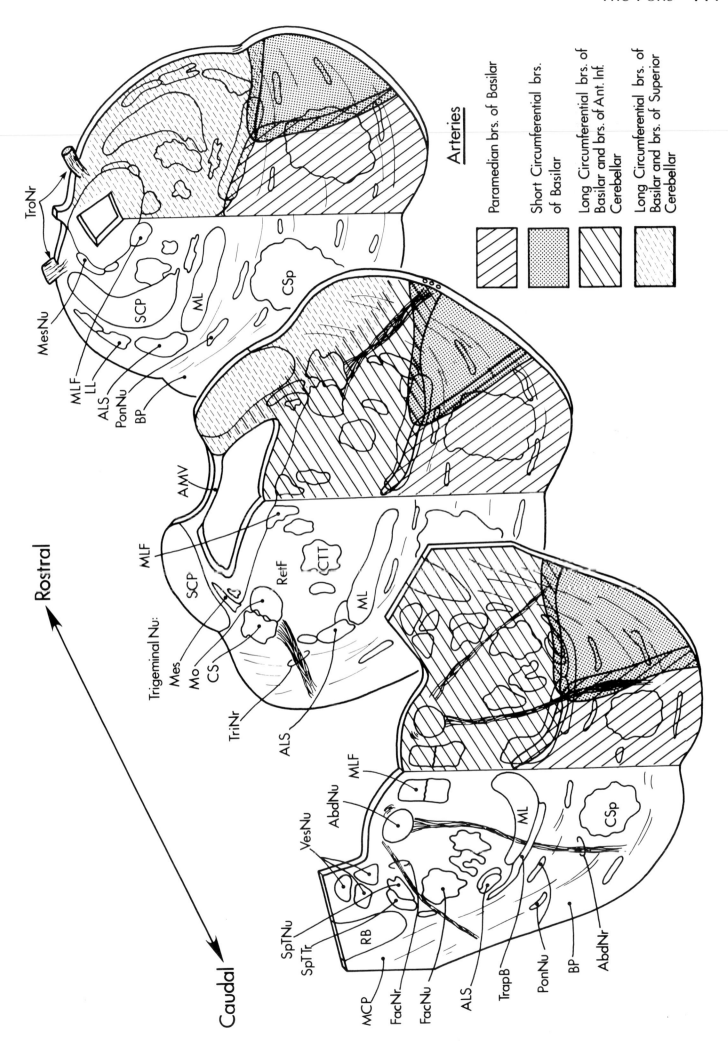

Rostral

Caudal

Arteries

Paramedian brs. of Basilar

Short Circumferential brs. of Basilar

Long Circumferential brs. of Basilar and brs. of Ant. Inf. Cerebellar

Long Circumferential brs. of Basilar and brs. of Superior Cerebellar

TroNr
MesNu
MLF
LL
ALS
PonNu
BP
SCP
ML
CSp

AMV
MLF
Trigeminal Nu:
Mes
Mo
CS
TriNr
ALS
SCP
RetF
CTT
ML

MLF
AbdNu
VesNu
SpTNu
SpTTr
RB
MCP
FacNr.
FacNu
ALS
TrapB
PonNu
BP
AbdNr.
ML
CSp

5-22   Transverse section of pons-midbrain junction through the *inferior colliculus*, caudal portions of the decussation of the *superior cerebellar peduncle*, and rostral parts of the *basilar pons*. The plane of section is just caudal to the *trochlear nucleus*.

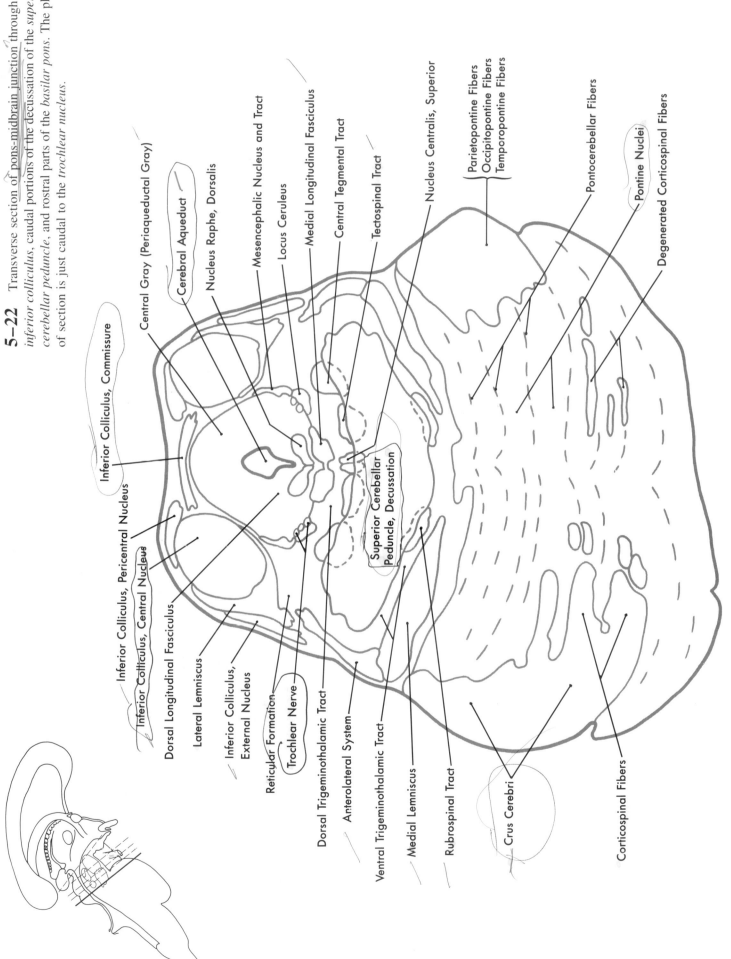

Central Gray (Periaqueductal Gray)

Cerebral Aqueduct

Nucleus Raphe, Dorsalis

Mesencephalic Nucleus and Tract

Locus Ceruleus

Medial Longitudinal Fasciculus

Central Tegmental Tract

Tectospinal Tract

Nucleus Centralis, Superior

Parietopontine Fibers
Occipitopontine Fibers
Temporopontine Fibers

Pontocerebellar Fibers

Pontine Nuclei

Degenerated Corticospinal Fibers

Inferior Colliculus, Commissure

Inferior Colliculus, Pericentral Nucleus

Inferior Colliculus, Central Nucleus

Dorsal Longitudinal Fasciculus

Lateral Lemniscus

Inferior Colliculus, External Nucleus

Reticular Formation

Trochlear Nerve

Dorsal Trigeminothalamic Tract

Anterolateral System

Ventral Trigeminothalamic Tract

Medial Lemniscus

Rubrospinal Tract

Superior Cerebellar Peduncle, Decussation

Crus Cerebri

Corticospinal Fibers

Two Levels of Neuro Axis

Midbrain

Pons Better Half

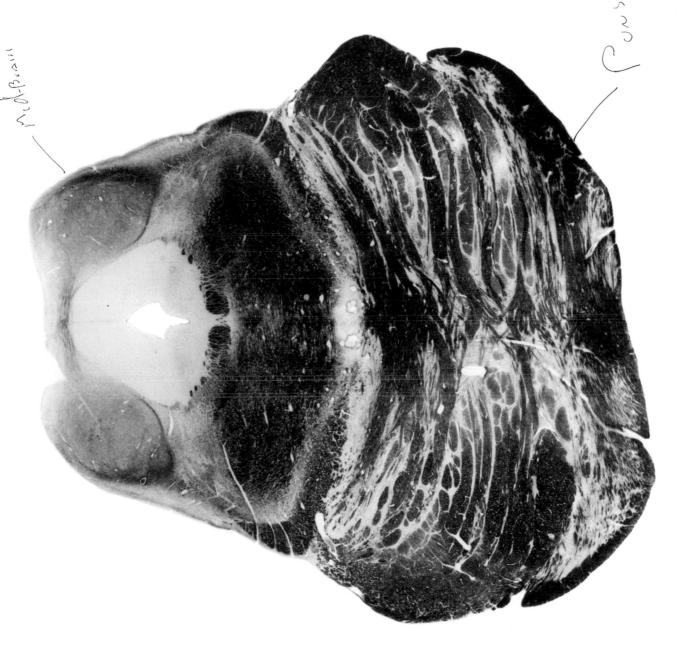

5-23 Transverse section of midbrain through the *trochlear nucleus* and *decussation of the superior cerebellar peduncle*. The section also includes caudal parts of the *superior colliculus* and the rostral tip of the *basilar pons*.

Dorsal Longitudinal Fasciculus

Nucleus Raphe, Dorsalis

Trochlear Nucleus

Spinotectal Tract

Spinothalamic Tract

Anterolateral System

Tectospinal Tract

Medial Lemniscus

Ventral Trigeminothalamic Tract

Substantia Nigra, pars compacta

Parietopontine Fibers (PPon)
Occipitopontine Fibers (OPon)
Temporopontine Fibers (TPon)

Degenerated Corticospinal Fibers

Frontopontine Fibers (FPon)

Interpeduncular Nucleus

Interpeduncular Fossa

Cerebral Aqueduct

Central Gray (Periaqueductal Gray)

Superior Colliculus

Mesencephalic Nucleus and Tract

Inferior Colliculus, Brachium

Reticular Formation

Dorsal Trigeminothalamic Tract

Central Tegmental Tract

Medial Longitudinal Fasciculus

Superior Cerebellar Peduncle, Decussation

PPon
OPon
TPon

Corticospinal Fibers

FPon

Corticobulbar Fibers

Crus Cerebri

Pontine Nuclei

Rubrospinal Tract

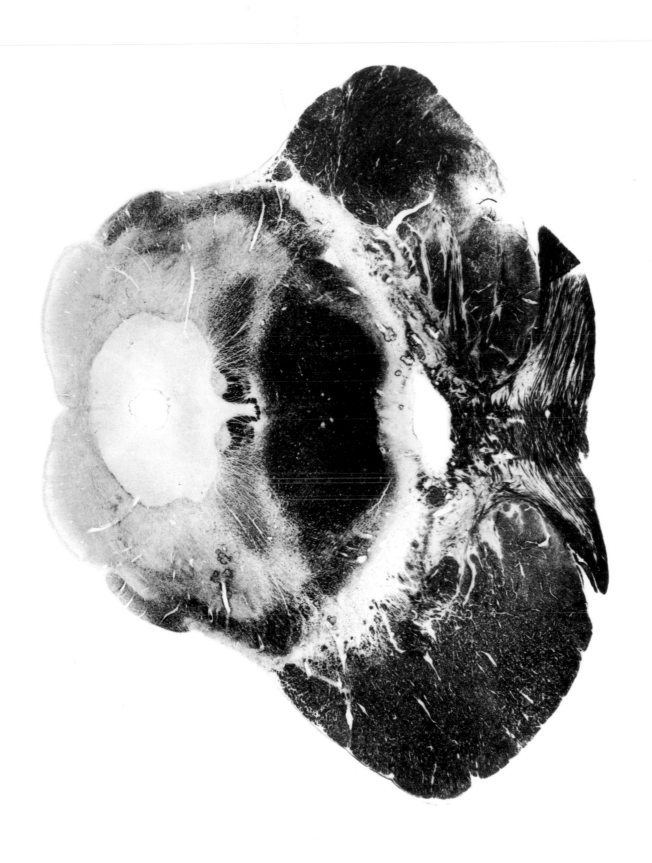

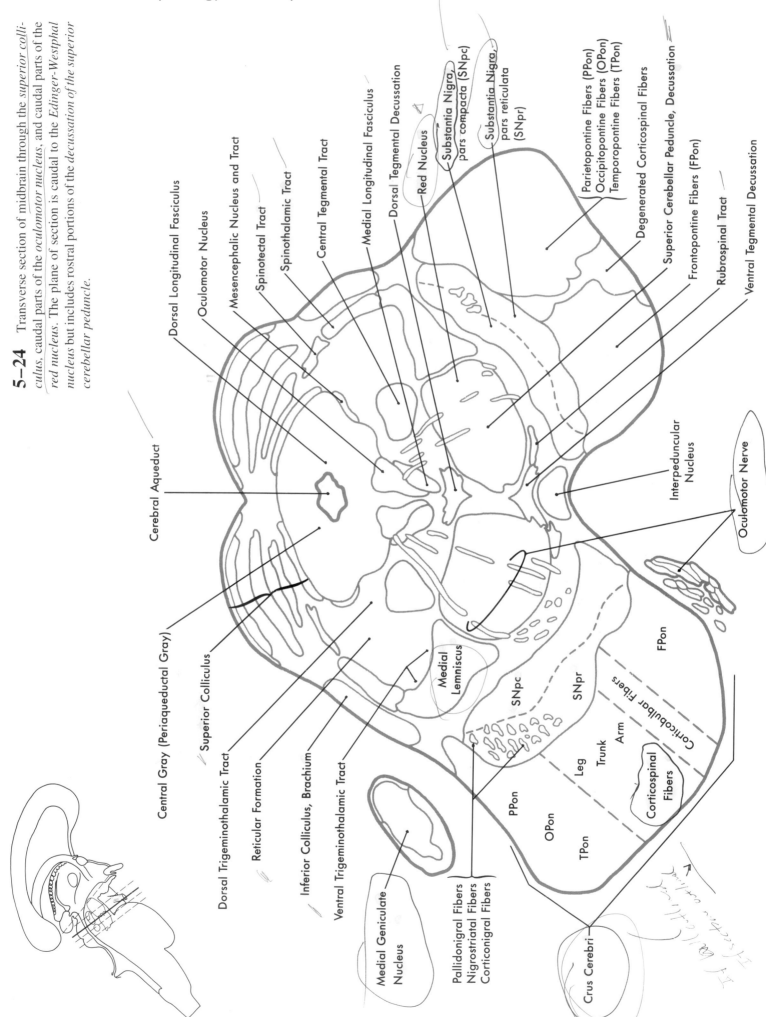

5-24   Transverse section of midbrain through the *superior colliculus*, caudal parts of the *oculomotor nucleus*, and caudal parts of the *red nucleus*. The plane of section is caudal to the *Edinger-Westphal nucleus* but includes rostral portions of the *decussation of the superior cerebellar peduncle*.

Dorsal Longitudinal Fasciculus

Oculomotor Nucleus

Mesencephalic Nucleus and Tract

Spinotectal Tract

Spinothalamic Tract

Central Tegmental Tract

Medial Longitudinal Fasciculus

Dorsal Tegmental Decussation

Red Nucleus

Substantia Nigra, pars compacta (SNpc)

Substantia Nigra, pars reticulata (SNpr)

Parietopontine Fibers (PPon)
Occipitopontine Fibers (OPon)
Temporopontine Fibers (TPon)

Degenerated Corticospinal Fibers

Superior Cerebellar Peduncle, Decussation

Frontopontine Fibers (FPon)

Rubrospinal Tract

Ventral Tegmental Decussation

Cerebral Aqueduct

Interpeduncular Nucleus

Oculomotor Nerve

Central Gray (Periaqueductal Gray)

Superior Colliculus

Dorsal Trigeminothalamic Tract

Reticular Formation

Inferior Colliculus, Brachium

Ventral Trigeminothalamic Tract

Medial Lemniscus

SNpc

SNpr

FPon

Corticobulbar Fibers

Leg

Trunk

Arm

Corticospinal Fibers

PPon

OPon

TPon

Medial Geniculate Nucleus

Pallidonigral Fibers
Nigrostriatal Fibers
Corticonigral Fibers

Crus Cerebri

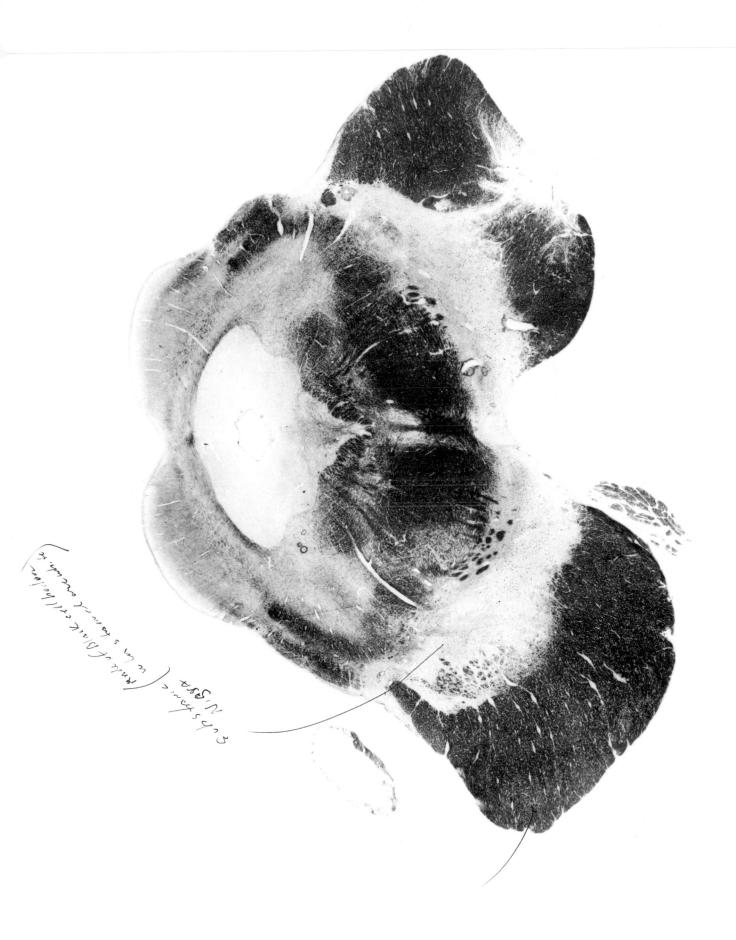

Substantia Nigra
(medial cell column believed
to be a strict homolog of...)

5-25   Transverse section of midbrain through the *superior colliculus*, rostral portions of the *oculomotor nucleus*, including the *Edinger-Westphal nucleus*, and the exit of fibers of the *oculomotor nerve.*

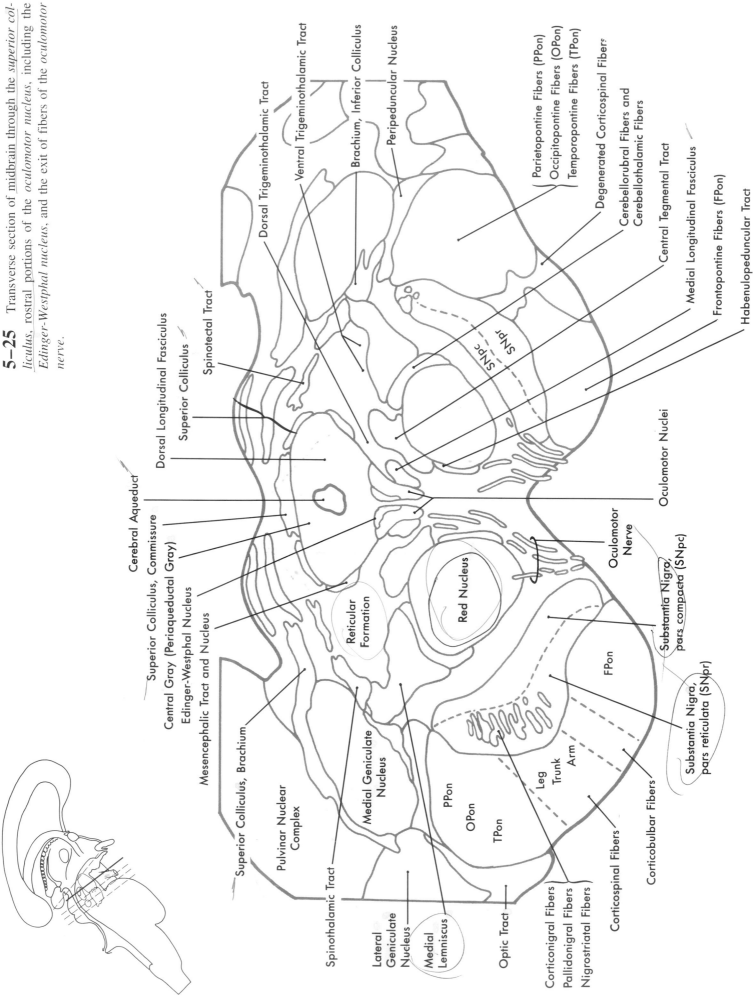

Dorsal Trigeminothalamic Tract

Ventral Trigeminothalamic Tract

Brachium, Inferior Colliculus

Peripeduncular Nucleus

Parietopontine Fibers (PPon)
Occipitopontine Fibers (OPon)
Temporopontine Fibers (TPon)

Degenerated Corticospinal Fibers

Cerebellorubral Fibers and
Cerebellothalamic Fibers

Central Tegmental Tract

Medial Longitudinal Fasciculus

Frontopontine Fibers (FPon)

Habenulopeduncular Tract

Spinotectal Tract

Dorsal Longitudinal Fasciculus

Superior Colliculus

Cerebral Aqueduct

Central Gray (Periaqueductal Gray)

Superior Colliculus, Commissure

Edinger-Westphal Nucleus

Mesencephalic Tract and Nucleus

Superior Colliculus, Brachium

Pulvinar Nuclear Complex

Spinothalamic Tract

Lateral Geniculate Nucleus

Medial Lemniscus

Optic Tract

Medial Geniculate Nucleus

Corticonigral Fibers
Pallidonigral Fibers
Nigrostriatal Fibers

Corticospinal Fibers

Corticobulbar Fibers

Reticular Formation

Red Nucleus

Oculomotor Nuclei

Oculomotor Nerve

Substantia Nigra, pars compacta (SNpc)

Substantia Nigra, pars reticulata (SNpr)

SNpr

SNpc

PPon
OPon
TPon

Leg
Trunk
Arm

FPon

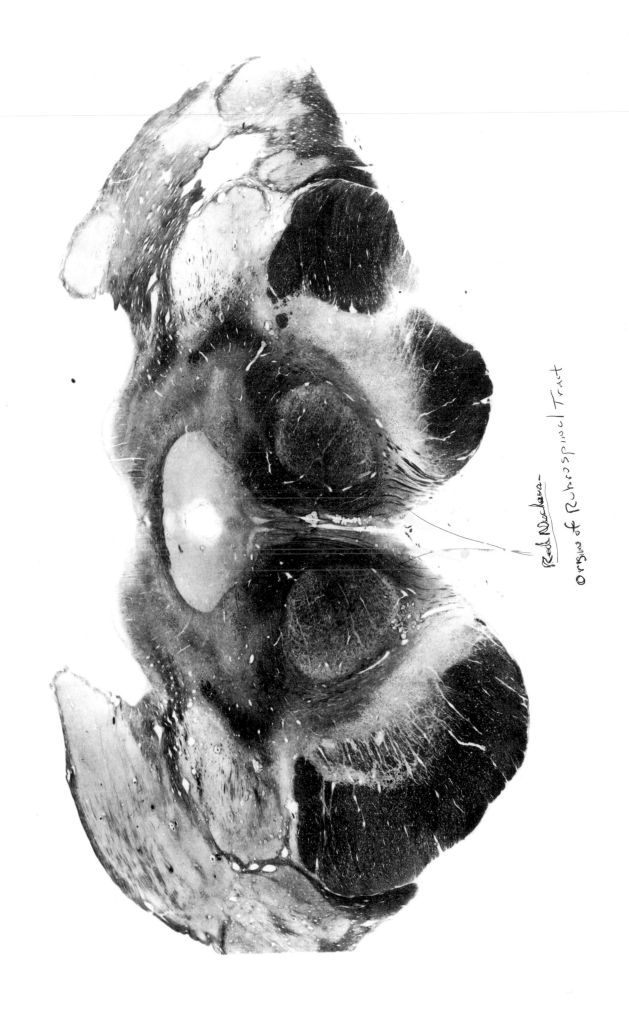

Red Nucleus

Origin of Rubospinal Tract

5-26 Slightly oblique section through the midbrain-diencephalon junction. The section passes through the *posterior commissure*, the rostral end of the *red nucleus*, and ends just dorsal to the *mammillary body*. At this level, the structure labeled *mammillothalamic tract* probably also contains some *mammillotegmental fibers*.

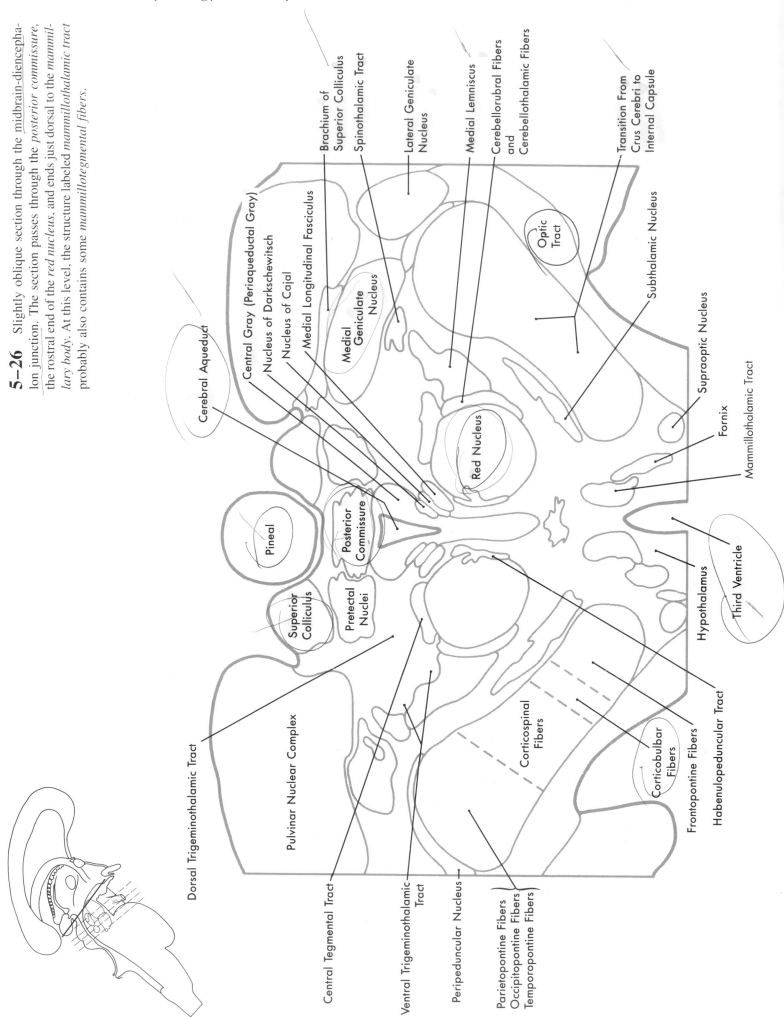

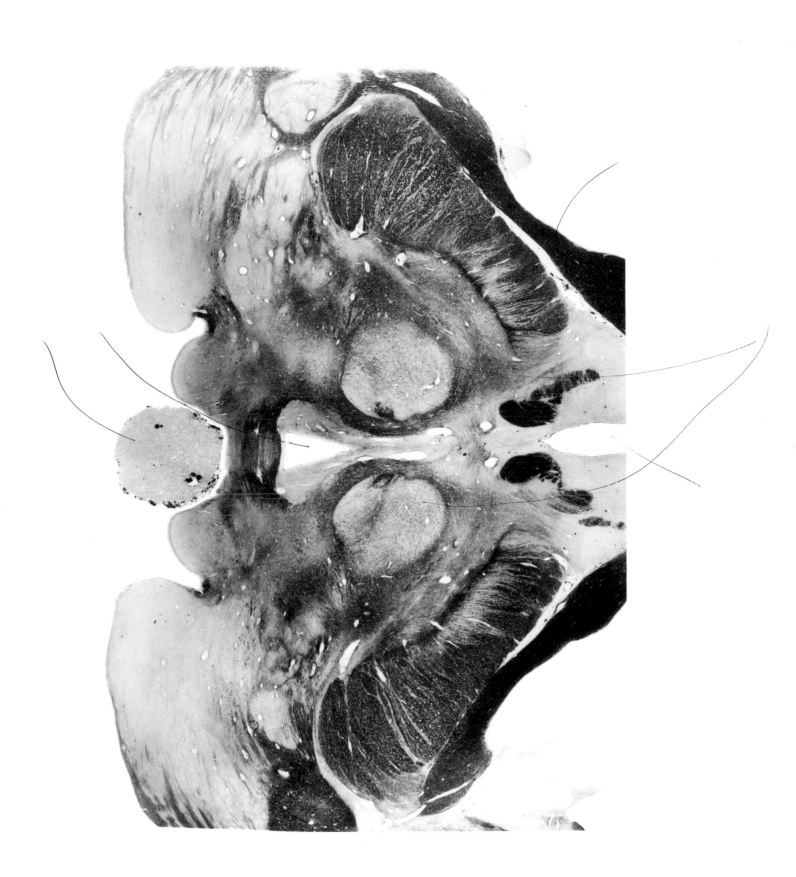

5–27 Semi-diagrammatic representation of the internal distribution of arteries in the midbrain. Selected main structures are labeled on the left side of each section; the general pattern of arterial distribution overlies these structures on the right.

Abbreviations

ALS	Anterolateral System
BP	Basilar Pons
CC	Crus Cerebri
EWNu	Edinger-Westphal Nucleus
IC	Inferior Colliculus
LGB	Lateral Geniculate Body (Nucleus)
LL	Lateral Lemniscus
MesNu	Mesencephalic Nucleus
MGB	Medial Geniculate Body (Nucleus)
ML	Medial Lemniscus
MLF	Medial Longitudinal Fasciculus
OcNr	Oculomotor Nerve
OcNu	Oculomotor Nucleus
RNu	Red Nucleus
SC	Superior Colliculus
SCP	Superior Cerebellar Peduncle
SCP,Dec	Superior Cerebellar Peduncle, Decussation
SN	Substantia Nigra
TriTh	Trigeminothalamic Tracts
TroNu	Trochlear Nucleus

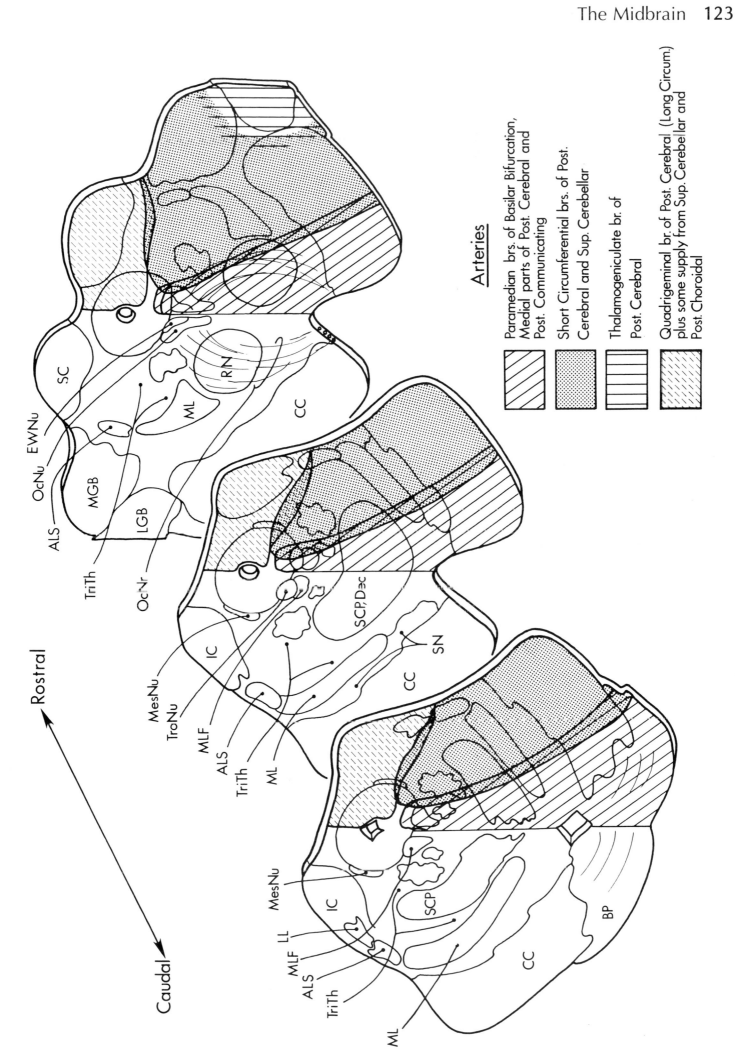

Rostral

Caudal

SC

RN

EWNu

OcNu

ML

CC

ALS

MGB

LGB

TriTh

OcNr

MesNu

TroNu

MLF

ALS

TriTh

ML

IC

SCP;Dec

SN

CC

CC

MesNu

IC

LL

MLF

ALS

TriTh

ML

SCP

CC

BP

<u>Arteries</u>

Paramedian brs. of Basilar Bifurcation, Medial parts of Post. Cerebral and Post. Communicating

Short Circumferential brs. of Post. Cerebral and Sup. Cerebellar

Thalamogeniculate br. of Post. Cerebral

Quadrigeminal br. of Post. Cerebral (Long Circum,) plus some supply from Sup. Cerebellar and Post. Choroidal

5-28   Coronal section of forebrain through the *splenium of the corpus callosum* and *crus of fornix*, and extending into the *inferior colliculus* and exit of the *trochlear nerve*. Many of the structures labeled in this figure can be easily identified in the MRI.

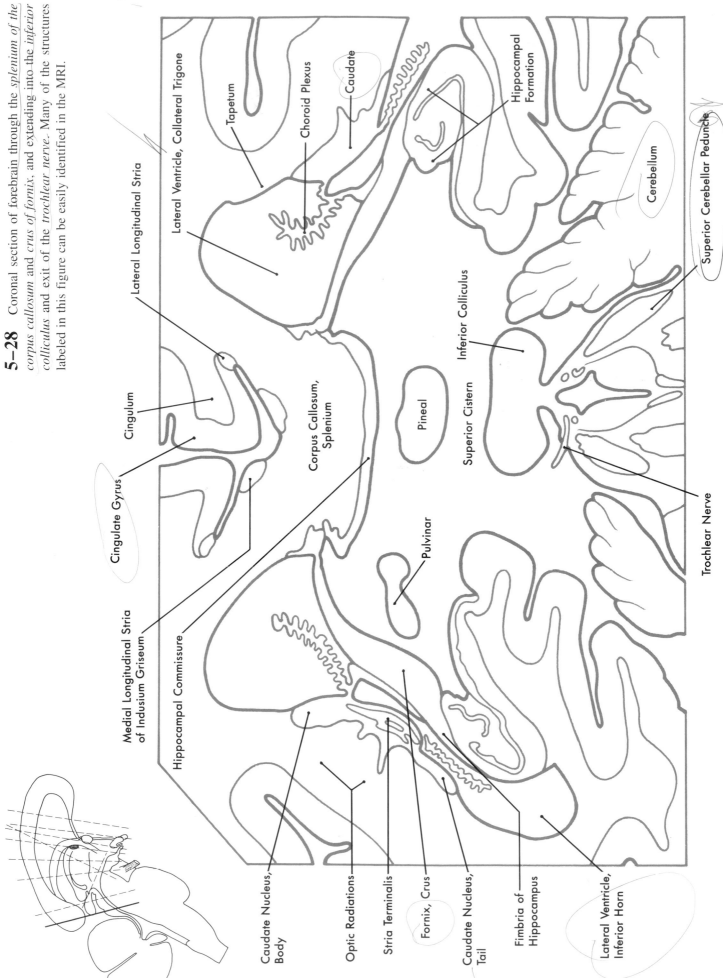

Tapetum

Lateral Ventricle, Collateral Trigone

Choroid Plexus

Caudate

Hippocampal Formation

Cerebellum

Superior Cerebellar Peduncle

Lateral Longitudinal Stria

Cingulum

Cingulate Gyrus

Corpus Callosum, Splenium

Pineal

Superior Cistern

Inferior Colliculus

Trochlear Nerve

Medial Longitudinal Stria of Indusium Griseum

Hippocampal Commissure

Pulvinar

Caudate Nucleus, Body

Optic Radiations

Stria Terminalis

Fornix, Crus

Caudate Nucleus, Tail

Fimbria of Hippocampus

Lateral Ventricle, Inferior Horn

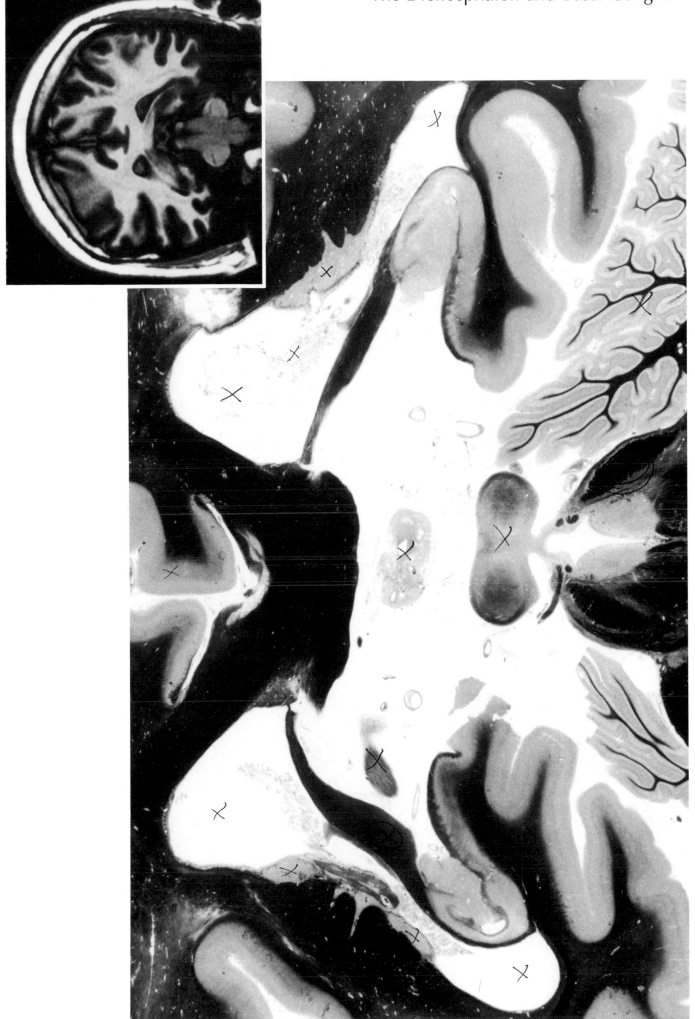

5-29 Coronal section of forebrain through the *pulvinar* and *medial* and *lateral geniculate bodies* (nuclei). The section extends into upper portions of the *midbrain tegmentum*. Many of the structures labeled in this figure can be easily identified in the MRI.

Cingulum

Lateral Longitudinal Stria
of Indusium Griseum

External Medullary Lamina

Insula

Internal Capsule:
Retrolenticular Part
Sublenticular Part

Hippocampal
Formation

Hippocampus,
Fimbria of

Lateral
Nucleus

Central Gray (Periaqueductal Gray)

Choroid
Plexus

Pulvinar
Nuclear
Complex

Medial
Nucleus

Cingulate Gyrus

Medial Longitudinal Stria

Corpus Callosum,
Body

Superior Cistern

Trochlear Nucleus

Fornix, Body

Inferior Colliculus, Brachium

Lateral Ventricle, Body

Caudate Nucleus, Body

Inferior Colliculus, Brachium

Superior Colliculus, Brachium

Stria Terminalis (StTer)

Medial Geniculate
Nucleus

Inferior Pulvinar
Nucleus

Optic Radiations

Lateral Geniculate
Nucleus

StTer and
Bed Nucleus

Caudate Nucleus,
Tail

Alveus of
Hippocampus

Lateral Ventricle, Inferior Horn

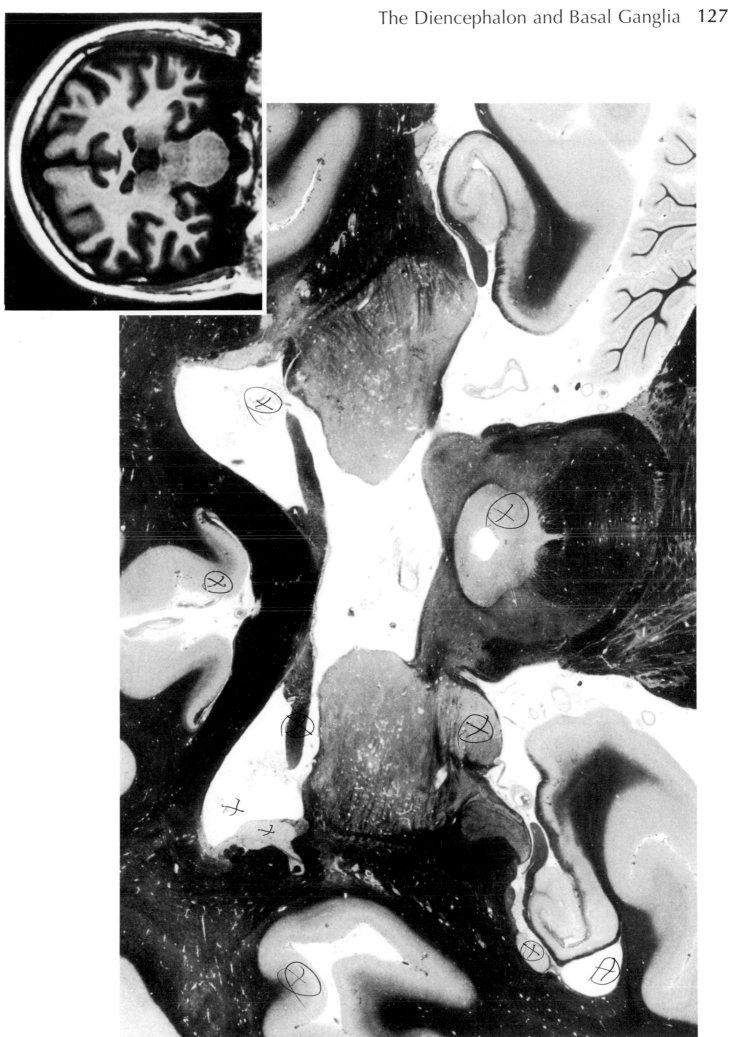

5-30 Slightly oblique section of forebrain through the *pulvinar, ventral posteromedial,* and *ventral posterolateral nuclei.* The section extends rostrally through the *subthalamic nucleus* and ends in the caudal hypothalamus just dorsal to the *mammillary bodies.*

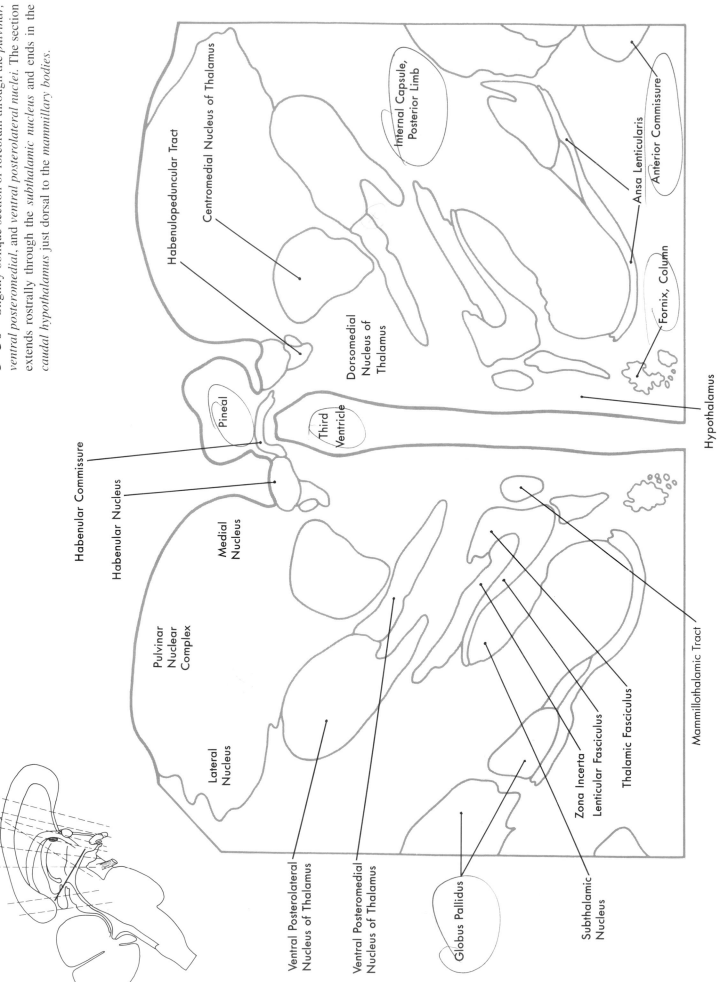

Habenulopeduncular Tract

Centromedial Nucleus of Thalamus

Internal Capsule, Posterior Limb

Ansa Lenticularis

Anterior Commissure

Dorsomedial Nucleus of Thalamus

Fornix, Column

Pineal

Third Ventricle

Hypothalamus

Habenular Commissure

Habenular Nucleus

Medial Nucleus

Pulvinar Nuclear Complex

Lateral Nucleus

Zona Incerta

Lenticular Fasciculus

Thalamic Fasciculus

Mammillothalamic Tract

Ventral Posterolateral Nucleus of Thalamus

Ventral Posteromedial Nucleus of Thalamus

Globus Pallidus

Subthalamic Nucleus

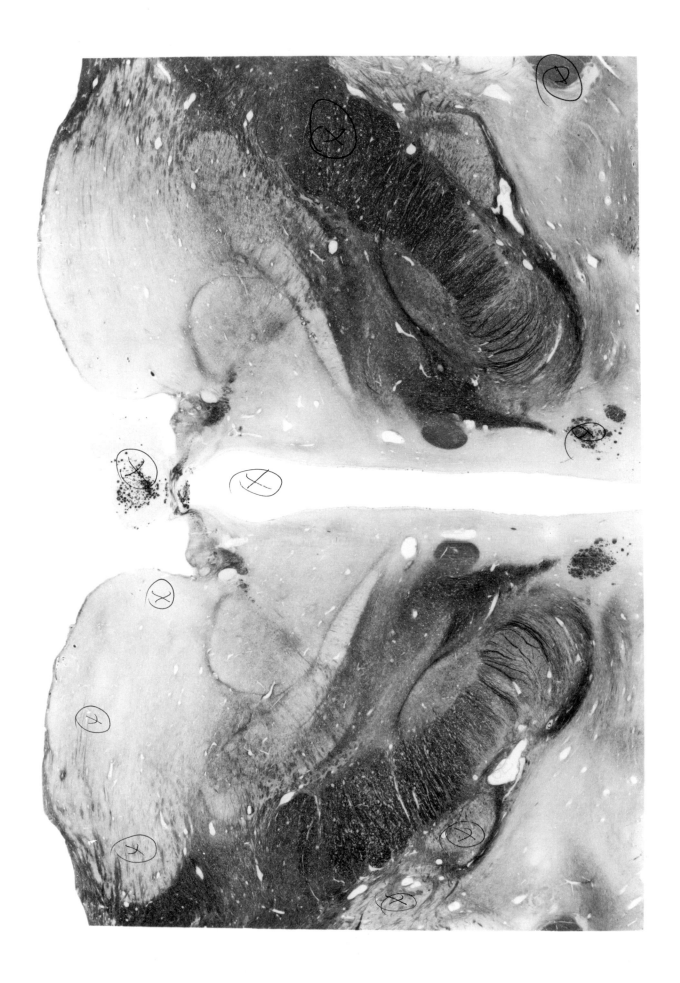

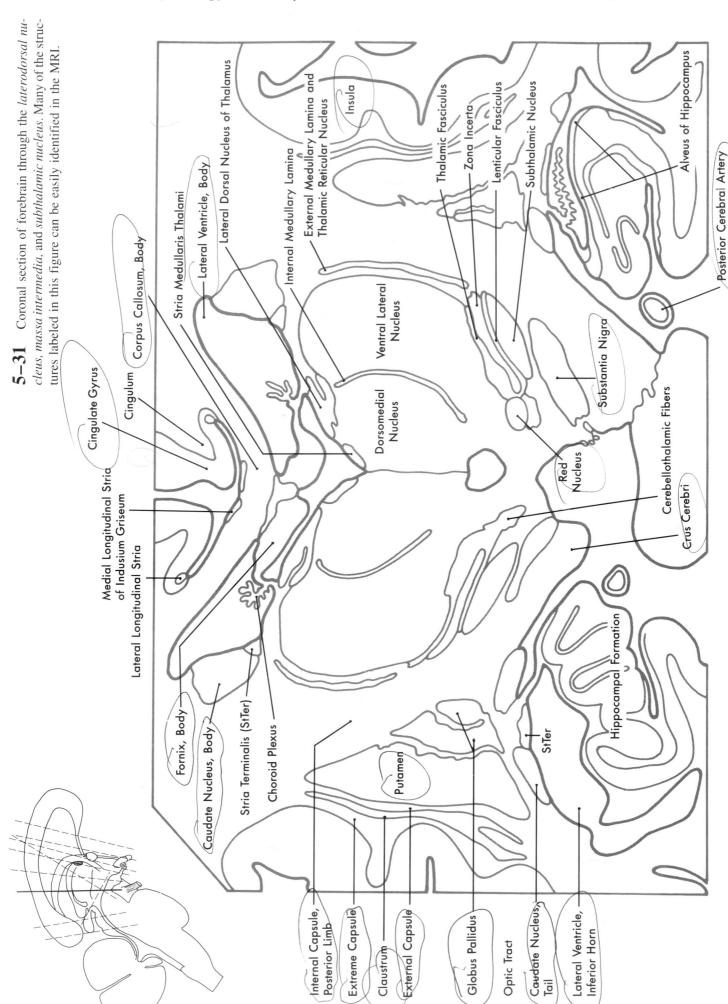

5-31 Coronal section of forebrain through the *laterodorsal nucleus, massa intermedia,* and *subthalamic nucleus.* Many of the structures labeled in this figure can be easily identified in the MRI.

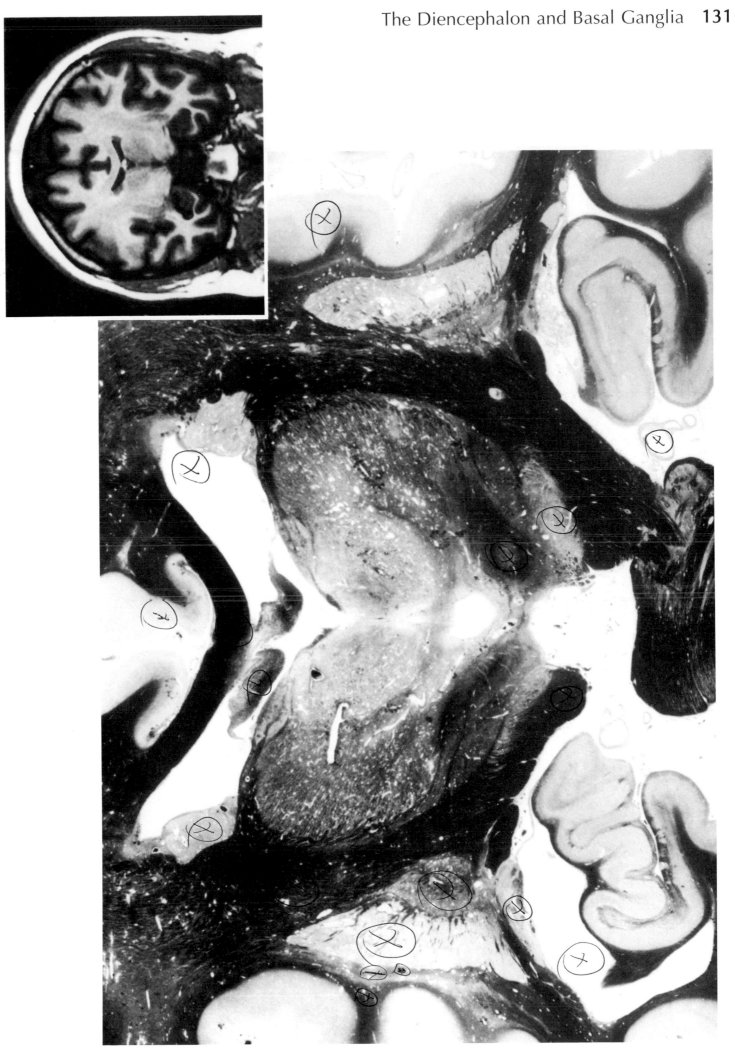

5–32 Coronal section of forebrain through the *anterior nucleus of the thalamus and mammillary body.*

Corpus Callosum, Body

Lateral Ventricle, Body

Choroid Plexus

Stria Medullaris Thalami

Dorsomedial Nucleus of Thalamus

External Medullary Lamina and Thalamic Reticular Nucleus

Internal Medullary Lamina

Thalamic Fasciculus

Zona Incerta

Lenticular Fasciculus

Subthalamic Nucleus

Mammillothalamic Tract

Alveus of Hippocampus

Hippocampal Formation

Cingulum

Cingulate Gyrus

Medial Longitudinal Stria

Lateral Longitudinal Stria of Indusium Griseum

Fornix, Body

Caudate Nucleus, Body

Stria Terminalis

Anterior Nucleus

Ventral Lateral Nucleus

Third Ventricle

Posterior Hypothalamus

Mammillary Body

Internal Capsule, Posterior Limb

Extreme Capsule

Claustrum

External Capsule

Putamen

Globus Pallidus

Insula

Optic Tract

Amygdaloid Nuclear Complex

Lateral Ventricle, Inferior Horn

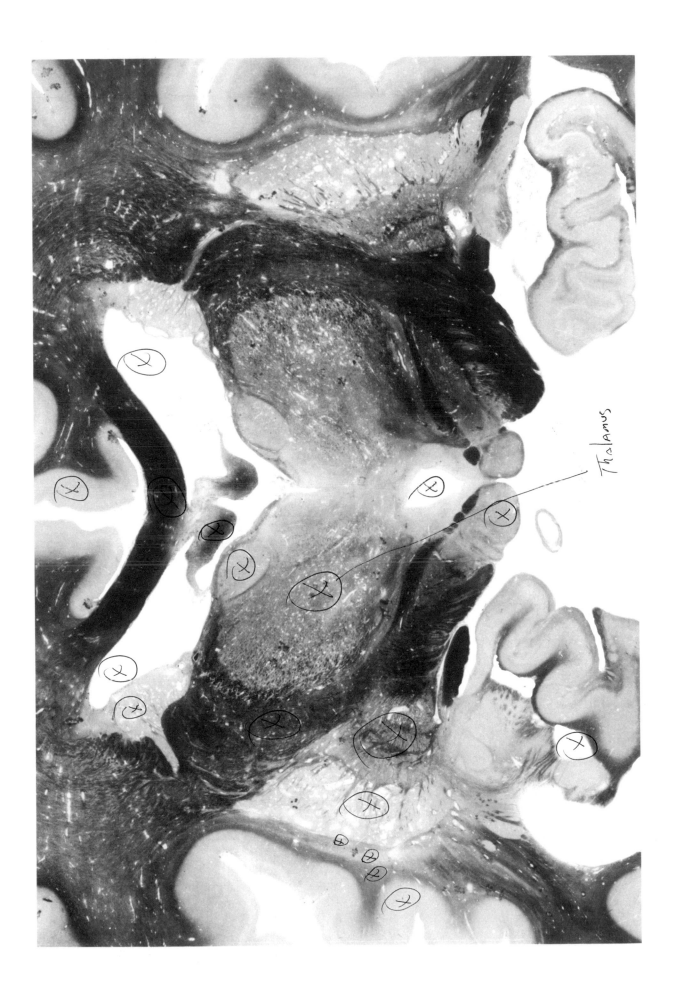

Thalamus

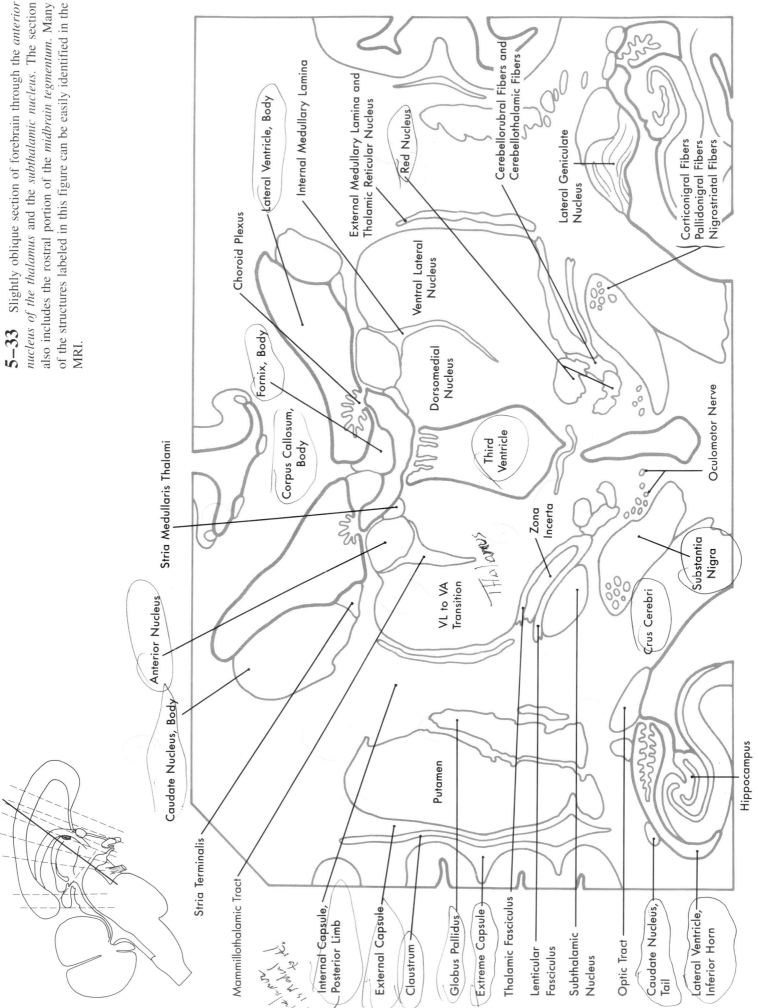

5–33 Slightly oblique section of forebrain through the *anterior nucleus of the thalamus* and the *subthalamic nucleus*. The section also includes the rostral portion of the *midbrain tegmentum*. Many of the structures labeled in this figure can be easily identified in the MRI.

Lateral Ventricle, Body

Internal Medullary Lamina

External Medullary Lamina and Thalamic Reticular Nucleus

Red Nucleus

Cerebellorubral Fibers and Cerebellothalamic Fibers

Lateral Geniculate Nucleus

Corticonigral Fibers
Pallidonigral Fibers
Nigrostriatal Fibers

Choroid Plexus

Fornix, Body

Ventral Lateral Nucleus

Corpus Callosum, Body

Dorsomedial Nucleus

Third Ventricle

Oculomotor Nerve

Stria Medullaris Thalami

Thalamus

Zona Incerta

Substantia Nigra

Anterior Nucleus

VL to VA Transition

Crus Cerebri

Caudate Nucleus, Body

Mammillothalamic Tract

Stria Terminalis

Putamen

Hippocampus

Internal Capsule, Posterior Limb

External Capsule

Claustrum

Globus Pallidus

Extreme Capsule

Thalamic Fasciculus

Lenticular Fasciculus

Subthalamic Nucleus

Optic Tract

Caudate Nucleus, Tail

Lateral Ventricle, Inferior Horn

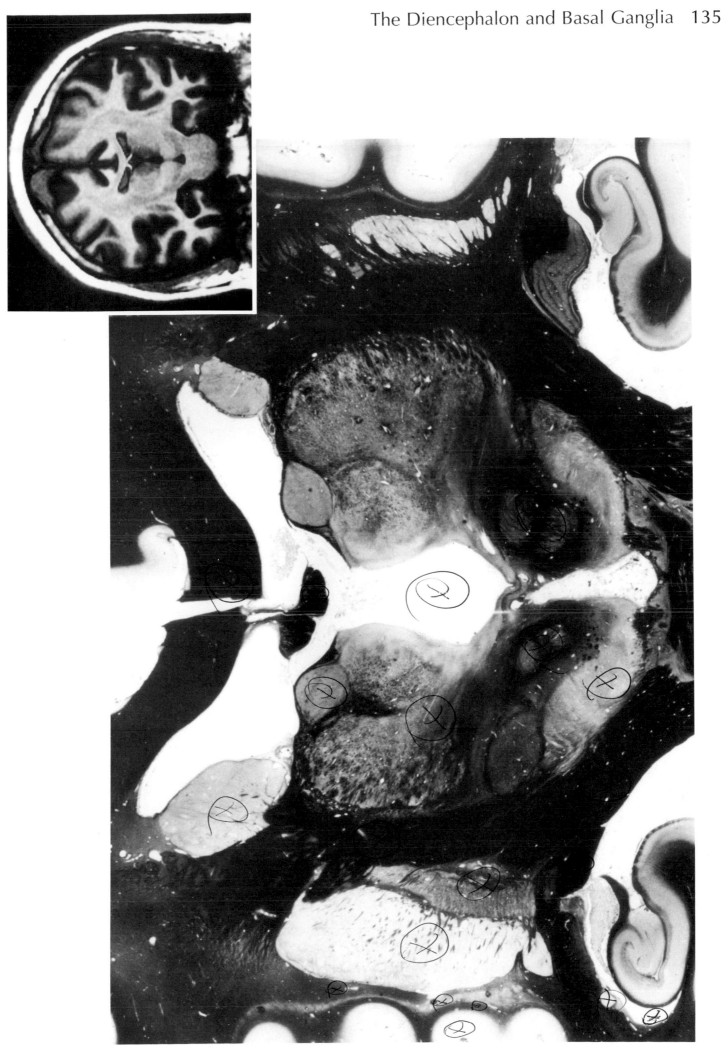

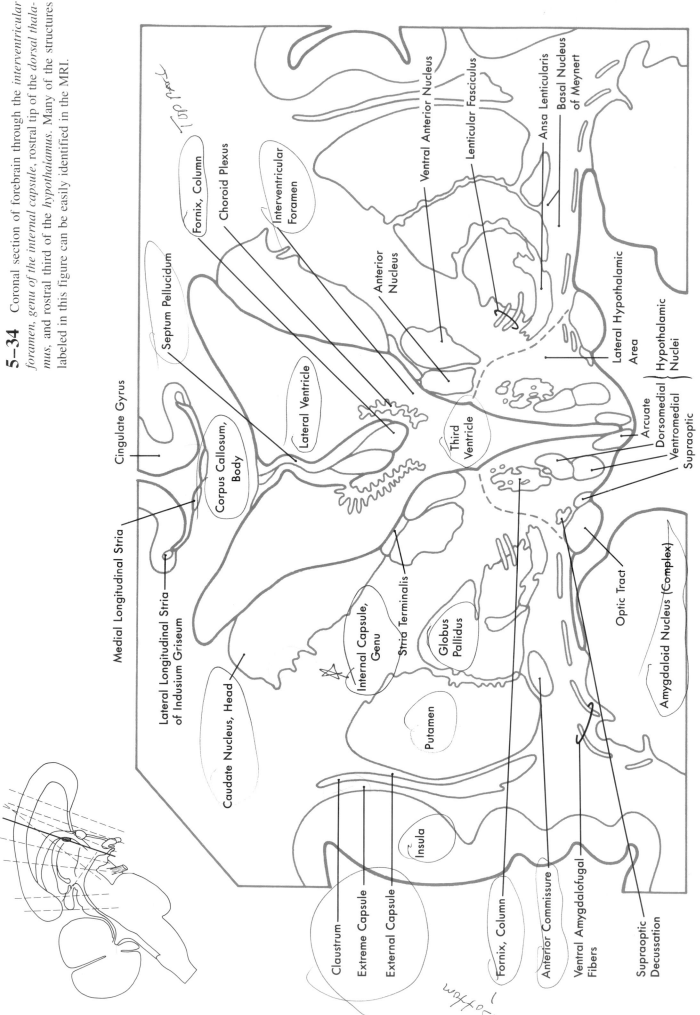

5-34   Coronal section of forebrain through the *interventricular foramen, genu of the internal capsule, rostral tip of the dorsal thalamus,* and rostral third of the *hypothalamus.* Many of the structures labeled in this figure can be easily identified in the MRI.

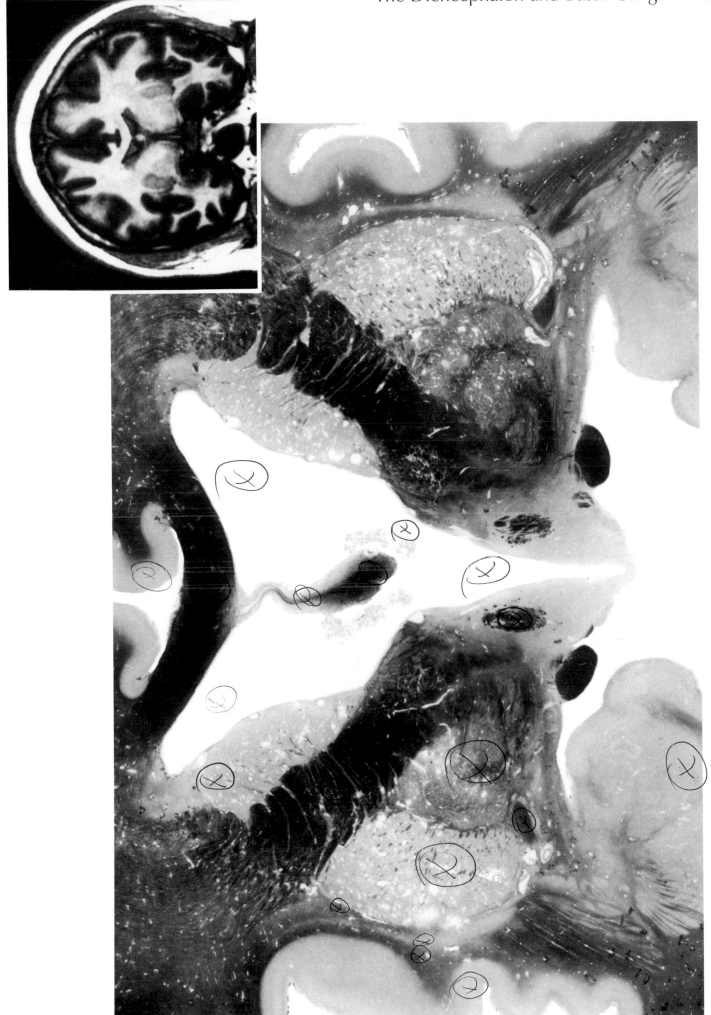

5–35 Coronal section of forebrain through the *anterior commissure* and rostral aspects of the *hypothalamus*.

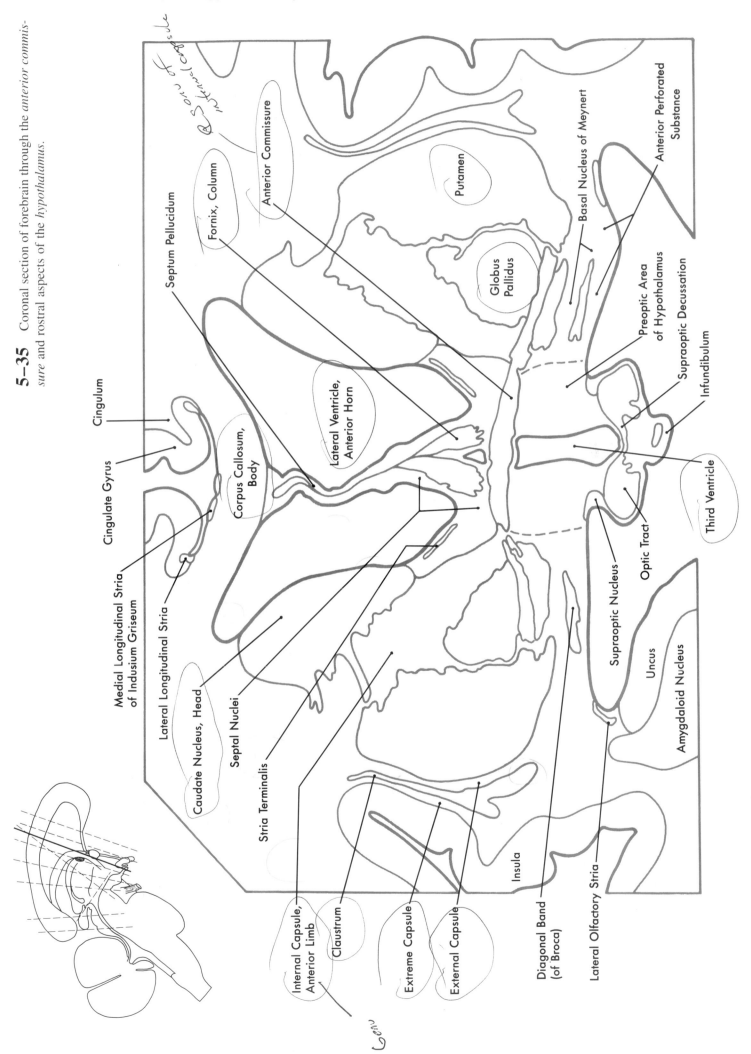

Cingulum

Cingulate Gyrus

Medial Longitudinal Stria
of Indusium Griseum

Lateral Longitudinal Stria

Caudate Nucleus, Head

Septal Nuclei

Stria Terminalis

Septum Pellucidum

Fornix, Column

Anterior Commissure

Corpus Callosum, Body

Lateral Ventricle, Anterior Horn

Putamen

Globus Pallidus

Basal Nucleus of Meynert

Anterior Perforated Substance

Preoptic Area of Hypothalamus

Supraoptic Decussation

Infundibulum

Third Ventricle

Optic Tract

Supraoptic Nucleus

Uncus

Amygdaloid Nucleus

Diagonal Band (of Broca)

Lateral Olfactory Stria

Insula

External Capsule

Extreme Capsule

Claustrum

Internal Capsule, Anterior Limb

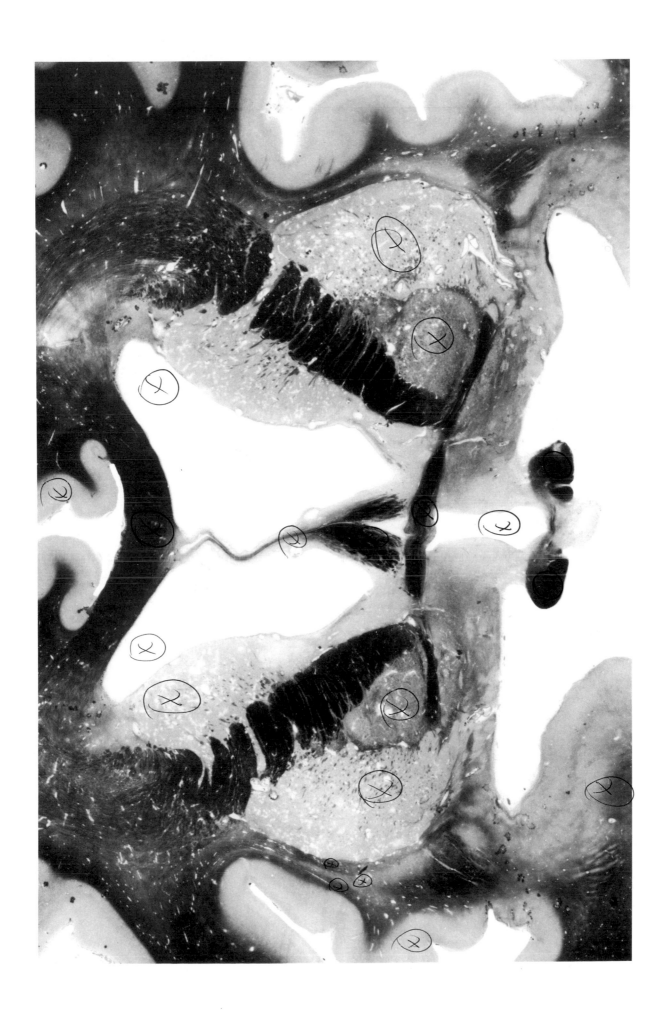

5-36 Coronal section of forebrain through the *head of the caudate nucleus* and the *optic chiasm*. Many of the structures labeled in this figure can be easily identified in the MRI.

Insula

Internal Capsule, Anterior Limb

Putamen

Middle Cerebral Artery

Nucleus Accumbens Septi

Cingulum

Lateral Longitudinal Stria

Septum Pellucidum

Medial Olfactory Stria

Paraterminal Gyrus

Cingulate Gyrus

Corpus Callosum, Body

Anterior Cerebral Arteries

Lateral Ventricle, Anterior Horn

Optic Chiasm

Diagonal Band (of Broca)

Medial Longitudinal Stria of Indusium Griseum

Caudate Nucleus, Head

Anterior Cerebral Artery

Globus Pallidus

Lateral Olfactory Stria

Extreme Capsule

External Capsule

Claustrum

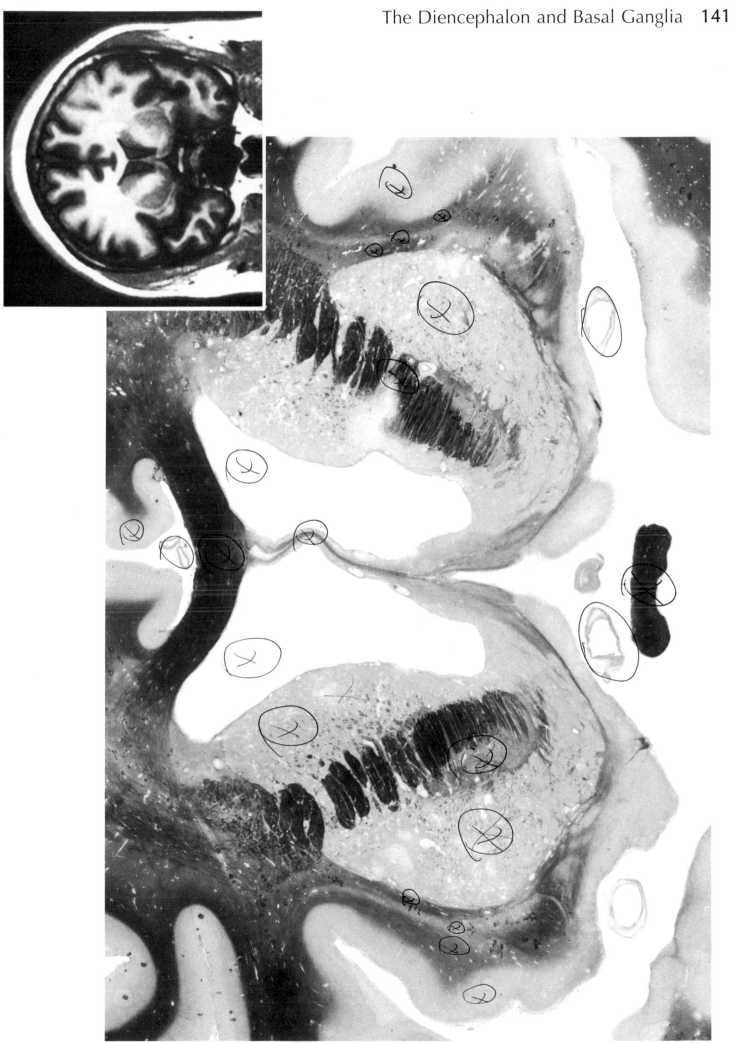

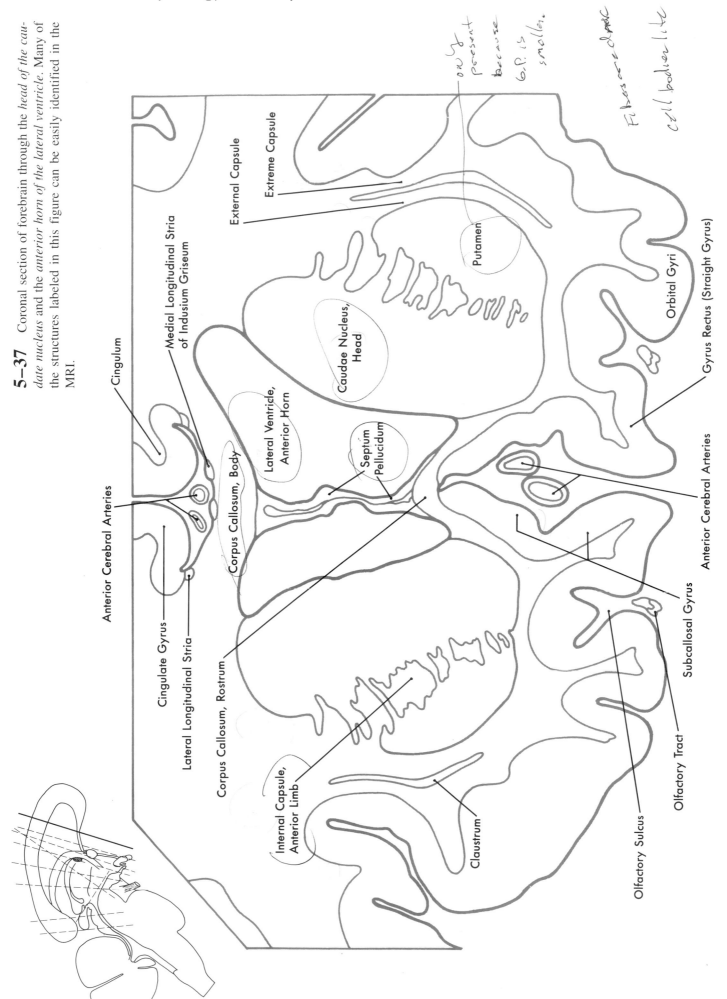

5-37 Coronal section of forebrain through the *head of the caudate nucleus* and the *anterior horn of the lateral ventricle*. Many of the structures labeled in this figure can be easily identified in the MRI.

Cingulum

Medial Longitudinal Stria
of Indusium Griseum

External Capsule

Extreme Capsule

Caudae Nucleus,
Head

Putamen

Lateral Ventricle,
Anterior Horn

Septum
Pellucidum

Orbital Gyri

Gyrus Rectus (Straight Gyrus)

Anterior Cerebral Arteries

Anterior Cerebral Arteries

Cingulate Gyrus

Lateral Longitudinal Stria

Corpus Callosum, Body

Corpus Callosum, Rostrum

Internal Capsule,
Anterior Limb

Claustrum

Subcallosal Gyrus

Olfactory Tract

Olfactory Sulcus

only
present
because
G.P. is
smaller.

Fibers are darker

cell bodies lite

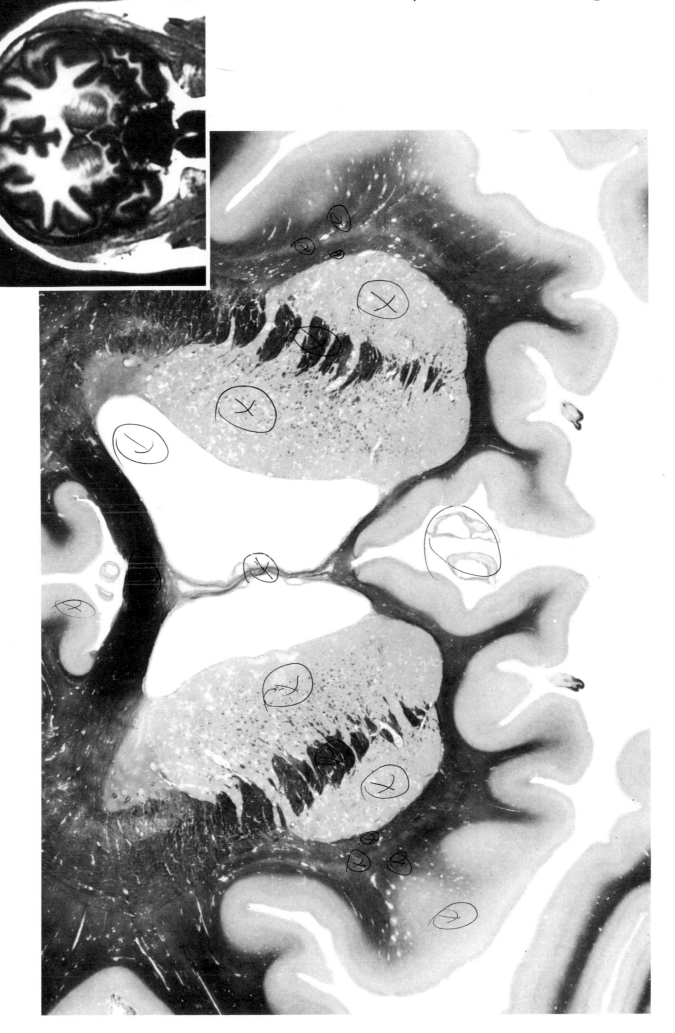

5-38 Semi-diagrammatic representation of the internal distribution of arteries to the diencephalon, basal ganglia, and internal capsule. Selected main structures are labeled on the left side of each section; the general pattern of arterial distribution overlies these structures on the right.

Abbreviations

AC	Anterior Commissure
AmyNu	Amygdaloid Nucleus (Complex)
AntNu	Anterior Nucleus of Thalamus
APS	Anterior Perforated Substance
CaNu,B	Caudate Nucleus, Body
CaNu,H	Caudate Nucleus, Head
CaNu,T	Caudate Nucleus, Tail
CC	Crus Cerebri
Cl	Claustrum
CM	Centromedian Nucleus of Thalamus
CorCl,B	Corpus Callosum, Body
CorCl,Spl	Corpus Callosum, Splenium
DMNu	Dorsomedial Nucleus of Thalamus
For,B	Fornix, Body
For,Col	Fornix, Column
For,Cr	Fornix, Crus
GP	Globus Pallidus
Hip	Hippocampal Formation
HyTh	Hypothalamus
IntCap,AL	Internal Capsule, Anterior Limb
IntCap,PL	Internal Capsule, Posterior Limb
IntCap,RL	Internal Capsule, Retrolenticular Limb
LDNu	Lateral Dorsal Nucleus of Thalamus
LGB	Lateral Geniculate Body (Nucleus)
MB	Mammillary Body
MGB	Medial Geniculate Body (Nucleus)
OpTr	Optic Tract
Pi	Pineal
PulNu	Pulvinar Nuclear Complex
Put	Putamen
RNu	Red Nucleus
Sep	Septum Pellucidum
SN	Substantia Nigra
SThNu	Subthalamic Nucleus
StTer	Stria Terminalis
VA	Ventral Anterior Nucleus of Thalamus
VL	Ventral Lateral Nucleus of Thalamus

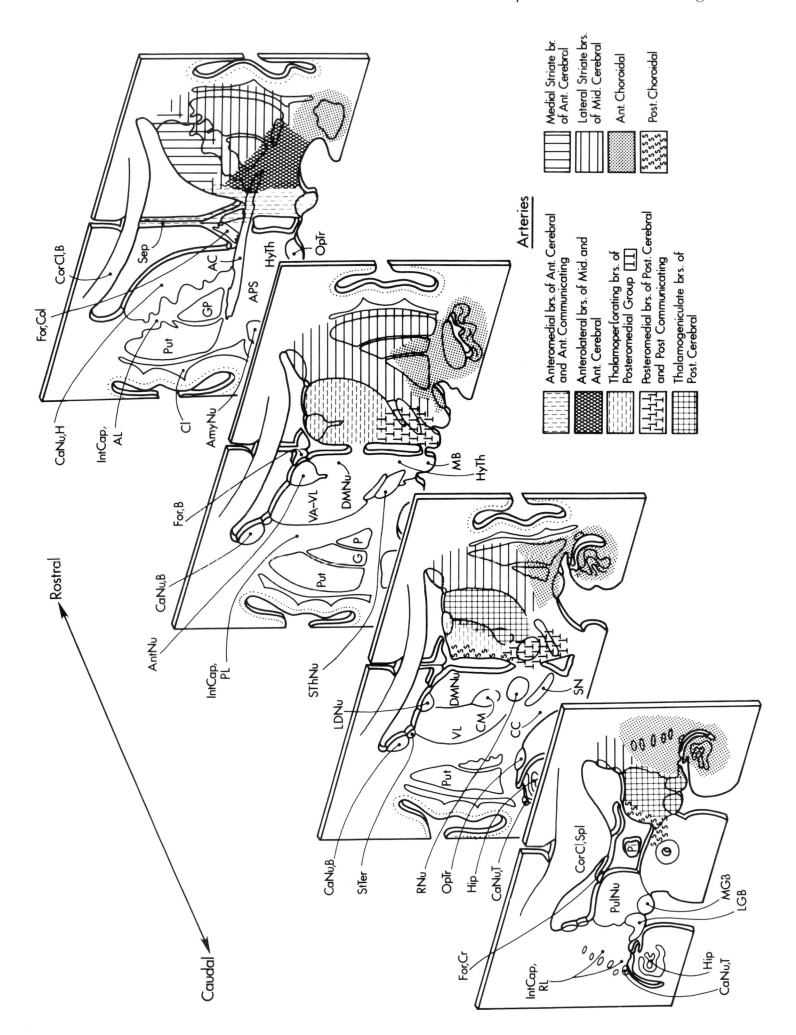

Rostral

Caudal

Arteries

Medial Striate br. of Ant. Cerebral

Lateral Striate brs. of Mid. Cerebral

Ant. Choroidal

Post. Choroidal

Anteromedial brs. of Ant. Cerebral and Ant. Communicating

Anterolateral brs. of Mid. and Ant. Cerebral

Thalamoperforating brs. of Posteromedial Group II

Posteromedial brs. of Post. Cerebral and Post Communicating

Thalamogeniculate brs. of Post. Cerebral

Chapter 6

Internal Morphology of the Brain in Stained Sections: Axial-Sagittal Correlations with MRI

Although the general organization of Chapter 6 has been described in the Preface and in Chapter 1 (the reader may wish to refer back to these sections), it is entirely appropriate to reiterate its unique features at this point. Each set of facing pages has photographs of an axial stained section (left hand page) and a sagittal stained section (right hand page); appropriate structures are labeled on each. In addition to individually labeled structures, a heavy line appears on each photograph. This prominent line on the axial section represents the approximate plane of the sagittal section located on the facing page. On the sagittal section this line signifies the approximate plane of the corresponding axial section. The reader can identify features in each photograph and then, using this line as a reference point, visualize structures that are located either above or below that plane (axial to sagittal comparison) or medial or lateral to that plane (sagittal to axial comparison). This method of presentation provides a format for easily reconstructing and understanding three-dimensional relationships within the central nervous system (CNS).

The magnetic resonance imaging (MRI) scans placed on every other set of pages in this chapter give the user an opportunity to compare internal brain anatomy, as seen in stained sections, with those structures visualized in clinical images generated in the same plane. Even a general comparison reveals that many anatomical features and structures, as labeled in the stained section, can be readily identified in the adjacent MRI scan.

This chapter is also organized so that one can view structures in either the axial or the sagittal plane only. Axial photographs appear on left-hand pages and are sequenced from dorsal to ventral (Figs. 6-1 through 6-9), while sagittal photographs are on the right-hand pages and progress from medial to lateral (Figs. 6-2 through 6-10). Consequently, the user can identify and follow structures through an axial series by simply flipping through the left-hand pages or through a sagittal series by flipping through the right-hand pages. The inherent flexibility in this chapter should prove useful in a wide variety of instructional/learning situations. The drawings shown below illustrate, in relation to gross brain structures, the axial and sagittal planes of the photographs in this chapter.

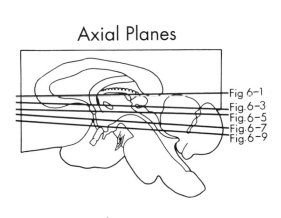

Axial Planes

Fig 6-1
Fig. 6-3
Fig. 6-5
Fig. 6-7
Fig. 6-9

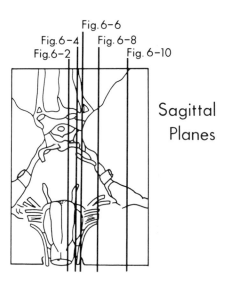

Fig. 6-6
Fig. 6-4   Fig. 6-8
Fig. 6-2   Fig. 6-10

Sagittal Planes

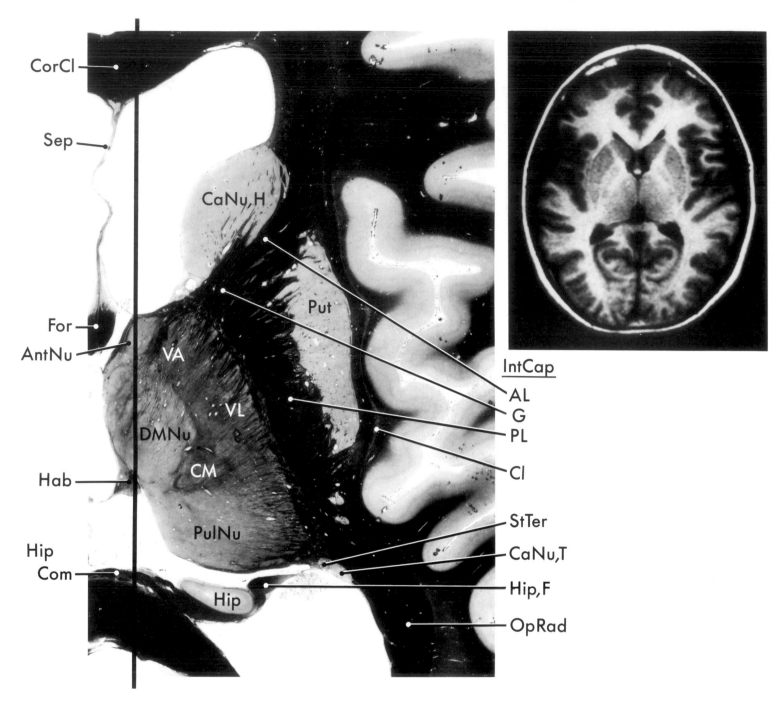

6-1   Axial (horizontal) section through the *head of the caudate nucleus* and several key *thalamic nuclei (anterior, centromedian, pulvinar, habenular)*. The heavy line represents the approximate plane of the sagittal section shown in Figure 6-2 (facing page). Many of the structures labeled in this figure can be easily identified in the MRI scan.

Abbreviations

AntNu	Anterior Nucleus of Thalamus	**HipCom**	Hippocampal Commissure
CaNu,H	Caudate Nucleus, Head	**IntCap,AL**	Internal Capsule, Anterior Limb
CaNu,T	Caudate Nucleus, Tail	**IntCap,G**	Internal Capsule, Genu
Cl	Claustrum	**IntCap,PL**	Internal Capsule, Posterior Limb
CM	Centromedial Nucleus of Thalamus	**OpRad**	Optic Radiations
CorCl	Corpus Callosum	**PulNu**	Pulvinar Nuclear Complex
DMNu	Dorsomedial Nucleus of Thalamus	**Put**	Putamen
For	Fornix, Column	**Sep**	Septum Pellucidum
Hab	Habenular Nucleus	**StTer**	Stria Terminalis
Hip	Hippocampal Formation	**VA**	Ventral Anterior Nucleus of Thalamus
Hip,F	Hippocampus, Fimbria	**VL**	Ventral Lateral Nucleus of Thalamus

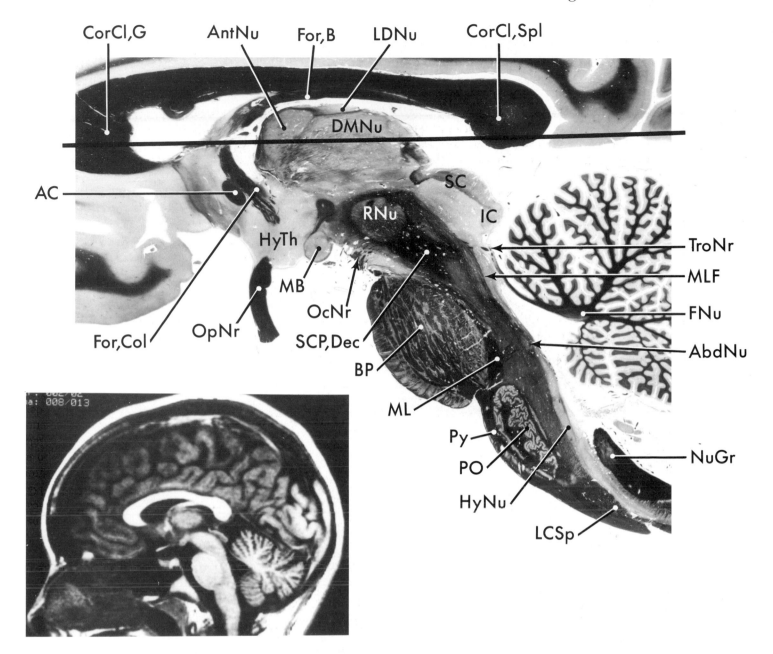

6-2   Sagittal section through the *column of the fornix, anterior thalamic nucleus, red nucleus,* and medial portions of the *pons (abducens nucleus), cerebellum (fastigial nucleus),* and *medulla (nucleus gracilis).* The heavy line represents the approximate plane of the axial section shown in Figure 6-1 (facing page). Many of the structures labeled in this figure can be easily identified in the MRI scan.

Abbreviations

AbdNu	Abducens Nucleus	**LDNu**	Lateral Dorsal Nucleus
AC	Anterior Commissure	**MB**	Mammillary Body
AntNu	Anterior Nucleus of Thalamus	**ML**	Medial Lemniscus
BP	Basilar Pons	**MLF**	Medial Longitudinal Fasciculus
CorCl,G	Corpus Callosum, Genu	**NuGr**	Nucleus Gracilis
CorCl,Spl	Corpus Callosum, Splenium	**OcNr**	Oculomotor Nerve
DMNu	Dorsomedial Nucleus of Thalamus	**OpNr**	Optic Nerve
FNu	Fastigial Nucleus (Medial Cerebellar Nucleus)	**PO**	Principal (Inferior) Olivary Nucleus
For,B	Fornix, Body	**Py**	Pyramid
For,Col	Fornix, Column	**RNu**	Red Nucleus
HyNu	Hypoglossal Nucleus	**SC**	Superior Colliculus
HyTh	Hypothalamus	**SCP,Dec**	Superior Cerebellar Peduncle, Decussation
IC	Inferior Colliculus	**TroNr**	Trochlear Nerve
LCsp	Lateral Corticospinal Tract		

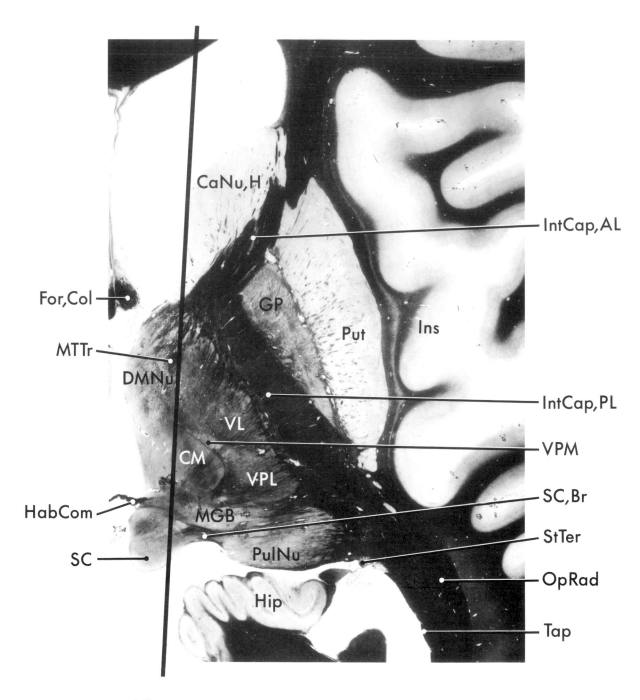

6-3 Axial (horizontal) section through the *head of the caudate nucleus, centromedian nucleus, medial geniculate body*, and *superior colliculus*. The heavy line represents the approximate plane of the sagittal section shown in Figure 6-4 (facing page).

Abbreviations

CaNu,H	Caudate Nucleus, Head		**OpRad**	Optic Radiations
CM	Centromedian Nucleus of Thalamus		**PulNu**	Pulvinar Nuclear Complex
DMNu	Dorsomedial Nucleus of Thalamus		**Put**	Putamen
For,Col	Fornix, Column		**SC**	Superior Colliculus
GP	Globus Pallidus		**SC,Br**	Superior Colliculus, Brachium
Hab,Com	Habenular Commissure		**StTer**	Stria Terminalis
Hip	Hippocampal Formation		**VL**	Ventral Lateral Nucleus of Thalamus
Ins	Insula		**VPL**	Ventral Posterolateral Nucleus of Thalamus
IntCap,AL	Internal Capsule, Anterior Limb		**VPM**	Ventral Posteromedial Nucleus of
IntCap,PL	Internal Capsule, Posterior Limb			Thalamus
MGB	Medial Geniculate Body		**Tap**	Tapetum
MTTr	Mammillothalamic Tract			

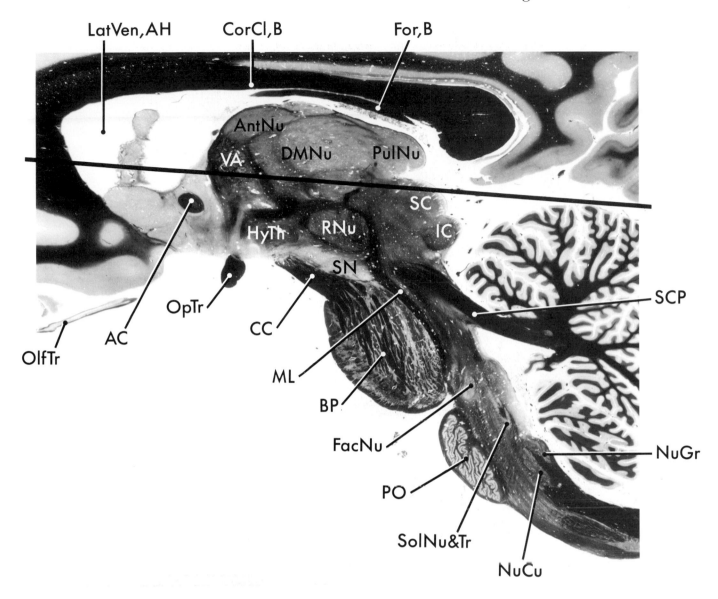

6-4 Sagittal section through *anterior* and *ventral anterior thalamic nuclei, red nucleus* and central areas of the *pons, cerebellum (superior peduncle),* and *medulla (solitary nucleus and tract).* Note the position of the *facial nucleus* at the pons-medulla junction. The heavy line represents the approximate plane of the axial section shown in Figure 6-3 (facing page).

Abbreviations

AC	Anterior Commissure		**NuGr**	Nucleus Gracilis
AntNu	Anterior Nucleus of Thalamus		**OlfTr**	Olfactory Tract
BP	Basilar Pons		**OpTr**	Optic Tract
CC	Crus Cerebri		**PO**	Principal (Inferior) Olivary Nucleus
CorCl,B	Corpus Callosum, Body		**PulNu**	Pulvinar Nuclear Complex
DMNu	Dorsomedial Nucleus of Thalamus		**RNu**	Red Nucleus
FacNu	Facial Nucleus		**SC**	Superior Colliculus
For,B	Fornix, Body		**SCP**	Superior Cerebellar Peduncle (Brachium Conjunctivum)
HyTh	Hypothalamus		**SN**	Substantia Nigra
IC	Inferior Colliculus		**SolNu&Tr**	Solitary Nucleus and Tract
LatVen,AH	Lateral Ventricle, Anterior Horn		**VA**	Ventral Anterior Nucleus of Thalamus
ML	Medial Lemniscus			
NuCu	Nucleus Cuneatus			

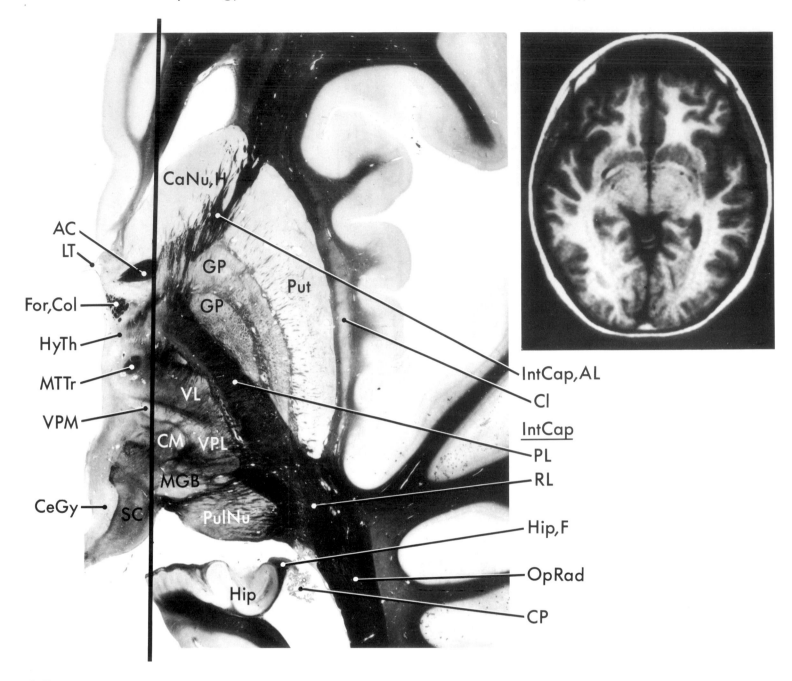

6-5 Axial (horizontal) section through the *head of the caudate nucleus, ventral posteromedial nucleus, medial geniculate body,* and ventral parts of the *pulvinar.* The heavy line represents the approximate plane of the sagittal section shown in Figure 6-6 (facing page). Many of the structures labeled in this figure can be easily identified in the MRI scan.

Abbreviations

AC	Anterior Commissure	**IntCap,RL**	Internal Capsule, Retrolenticular Limb
CaNu,H	Caudate Nucleus, Head	**LT**	Lamina Terminalis
CeGy	Central Gray (Periaqueductal Gray)	**MGB**	Medial Geniculate Body (Nucleus)
Cl	Claustrum	**MTTr**	Mammillothalamic Tract
CM	Centromedian Nucleus of Thalamus	**OpRad**	Optic Radiations
CP	Choroid Plexus	**PulNu**	Pulvinar Nuclear Complex
For,Col	Fornix, Column	**Put**	Putamen
GP	Globus Pallidus	**SC**	Superior Colliculus
Hip	Hippocampal Formation	**VL**	Ventral Lateral Nucleus of Thalamus
Hip,F	Hippocampus, Fimbria	**VPL**	Ventral Posterolateral Nucleus of Thalamus
HyTh	Hypothalamus	**VPM**	Ventral Posteromedial Nucleus of
IntCap,AL	Internal Capsule, Anterior Limb		Thalamus
IntCap,Pl	Internal Capsule, Posterior Limb		

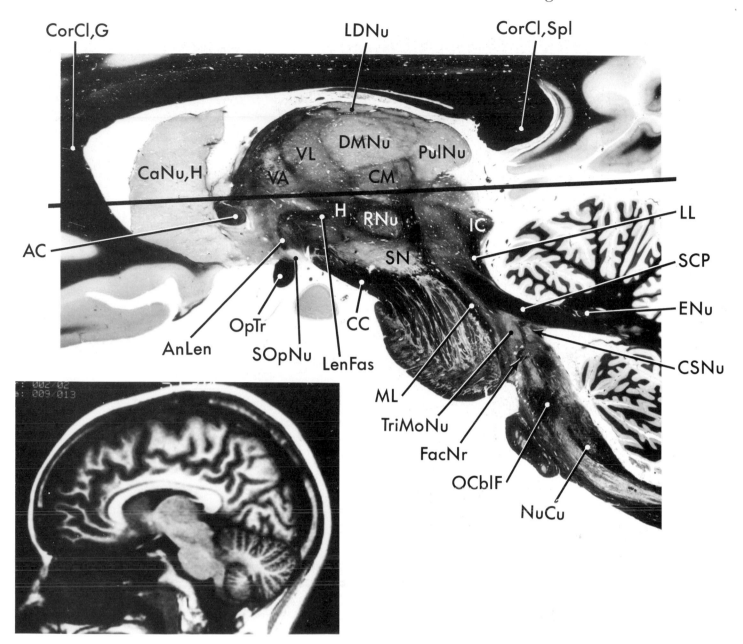

6-6 Sagittal section through central regions of the *diencephalon (centromedian nucleus)* and *midbrain (red nucleus)*, and through lateral areas of the *pons (trigeminal motor nucleus)* and *medulla (nucleus cuneatus).* The heavy line represents the approximate plane of the axial section shown in Figure 6-5 (facing page). Many of the structures labeled in this figure can be easily identified in the MRI scan.

Abbreviations

AC	Anterior Commissure	**LDNu**	Lateral Dorsal Nucleus of Thalamus
AnLen	Ansa Lenticularis	**LL**	Lateral Lemniscus
CaNu,H	Caudate Nucleus, Head	**ML**	Medial Lemniscus
CC	Crus Cerebri	**NuCu**	Nucleus Cuneatus
CM	Centromedian Nucleus of Thalamus	**OCblF**	Olivocerebellar Fibers
CorCl,G	Corpus Callosum, Genu	**OpTr**	Optic Tract
CorCl,Spl	Corpus Callosum, Splenium	**PulNu**	Pulvinar Nuclear Complex
CSNu	Chief Sensory Nucleus (Trigeminal)	**RNu**	Red Nucleus
DMNu	Dorsomedial Nucleus of Thalamus	**SCP**	Superior Cerebellar Peduncle (Brachium Conjunctivum)
ENu	Emboliform Nucleus (Anterior Interposed Cerebellar Nucleus)	**SN**	Substantia Nigra
		SOpNu	Supraoptic Nucleus
FacNr	Facial Nerve	**TriMoNu**	Trigeminal Motor Nucleus
H	H Field of Forel (Prerubral Field)	**VA**	Ventral Anterior Nucleus of Thalamus
IC	Inferior Colliculus	**VL**	Ventral Lateral Nucleus of Thalamus
LenFas	Lenticular Fasciculus		

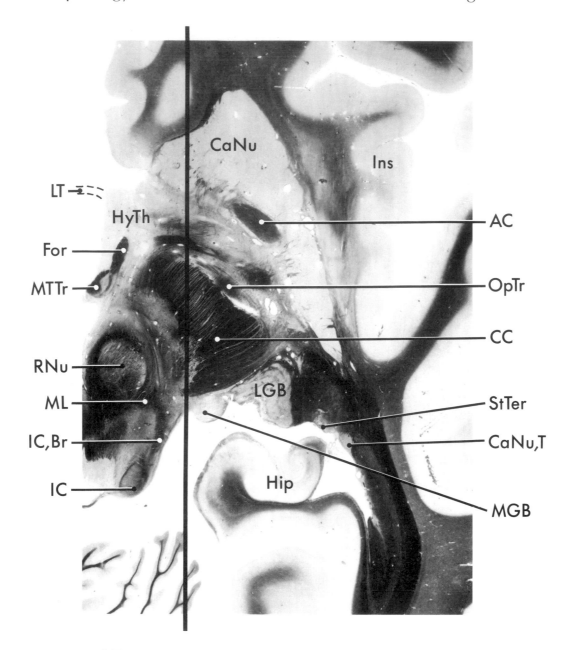

6-7   Axial (horizontal) section through the *hypothalamus, red nucleus, inferior colliculus*, and *lateral geniculate body*. The heavy line represents the approximate plane of the sagittal section shown in Figure 6-8 (facing page). The axial plane through the hemisphere, when continued into the intact midbrain, represents a somewhat oblique section through the mesencephalon. Although the lamina terminalis was missing from this slice of brain, its position is indicated by the double dashed lines.

Abbreviations

AC	Anterior Commissure		**LGB**	Lateral Geniculate Body (Nucleus)
CaNu	Caudate Nucleus		**LT**	Lamina Terminalis
CaNu,T	Caudate Nucleus, Tail		**MGB**	Medial Geniculate Body (Nucleus)
CC	Crus Cerebri			
For	Fornix		**ML**	Medial Lemniscus
Hip	Hippocampal Formation		**MTTr**	Mammillothalamic Tract
HyTh	Hypothalamus		**OpTr**	Optic Tract
IC	Inferior Colliculus		**RNu**	Red Nucleus
IC,Br	Inferior Colliculus, Brachium		**StTer**	Stria Terminalis
Ins	Insula			

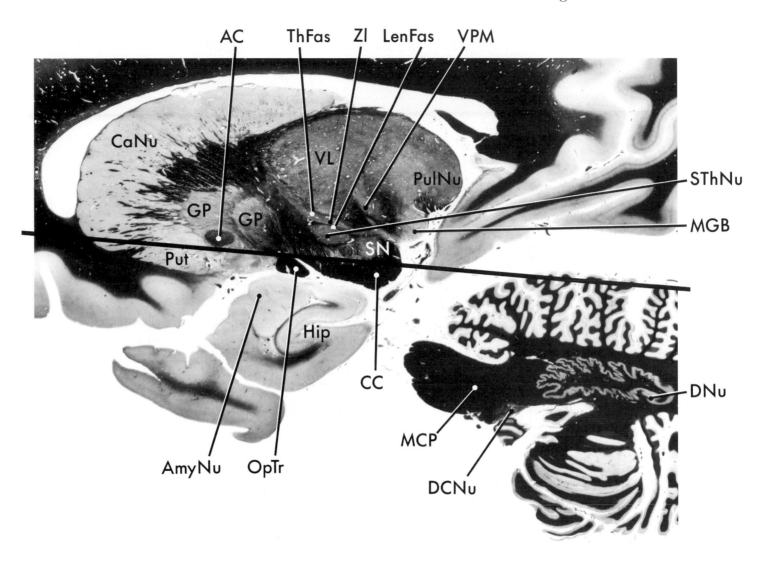

6-8 Sagittal section through the *caudate nucleus*, central parts of the *diencephalon (ventral posteromedial nucleus)*, and lateral portions of the *pons* and *cerebellum (dentate nucleus)*. The heavy line represents the approximate plane of the axial section shown in Figure 6-7 (facing page).

Abbreviations

AC	Anterior Commissure
AmyNu	Amygdaloid Nucleus (Complex)
CaNu	Caudate Nucleus
CC	Crus Cerebri
DCNu	Dorsal Cochlear Nucleus
DNu	Dentate Nucleus (Lateral Cerebellar Nucleus)
GP	Globus Pallidus
Hip	Hippocampal Formation
LenFas	Lenticular Fasciculus
MCP	Middle Cerebellar Peduncle (Brachium Pontis)
MGB	Medial Geniculate Body (Nucleus)
OpTr	Optic Tract
PulNu	Pulvinar Nuclear Complex
Put	Putamen
SN	Substantia Nigra
SThNu	Subthalamic Nucleus
ThFas	Thalamic Fasciculus
VL	Ventral Lateral Nucleus of Thalamus
VPM	Ventral Posteromedial Nucleus of Thalamus
ZI	Zona Incerta

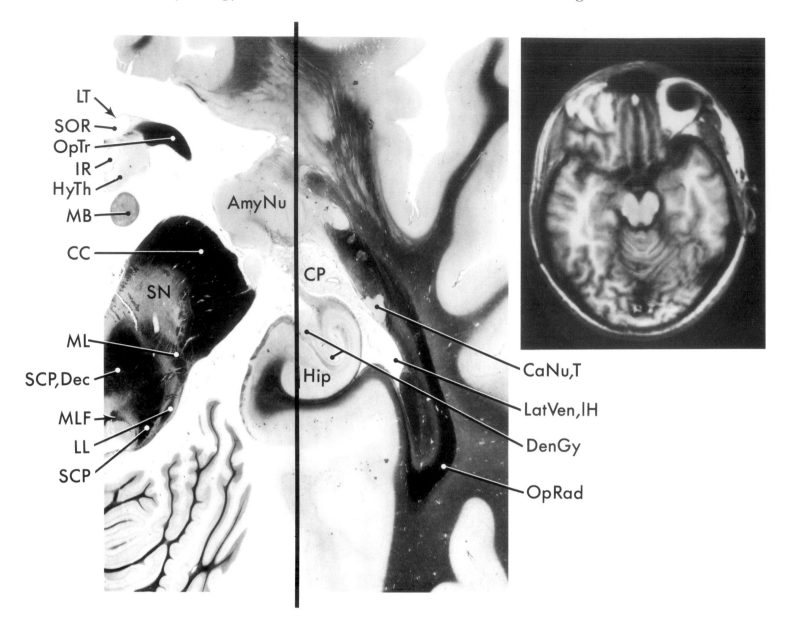

6-9 Axial (horizontal) section through ventral portions of the *hy-pothalamus (supraoptic recess* and *mammillary body)* and forebrain *(amygdaloid nucleus)*, and through the *superior cerebellar peduncle decussation* in the midbrain. The heavy line represents the approximate plane of the sagittal section shown in Figure 6-10 (facing page).

The axial plane through the hemisphere, when continued into the intact midbrain, represents a somewhat oblique section through the mesencephalon. Many of the structures labeled in this figure can be easily identified in the MRI scan.

Abbreviations

AmyNu	Amygdaloid Nucleus (Complex)		**MB**	Mammillary Body
CaNu,T	Caudate Nucleus, Tail		**ML**	Medial Lemniscus
CC	Crus Cerebri		**MLF**	Medial Longitudinal Fasciculus
CP	Choroid Plexus		**OpRad**	Optic Radiations
DenGy	Dentate Gyrus		**OpTr**	Optic Tract
Hip	Hippocampal Formation		**SCP**	Superior Cerebellar Peduncle (Brachium Conjunctivum)
HyTh	Hypothalamus			
IR	Infundibular Recess of Third Ventricle		**SCP,Dec**	Superior Cerebellar Peduncle, Decussation
LatVen,IH	Lateral Ventricle, Inferior (Temporal) Horn		**SN**	Substantia Nigra
LL	Lateral Lemniscus		**SOR**	Supraoptic Recess of Third Ventricle
LT	Lamina Terminalis			

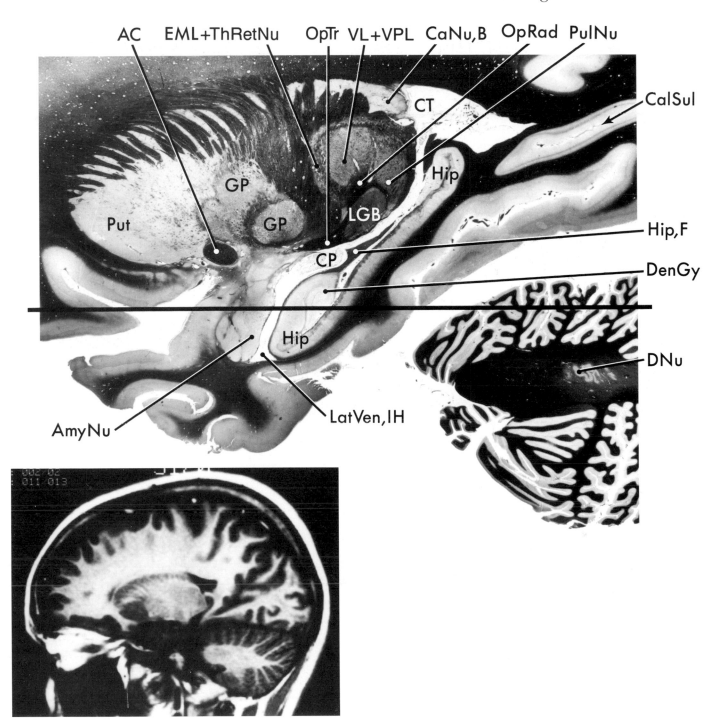

6-10   Sagittal section through the *putamen, amygdaloid nucleus,* and *hippocampus* and through the most lateral portions of the *diencephalon (external medullary lamina* and *ventral posterolateral nu-* *cleus).* The heavy line represents the approximate plane of the axial section shown in Figure 6-9 (facing page). Many of the structures labeled in this figure can be easily identified in the MRI scan.

Abbreviations

AC	Anterior Commissure		**Hip,F**	Hippocampus, Fimbria
AmyNu	Amygdaloid Nucleus (Complex)		**LatVen,IH**	Lateral Ventricle, Inferior (Temporal) Horn
CalSul	Calcarine Sulcus		**LGB**	Lateral Geniculate Body (Nucleus)
CaNu,B	Caudate Nucleus, Body		**OpRad**	Optic Radiations
CP	Choroid Plexus		**OpTr**	Optic Tract
CT	Collateral Trigone of Lateral Ventricular		**PulNu**	Pulvinar Nuclear Complex
DenGy	Dentate Gyrus		**Put**	Putamen
DNu	Dentate Nucleus		**ThRetNu**	Thalamic Reticular Nuclei
EML	External Medullary Lamina		**VL**	Ventral Lateral Nucleus of Thalamus
GP	Globus Pallidus		**VPL**	Ventral Posterolateral Nucleus of
Hip	Hippocampal Formation			Thalamus

Chapter 7

Synopsis of Functional Components, Tracts, Pathways, and Systems

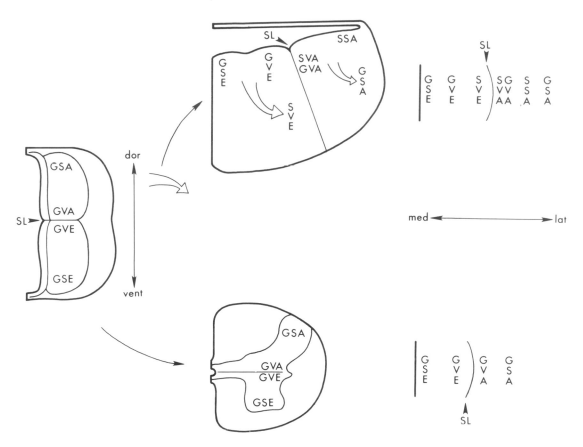

7-1 A semi-diagrammatic summary of the positions of functional components as seen in the developing neural tube (left) and in the spinal cord and brainstem of the adult (right). In the neural tube, the alar plate and its associated GSA and GVA components are dorsal to the sulcus limitans (SL) while the basal plate and its related GVE and GSE components are ventral to the SL. In the adult spinal cord this general dorsoventral relationship is maintained, although the neural canal (as central canal) is reduced and/or absent. Two major changes occur in the transition from spinal cord to brainstem in the adult. First, as the central canal of the cervical cord enlarges into the fourth ventricle and the cerebellum develops, the dorsal portion of the primitive neural tube is rotated laterally. Consequently, in the adult the sulcus limitans is present in the adult brainstem with motor components (adult derivatives of the basal plate) medial to it, and sensory components (adult derivatives of the alar plate) located laterally. Second, in the brainstem, special functional components (SVE to muscles of brachiomeric origin; SVA taste and olfaction; SSA vestibular, auditory, and visual systems) are intermingled with the rostral continuation of the general functional components as found in the spinal cord. In the brainstem, however, there is a slight transposition of the SVE and GSA functional components. Embryologically, SVE cell groups appear between those associated with GSE and GVE components. As development progresses, however, SVE cell groups migrate (open arrow) to ventrolateral areas of the tegmentum and, therefore, are diagrammatically shown here as being located lateral to GVE cell groups. Cell groups associated with the GSA functional component are displaced from their dorsolateral position in the developing brainstem by the newly acquired cell groups having SSA components (as well as other structures). Consequently, structures associated with the GSA component are located (open arrow) in more ventrolateral and lateral areas of the brainstem. The approximate border between motor and sensory regions of the brainstem is represented by an oblique line drawn through the brainstem beginning at the SL. The medial (from midline) to lateral positions of the various functional components, as shown on the far right of this figure, are taken from their representative diagrams of brainstem and cord, and are directly translatable to Figure 7-2 (facing page).

Abbreviations

		Other
GSA	General Somatic Afferent	
GSE	General Somatic Efferent	
GVA	General Visceral Afferent	**dor** dorsal
GVE	General Visceral Efferent	**lat** lateral
SSA	Special Somatic Afferent	**med** medial
SVA	Special Visceral Afferent	**SL** Sulcus Limitans
SVE	Special Visceral Efferent	**ven** ventral

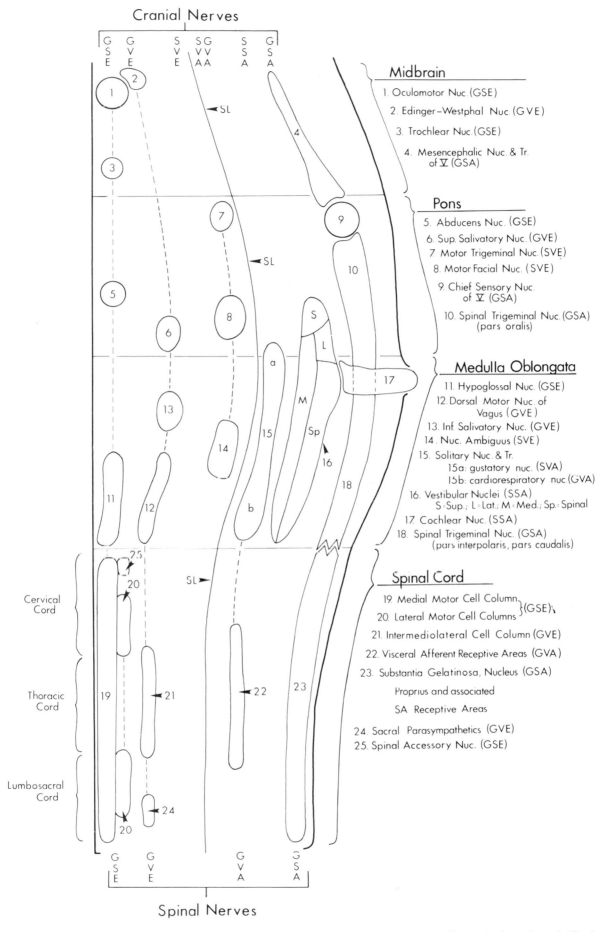

Cranial Nerves

G S E	G V E	S V E	S G V V A A	S S A	G S A

Midbrain

1. Oculomotor Nuc. (GSE)
2. Edinger–Westphal Nuc. (GVE)
3. Trochlear Nuc. (GSE)
4. Mesencephalic Nuc. & Tr. of V (GSA)

Pons

5. Abducens Nuc. (GSE)
6. Sup. Salivatory Nuc. (GVE)
7. Motor Trigeminal Nuc. (SVE)
8. Motor Facial Nuc. (SVE)
9. Chief Sensory Nuc. of V (GSA)
10. Spinal Trigeminal Nuc. (GSA) (pars oralis)

Medulla Oblongata

11. Hypoglossal Nuc. (GSE)
12. Dorsal Motor Nuc. of Vagus (GVE)
13. Inf. Salivatory Nuc. (GVE)
14. Nuc. Ambiguus (SVE)
15. Solitary Nuc. & Tr.
    15a: gustatory nuc. (SVA)
    15b: cardiorespiratory nuc. (GVA)
16. Vestibular Nuclei (SSA)
    S:Sup.; L:Lat.; M:Med.; Sp:Spinal
17. Cochlear Nuc. (SSA)
18. Spinal Trigeminal Nuc. (GSA) (pars interpolaris, pars caudalis)

Spinal Cord

19. Medial Motor Cell Column ⎱(GSE)
20. Lateral Motor Cell Columns ⎰
21. Intermediolateral Cell Column (GVE)
22. Visceral Afferent Receptive Areas (GVA)
23. Substantia Gelatinosa, Nucleus (GSA)
    Proprius and associated
    SA Receptive Areas
24. Sacral Parasympathetics (GVE)
25. Spinal Accessory Nuc. (GSE)

Cervical Cord

Thoracic Cord

Lumbosacral Cord

G S E	G V E	G V A	S S A

Spinal Nerves

7–2   The medial to lateral positions of brainstem cranial nerve and spinal cord nuclei shown here are the same as in Figure 7–1. This diagrammatic dorsal view shows (1) the relative positions and names of specific cell groups and their associated functional components, (2) the approximate location of particular nuclei in their specific division of brainstem and/or spinal cord, and (3) the rostro-caudal continuity of cell columns (either as continuous or discontinuous cell groups) from one division of the brainstem to the next or from brainstem to spinal cord. Nuclei associated with cranial nerves I (olfaction, SVA) and II (optic, SSA) are not shown.

7–3   Orientation drawing for pathways. The trajectory of most pathways illustrated in Chapter 7 appears on individualized versions of this representation of the central nervous system (CNS). Although slight changes are made in each drawing, so as to more clearly diagram a specific pathway, the basic configuration of the CNS is as represented here. The forebrain (telencephalon and diencephalon) is shown in the coronal plane, and the midbrain, pons, medulla, and spinal cord are represented through their longitudinal axes. The internal capsule is represented in the axial (horizontal) plane in an effort to show the rostrocaudal distribution of fibers located therein.

The reader should become familiar with the structures and regions as shown here since their locations and relationships are easily transferable to subsequent illustrations. It may also be helpful to refer back to this illustration when using subsequent sections of this chapter.

Neurotransmitters: Three important facts are self-evident in the descriptions of neurotransmitters that accompany each pathway drawing. These are illustrated by noting, as an example, that glutamate is found in corticospinal fibers (see Fig. 7–10). First, the *location of neuronal cell bodies* containing a specific transmitter is indicated (glutamate-containing cell bodies are found in cortical areas that project to the spinal cord). Second, the *trajectory of fibers* containing a particular neurotransmitter is obvious from the route taken by the tract (glutaminergic corticospinal fibers are found in the internal cap-

sule, crus cerebri, basilar pons, pyramid, and lateral corticospinal tract). Third, the *location of terminals* containing specific neurotransmitters is indicated by the site(s) of termination of each tract (glutaminergic terminals of corticospinal fibers are located in the spinal cord gray matter). In addition, the action of most neuroactive substances is indicated as excitatory (+) or inhibitory (-). This level of neurotransmitter information, as explained here for glutaminergic corticospinal fibers, is repeated for each pathway drawing.

Clinical Correlations: The clinical correlations are designed to give the user an overview of specific deficits (i.e. *hemiplegia, athetosis*) seen in lesions of each pathway and to provide examples of some syndromes or diseases (i.e. *Brown-Sequard syndrome, Wilson's disease*) in which these deficits are seen. Although purposefully brief, these correlations highlight examples of deficits for each pathway and provide a built-in mechanism for expanded study. For example, the words that appear in *italics* in each correlation are clinical terms and phrases that can be found in standard medical dictionaries and neurology textbooks. The user can not only glean important clinical points that correlate with the pathway under consideration, but can enlarge his or her knowledge and understanding by researching the italicized words and phrases in a medical dictionary or neurology text.

Abbreviations

CE	Cervical Enlargement of Spinal Cord	**LatSul**	Lateral Sulcus (Sylvian Sulcus)
Cer	Cervical Levels of Spinal Cord	**LatVen**	Lateral Ventricle
CinSul	Cingulate Sulcus	**LSE**	Lumbosacral Enlargement of Spinal Cord
CaNu	Caudate Nucleus (+ Put = Neostriatum)	**LumSac**	Lumbosacral Level of Spinal Cord
CM	Centromedian (and Intralaminar) Nuclei	**L-VTh**	Lateral and Ventral Thalamic Nuclei excluding VPM and VPL
CorCl	Corpus Callosum		
Dien	Diencephalon	**Mes**	Mesencephalon
DMNu	Dorsomedial Nucleus of Thalamus	**Met**	Metencephalon
For	Fornix	**Myelen**	Myelencephalon
GP	Globus Pallidus (paleostriatum)	**Put**	Putamen (+ CaNu = Neostriatum)
HyTh	Hypothalamic area	**SThNu**	Subthalamic Nucleus
IC	Internal Capsule	**Telen**	Telencephalon
IntCap,AL	Internal Capsule, Anterior Limb	**Thor**	Thoracic Levels of Spinal Cord
IntCap,G	Internal Capsule, Genu	**VPL**	Ventral Posterolateral Nucleus of Thalamus
IntCap,PL	Internal Capsule, Posterior Limb	**VPM**	Ventral Posteromedial Nucleus of Thalamus

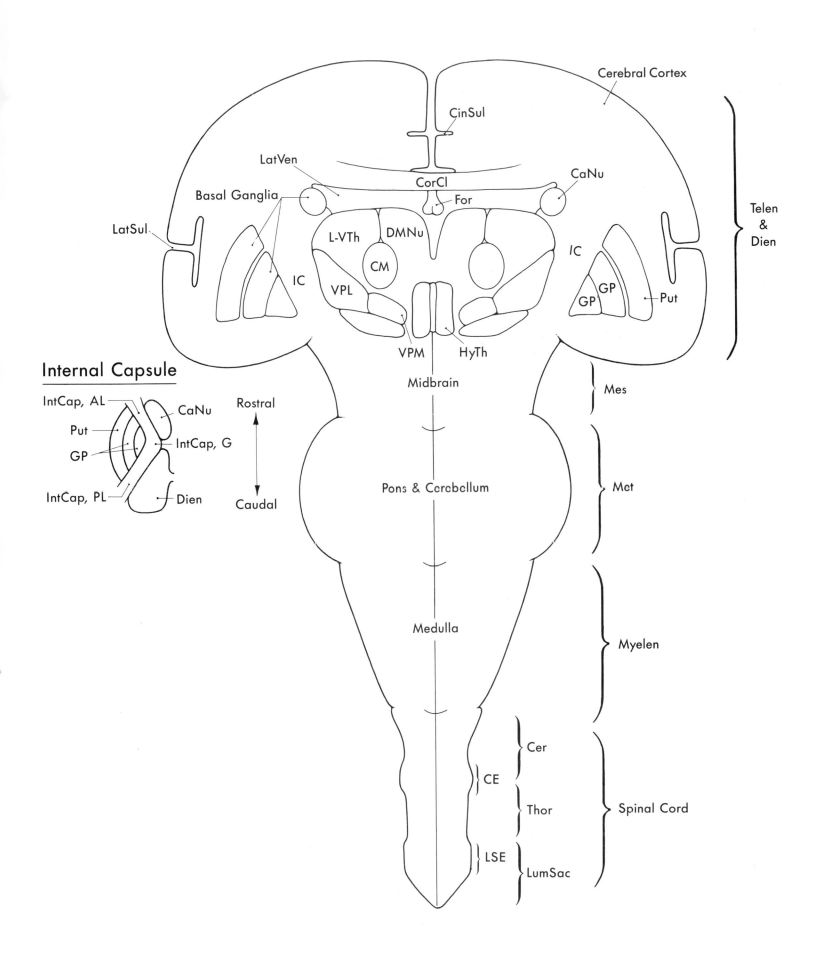

Cerebral Cortex

CinSul

LatVen

CorCl

CaNu

Basal Ganglia

For

Telen
&
Dien

LatSul

L-VTh

DMNu

IC

CM

IC

VPL

GP

GP

Put

VPM

HyTh

Midbrain

Mes

Internal Capsule

IntCap, AL

CaNu

Put

Rostral

IntCap, G

GP

Pons & Cerebellum

Met

IntCap, PL

Dien

Caudal

Medulla

Myelen

Cer

CE

Thor

Spinal Cord

LSE

LumSac

Dorsal Column-Medial Lemniscus System

7–4 The origin, course, and distribution of fibers composing the dorsal column (DC)-medial lemniscus (ML) system. This illustration shows the longitudinal extent, the positions in representative cross-sections of brainstem and spinal cord, and the somatotopy of fibers in DC and ML. The ML undergoes positional changes as it courses from the myelencephalon (medulla) rostrally toward the mesencephalic-diencephalic junction. In the medulla, ML and ALS fibers are widely separated and receive different blood supplies, while in the midbrain they are served by a common arterial source. As the ML makes positional changes, the somatotopy therein follows accordingly. Fibers of the postsynaptic dorsal column system (shown in green) are considered in detail in Fig. 7–6.

Neurotransmitters: Acetylcholine and the excitatory amino acids glutamate and aspartate are associated with some of the large diameter heavily myelinated fibers of the dorsal horn and dorsal columns.

Clinical Correlations: Damage to dorsal column fibers on one side of the spinal cord (as in the *Brown-Sequard syndrome*) results in an ipsilateral loss of vibratory sensations, position sense, and discriminative touch (*stereoagnosis, stereoanesthesia*) below the level of the lesion. Bilateral damage (as in *tabes dorsalis* or *subacute combined degeneration of the spinal cord*) produces bilateral losses. Rostral to the sensory decussation, lesions of medial lemniscus fibers produce contralateral losses that include the entire body. Brainstem lesions involving medial lemniscus fibers usually include adjacent structures, result in motor and sensory losses, and may reflect the distribution patterns of vessels (as in *medial medullary* or *medial pontine syndromes*). Large lesions in the forebrain may result in a complete contralateral loss of those modalities carried in the dorsal columns and anterolateral systems, or may produce *pain* (as in the *thalamic syndrome*).

Abbreviations

ALS	Anterolateral System		**NuCu**	Cuneate Nucleus
BP	Basilar Pons		**NuGr**	Gracile Nucleus
CC	Crus Cerebri		**OcNu**	Oculomotor Nucleus
CTT	Central Tegmental Tract		**PoCGy**	Postcentral Gyrus
DC	Dorsal Column		**PPL**	Posterior Paracentral Lobule
DRG	Dorsal Root Ganglia		**Py**	Pyramid
FCu	Cuneate Fasciculus		**RB**	Restiform Body
FGr	Gracile Fasciculus		**RNu**	Red Nucleus
IAF	Internal Arcuate Fibers		**SN**	Substantia Nigra
IC	Internal Capsule		**TecSp**	Tectospinal Tract
IO	Inferior Olivary Nucleus		**VesNu**	Vestibular Nuclei
ML	Medial Lemniscus		**VPL**	Ventral Posterolateral Nucleus of Thalamus
MLF	Medial Longitudinal Fasciculus			

Somatotopy of Body Areas

L	fibers conveying input from leg		**C₂**	fibers from about the second cervical level
N	fibers conveying input from neck		**S₅**	fibers from about the fifth sacral level
T	fibers conveying input from trunk		**T₅**	fibers from about the fifth thoracic level

Review of Blood Supply to **DC-ML** System

Structures	Arteries
DC in Spinal Cord	penetrating branches of arterial vasocorona (see Fig. 5–6)
ML in Medulla	anterior spinal (see Fig. 5–14)
ML in Pons	overlap of paramedian and long circumferential branches of basilar (see Fig. 5–21)
ML in Midbrain	short circumferential branches of posterior cerebral and superior cerebellar (see Fig. 5–27)
VPL	thalmogeniculate branches of posterior cerebral (see Fig. 5–38)
Posterior Limb of **IC**	lateral striate branches of middle cerebral (see Fig. 5–38)

Dorsal Column-Medial Lemniscus System

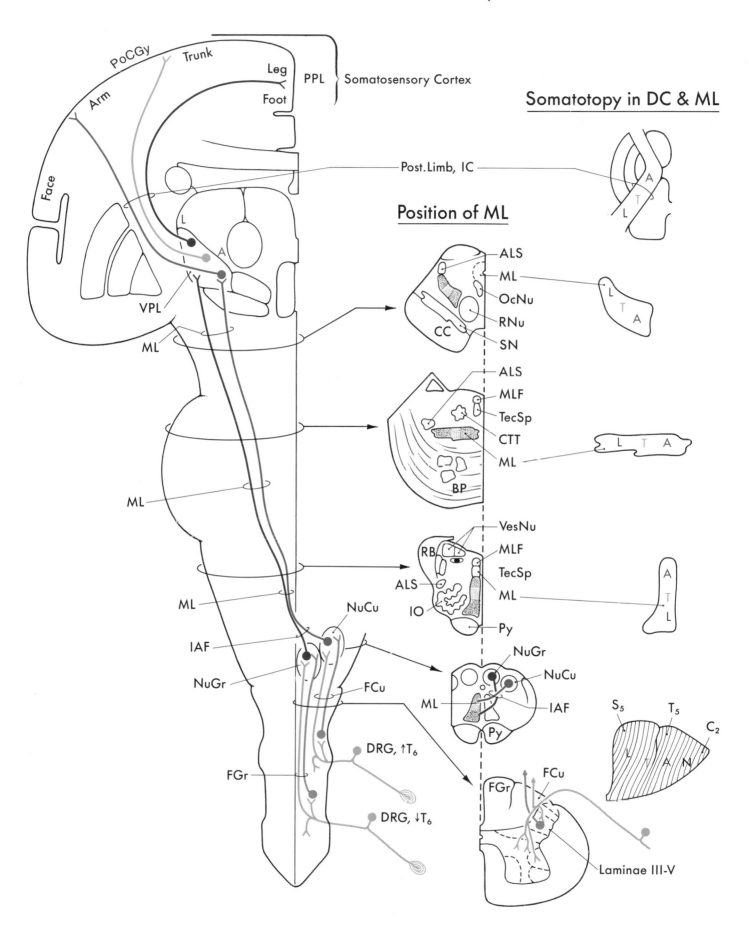

Somatotopy in DC & ML

Position of ML

Anterolateral System

7-5 The longitudinal extent and somatotopy of fibers composing the anterolateral system (ALS). The ALS is a composite bundle that terminates in the reticular formation (spinoreticular), deep layers of the superior colliculus (spinotectal), the periaqueductal gray, nucleus of Darkschewitsch, and midbrain reticular formation (spinomesencephalic), as well as in thalamic nuclei (spinothalamic). Spinotectal fibers are a subset of the overall spinomesencephalic projection. Spinothalamic fibers terminate in the VPL, in some intralaminar nuclei, and in medial areas of the posterior thalamic complex.

Fibers from the PAG and nucleus raphe dorsalis enter the nucleus raphe magnus and adjacent reticular area. These latter sites, in turn, project to laminae I, II, and V of the spinal cord via raphespinal and reticulospinal fibers.

Neurotransmitters: Glutamate(+), calcitonin gene-related peptide, and substance P(+)-containing dorsal root ganglion cells project into laminae I, II (heavy), V (moderate), and III, IV (sparse). Some spinoreticular and spinothalamic fibers contain enkephalin(-), somatostatin(-) and cholecystokinin(+). In addition to enkephalin and somatostatin, some spinomesencephalic fibers contain vasoactive intestinal polypeptide(+). Neurons in the PAG and nucleus raphe dor-

salis containing serotonin and neurotensin project into the nucleus raphe magnus and adjacent reticular formation. Cells in these latter centers that contain serotonin and enkephalin send processes to spinal cord laminae I, II, and V. Serotonergic raphespinal or enkephalinergic reticulospinal fibers may inhibit primary sensory fibers, or projection neurons, conveying nociceptive information.

Clinical Correlations: Spinal lesions that involve the anterolateral system (as in the *Brown-Sequard syndrome*) result in a loss of pain and temperature sensations on the contralateral side of the body beginning one level caudal to the lesion. *Syringomyelia* produces bilateral sensory losses restricted to adjacent dermatomes because of damage to the ventral white commissure. Vascular lesions in the lateral medulla (*posterior inferior cerebellar artery syndrome*) or lateral pons (anterior inferior cerebellar artery occlusion) result in a loss of pain and temperature over the entire contralateral body surface coupled with other motor and/or sensory deficits based on damage to structures served by these vessels. Profound loss of dorsal column and anterolateral system modalities, or intractable pain and/or paresthesias (as in the *thalamic syndrome*), results from vascular lesions in the posterolateral thalamus.

Abbreviations

A	input from arm regions		**Py**	Pyramid
ALS	Anterolateral System		**RaSp**	Raphespinal Fibers
BP	Basilar Pons		**RB**	Restiform Body
CC	Crus Cerebri		**RetF**	Reticular Formation (of midbrain)
DRG	Dorsal Root Ganglia		**RNu**	Red Nucleus
IC	Internal Capsule		**S**	input from sacral regions
IO	Inferior Olivary Nucleus		**SC**	Superior Colliculus
L	input from leg regions		**SN**	Substantia Nigra
MCP	Middle Cerebellar Peduncle		**SpRet**	Spinoreticular Fibers
ML	Medial Lemniscus		**SpTec**	Spinotectal Fibers
MLF	Medial Longitudinal Fasciculus		**SpTh**	Spinothalamic Fibers
Nu	Nucleus		**T**	input from thoracic regions
NuDark	Nucleus of Darkschewitsch		**TecSp**	Tectospinal Tract
NuRa,d	Nucleus Raphe, Dorsalis		**VesNu**	Vestibular Nuclei
NuRa,m	Nucleus Raphe, Magnus		**VPL**	Ventral Posterolateral Nucleus of Thalamus
PAG	Periaqueductal Gray		**VWCom**	Ventral White Commissure
PoCGy	Postcentral Gyrus		**I-VIII**	Laminae I-VIII of Rexed
PPL	Posterior Paracentral Lobule			

Review of Blood Supply to ALS

Structures	Arteries
ALS in Spinal Cord	penetrating branches of arterial vasocorona and branches of central (see Figs. 5-6, 5-14)
ALS in Medulla	caudal third, vertebral; rostral two-thirds, posterior inferior cerebellar (see Fig. 5-14)
ALS in Pons	long circumferential branches of basilar (see Fig. 5-21)
ALS in Midbrain	short circumferential branches of posterior cerebral, superior cerebellar (see Fig. 5-27)
VPL	thalmogeniculate branches of posterior cerebral (see Fig. 5-38)
Posterior Limb of **IC**	lateral striate branches of middle cerebral (see Fig. 5-38)

Anterolateral System

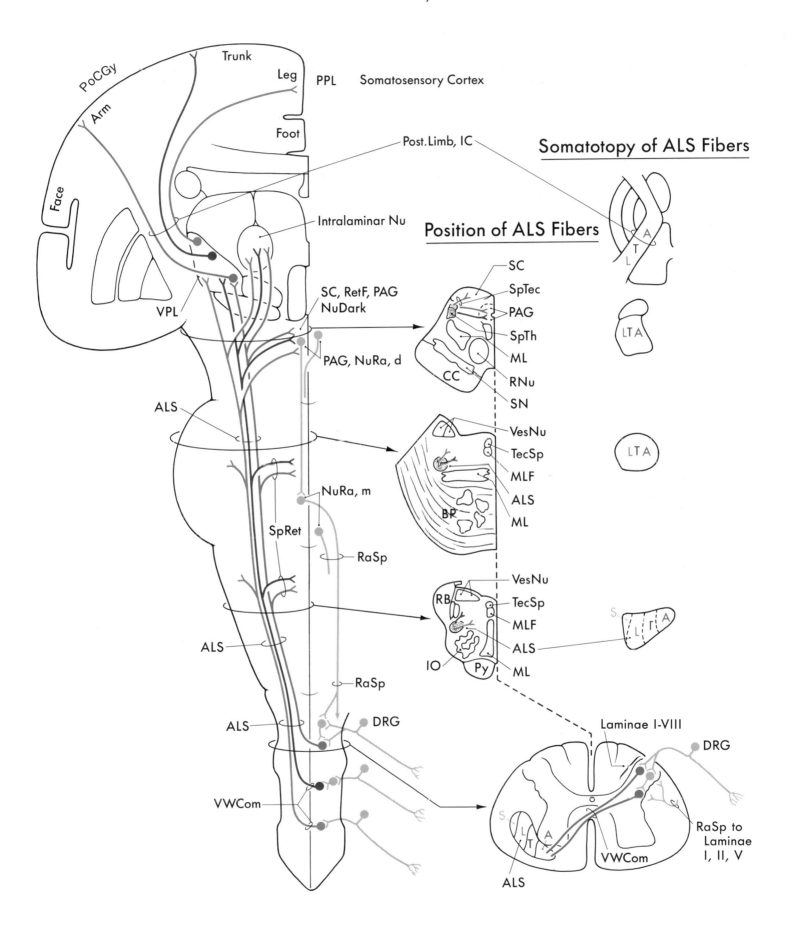

Somatotopy of ALS Fibers

Position of ALS Fibers

Somatosensory Cortex

PoCGy · Trunk · Leg · Arm · Face · PPL · Foot

Post. Limb, IC

Intralaminar Nu

SC, RetF, PAG NuDark

VPL

PAG, NuRa, d

ALS

NuRa, m

SpRet

RaSp

ALS

RaSp

ALS

DRG

VWCom

SC · SpTec · PAG · SpTh · ML · RNu · SN · CC

VesNu · TecSp · MLF · ALS · ML · BP

VesNu · TecSp · MLF · ALS · ML · RB · IO · Py

Laminae I–VIII · DRG · RaSp to Laminae I, II, V · VWCom · ALS

LTA

Postsynaptic-Dorsal Column System and the Spinocervicothalamic Pathway

7–6 The origin, course, and distribution of fibers composing the postsynaptic-dorsal column system (upper) and the spinocervicothalamic pathway (lower). Postsynaptic-dorsal column fibers originate primarily from cells in lamina IV (some cells in laminae III and V-VII also contribute), ascend in the ipsilateral dorsal fasciculi, and end in their respective nuclei in the caudal medulla. Moderate to sparse collaterals project to a few other medullary targets. Fibers of the spinocervical part of the spinocervicothalamic pathway also originate from cells in lamina IV (less so in III and V). The axons of these cells ascend in the dorsolateral part of the ipsilateral lateral funiculus (this is sometimes called the dorsolateral funiculus) and end in a topographic fashion in the lateral cervical nucleus: lumbosacral projections terminate dorsolaterally and cervical projections ventromedially. Cells of the dorsal column nuclei and the lateral cervical nucleus convey information to the contralateral thalamus via the medial lemniscus.

Neurotransmitters: Glutamate(+) and possibly substance P(+) are present in some spinocervical projections. Because some cells in laminae III-V have axons that collateralize to both the lateral cervical nucleus *and* the dorsal column nuclei, glutamate (and substance P) may also be present in some postsynaptic dorsal column fibers.

Clinical Correlations: The postsynaptic-dorsal column and spinocervicothalamic pathways are not known to be major circuits in the human nervous system. However, the occurrence of these fibers may explain a well known clinical observation. Patients that have received an *anterolateral cordotomy* (this lesion is placed just ventral to the denticulate ligament) for intractable pain may experience complete or partial relief, or there may be a recurrence of pain perception within days or weeks. While the cordotomy transects fibers of the anterolateral system (the main pain pathway), this lesion spares the dorsal horn, dorsal columns, and spinocervical fibers. Consequently, the recurrence of pain perception (or even the partial relief of pain) in these patients may be explained by these postsynaptic-dorsal column and spinocervicothalamic projections. Through these connections some nociceptive information may be transmitted to the ventral posterolateral nucleus, and on to the sensory cortex, via circuits that bypass the anterolateral system and are spared in a cordotomy.

Abbreviations

ALS	Anterolateral System
DRG	Dorsal Root Ganglion
FCu	Cuneate Fasciculus
FGr	Gracile Fasciculus
IAF	Internal Arcuate Fibers
LCerNu	Lateral Cervical Nucleus
ML	Medial Lemniscus
NuCu	Cuneate Nucleus
NuGr	Gracile Nucleus
VWCom	Ventral White Commissure

Review of Blood Supply to Dorsal Horn, **FGr, FCu, LCerNu**

Structures	Arteries
FGr, FCu in Spinal Cord	penetrating branches of arterial vasocorona and some branches from central (sulcal) (see Fig. 5–6)
LCerNu	penetrating branches of arterial vasocorona and branches from central (see Fig. 5–6)
NuGr NuCu	posterior spinal (see Fig. 5–14)

Postsynaptic - Dorsal Column

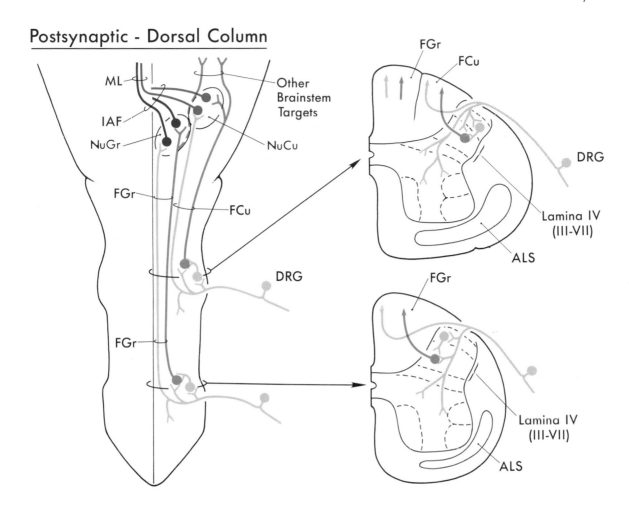

Spinocervicothalamic

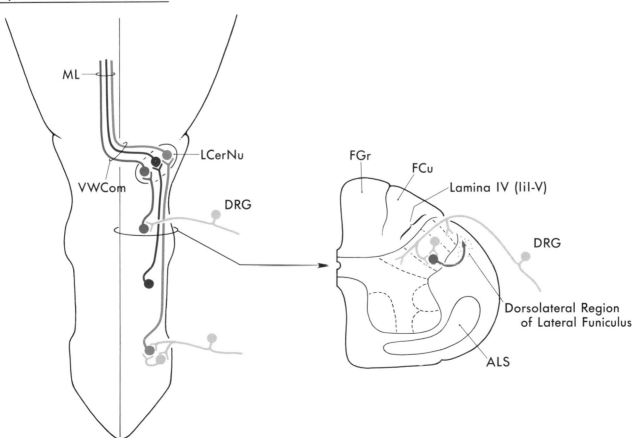

Trigeminal Pathways

7–7 The distribution of general sensory (GSA) information originating on cranial nerves V (trigeminal), VII (facial), IX (glossopharyngeal), and X (vagus). Some of these primary sensory fibers end in the chief sensory nucleus, while most form the spinal trigeminal tract and end in its nucleus. Neurons in the spinal nucleus and in ventral parts of the chief sensory nucleus give rise to crossed (ventral) trigeminothalamic fibers. Uncrossed (dorsal) trigeminothalamic fibers arise from dorsal regions of the chief sensory nucleus. Collaterals of these ascending fibers influence the hypoglossal, facial (corneal reflex), and trigeminal motor nuclei; mesencephalic collaterals are involved in the jaw-jerk reflex. Collaterals also enter the dorsal motor vagal nucleus (vomiting reflex), the superior salivatory nucleus (tearing/lacrimal reflex), and the nucleus ambiguus and adjacent reticular formation (sneezing reflex).

Neurotransmitters: Substance P(+) and cholecystokinin(+)-containing trigeminal ganglion cells project to the spinal trigeminal nucleus, especially its caudal part (pars caudalis). Glutamate(+) is found in many trigeminothalamic fibers arising from the chief sensory nucleus and the pars interpolaris of the spinal nucleus. It is present in fewer trigeminothalamic fibers from the pars caudalis and in almost none from the pars oralis. The locus ceruleus (noradrenergic fibers) and the raphe nuclei (serotonergic fibers) also project to the spinal nucleus. Enkephalin(-)-containing cells are present in caudal regions of the spinal nucleus, and enkephalinergic fibers are found in the nucleus ambiguus and in the hypoglossal, facial, and trigeminal motor nuclei.

Clinical Correlations: Lesions of the trigeminal ganglion or nerve proximal to the ganglion result in (1) a loss of pain, temperature, and tactile sensation from the ipsilateral face, oral cavity, and teeth, (2) ipsilateral paralysis of masticatory muscles, and (3) ipsilateral loss of the corneal reflex. *Trigeminal neuralgia (tic douloureux)* is a severe, but brief, pain restricted to the peripheral distribution of the trigeminal nerve, usually its V_2 (maxillary) division. This pain may be initiated by any contact to the face (e.g., shaving, putting makeup on), chewing, or even smiling.

In the medulla, fibers of the spinal trigeminal tract and ALS are served by the posterior inferior cerebellar artery (PICA). Consequently, an *alternating hemianesthesia* is one characteristic feature of the *PICA syndrome*. Pontine gliomas may produce a paralysis of masticatory muscles (motor trigeminal damage) and some loss of tactile input (chief sensory nucleus damage).

Abbreviations

ALS	Anterolateral System	**SpTNu**	Spinal Trigeminal Nucleus
CC	Crus Cerebri	**SpTTr**	Spinal Trigeminal Tract
CSNu	Chief (Principal) Sensory Nucleus	**TriMoNu**	Trigeminal Motor Nucleus
DTTr	Dorsal Trigeminothalamic Tract	**TMJ**	Temporomandibular Joint
FacNu	Facial Nucleus	**VPL**	Ventral Posterolateral Nucleus of Thalamus
GSA	General Somatic Afferent	**VPM**	Ventral Posteromedial Nucleus of Thalamus
HyNu	Hypoglossal Nucleus	**VTTr**	Ventral Trigeminothalamic Tract
IC	Internal Capsule		
Man.V	Mandibular Division of Trigeminal Nerve		
Max.V	Maxillary Division of Trigeminal Nerve		
MesNu	Mesencephalic Nucleus		
ML	Medial Lemniscus		
OpTh.V	Ophthalmic Division of Trigeminal Nerve		
Py	Pyramid		
RB	Restiform Body		
RetF	Reticular Formation		
RNu	Red Nucleus		
SN	Substantia Nigra		

Ganglia

1 Trigeminal Ganglion
2 Geniculate Ganglion
3 Superior of Glossopharyngeal
4 Superior of Vagus

Review of Blood Supply to **SpTT, SpTNu,** and Trigeminothalamic Tracts

Structures	Arteries
SpTTr and **SpTNu** in Medulla	caudal third, vertebral; rostral two-thirds, posterior inferior cerebellar (see Fig. 5–14)
SpTTr and **SpTNu** in Pons	long circumferential branches of basilar (see Fig. 5–21)
Trigeminothalamic Fibers in Midbrain	short circumferential branches of posterior cerebral and superior cerebellar (see Fig. 5–27)
VPM	thalmogeniculate branches of posterior cerebral (see Fig. 5–38)
Posterior Limb of **IC**	lateral striate branches of middle cerebral (see Fig. 5–38)

Trigeminal Pathways

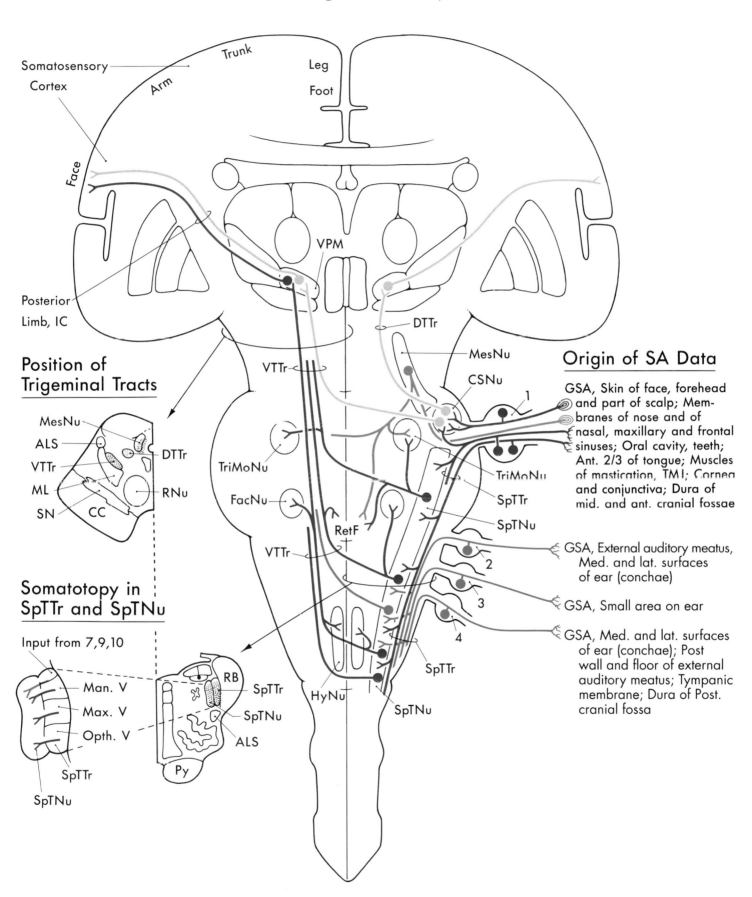

Position of Trigeminal Tracts

MesNu
ALS
VTTr
ML
SN
CC
DTTr
RNu

Somatotopy in SpTTr and SpTNu

Input from 7,9,10
Man. V
Max. V
Opth. V
SpTTr
SpTNu
RB
SpTTr
SpTNu
ALS
Py

Somatosensory Cortex
Trunk
Arm
Leg
Foot
Face
Posterior Limb, IC
VPM
DTTr
VTTr
TriMoNu
FacNu
VTTr
RetF
MesNu
CSNu
TriMoNu
SpTTr
SpTNu
HyNu
SpTTr
SpTNu

Origin of SA Data

GSA, Skin of face, forehead and part of scalp; Membranes of nose and of nasal, maxillary and frontal sinuses; Oral cavity, teeth; Ant. 2/3 of tongue; Muscles of mastication, TMJ; Cornea and conjunctiva; Dura of mid. and ant. cranial fossae

GSA, External auditory meatus, Med. and lat. surfaces of ear (conchae)

GSA, Small area on ear

GSA, Med. and lat. surfaces of ear (conchae); Post wall and floor of external auditory meatus; Tympanic membrane; Dura of Post. cranial fossa

1
2
3
4

Solitary Pathways

7–8   Visceral afferent input (SVA-taste; GVA general visceral sensation) on cranial nerves VII (facial), IX (glossopharyngeal), and X (vagus) enters the solitary nucleus via the solitary tract. Solitary cells project to the salivatory, hypoglossal, and dorsal motor vagal nuclei and the nucleus ambiguus. Solitary projections to the nucleus ambiguus are largely bilateral and are the intermediate neurons in the pathway for the gag reflex. Solitariospinal fibers are bilateral with a contralateral preponderance and project to the phrenic nucleus, the intermediolateral cell column, and the ventral horn. The VPM is the thalamic center through which visceral afferent information is relayed onto the cortex.

Neurotransmitters: Substance P(+) and cholecystokinin(+)-containing cells in the geniculate ganglion (facial nerve) and in the inferior ganglia of the glossopharyngeal and vagus nerves project to the solitary nucleus. Enkephalin(-), neurotensin, and GABA(+) are present in some solitary neurons that project into the adjacent dorsal motor vagal nucleus. Cholecystokinin(+), somatostatin(-), and enkephalin(-) are present in solitary neurons, in cells of the parabrachial nuclei, and in some thalamic neurons that project to taste, and other visceral areas, of the cortex.

Clinical Correlations: Lesions of the geniculate ganglion, or facial nerve proximal to the ganglion, result in (1) ipsilateral loss of taste (*ageusia*) from the anterior two-thirds of the tongue, and (2) an ipsilateral *facial (Bell's) palsy*. While a glossopharyngeal nerve lesion will result in *ageusia* from the posterior third of the tongue on the ipsilateral side, this loss is difficult to test. On the other hand, *glossopharyngeal neuralgia* is an idiopathic pain localized to the peripheral sensory branches of the IXth nerve in the posterior pharynx, posterior tongue, and tonsillar area. Occlusion of the posterior inferior cerebellar artery (as in the *lateral medullary syndrome*), in addition to producing an *alternate hemianesthesia* will also result in *ageusia* from the ipsilateral side of the tongue since the posterior inferior cerebellar artery serves the solitary tract and nucleus in the medulla.

Interestingly, lesions of the olfactory nerves or tract (*anosmia*, loss of olfactory sensation; *dysosmia*, distorted olfactory sense) may affect how the patient perceives taste. Witness the fact that the nasal congestion accompanying a severe cold will markedly affect the sense of taste.

Abbreviations

AmyNu	Amygdaloid Nucleus (Complex)	**SVA**	Special Visceral Afferent
CardResp	Cardiorespiratory portion (caudal) of solitary nucleus	**SpVNu**	Spinal (or Inferior) Vestibular Nucleus
GustNu	Gustatory Nucleus (rostral portion of solitary nucleus)	**Tr**	Tract
		VA	Visceral Afferent
		VPM	Ventral Posteromedial Nucleus of Thalamus
GVA	General Visceral Afferent		
HyNu	Hypoglossal Nucleus		
HyTh	Hypothalamus		
MVNu	Medial Vestibular Nucleus		
NuAm	Nucleus Ambiguus		
PBNu	Parabrachial Nucleus		
RB	Restiform Body		
SalNu	Salivatory Nuclei		
SolTr & Nu	Solitary Tract and Nucleus		

Number Key

1   geniculate ganglion of facial
2   inferior ganglion of glossopharyngeal
3   inferior ganglion of vagus
4   dorsal motor vagal nucleus

Review of Blood Supply to **SolNu** and **SolTr**

Structures	Arteries
SolNu and **Tr** in Medulla	caudal medulla, anterior spinal; rostral medulla, posterior inferior cerebellar (see Fig. 5–14)
Ascending Fibers in Pons	long circumferential branches of basilar and branches of superior cerebellar (see Fig. 5–21)
VPM	thalmogeniculate branches of posterior cerebral (see Fig. 5–38)
Posterior Limb of **IC**	lateral striate branches of middle cerebral (see Fig. 5–38)

Solitary Pathways

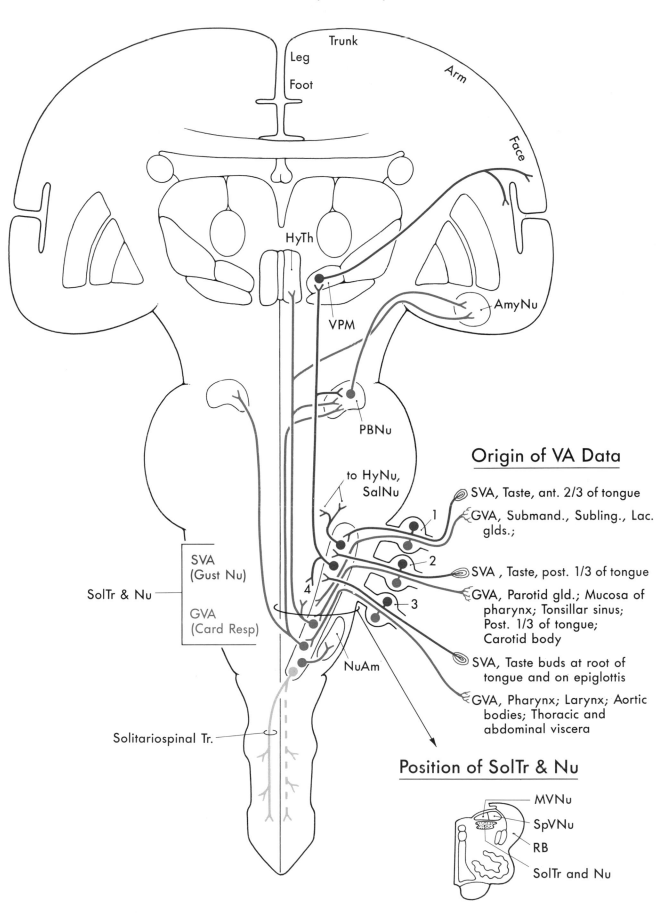

Trunk
Leg
Foot
Arm
Face

HyTh

VPM

AmyNu

PBNu

to HyNu,
SalNu

SVA
(Gust Nu)

SolTr & Nu

GVA
(Card Resp)

1

2

3

4

NuAm

Solitariospinal Tr.

Origin of VA Data

SVA, Taste, ant. 2/3 of tongue

GVA, Submand., Subling., Lac. glds.;

SVA , Taste, post. 1/3 of tongue

GVA, Parotid gld.; Mucosa of pharynx; Tonsillar sinus; Post. 1/3 of tongue; Carotid body

SVA, Taste buds at root of tongue and on epiglottis

GVA, Pharynx; Larynx; Aortic bodies; Thoracic and abdominal viscera

Position of SolTr & Nu

MVNu
SpVNu
RB
SolTr and Nu

7–9   Blank master drawing for sensory pathways. This illustration is provided for self-evaluation of sensory pathway understanding, for the instructor to expand on sensory pathways not covered in the atlas, or both.

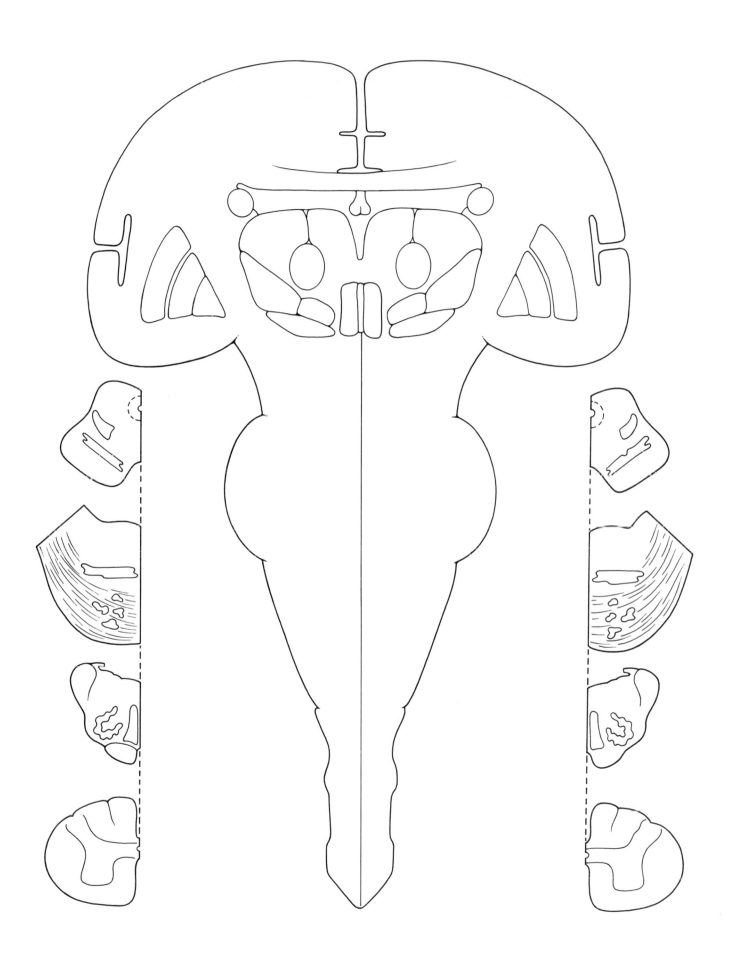

Corticospinal Tracts

7–10 The longitudinal extent of corticospinal fibers and their position and somatotopy at representative levels. The somatotopy of corticospinal fibers in the basilar pons is less obvious than in the internal capsule, crus cerebri, pyramid, or spinal cord. In the pyramidal decussation, fibers originating from arm areas of cortex cross rostral to those that arise from leg areas. In addition to fibers arising from the somatomotor cortex (area 4), a significant contingent also originates from the postcentral gyrus (areas 3, 1, 2); the former terminate primarily in laminae VI-IX, while the latter end mainly in laminae IV and V. Prefrontal regions, especially area 6, and parietal areas 5 and 7 also contribute to the corticospinal tract.

Neurotransmitters: Acetylcholine, gamma-aminobutyric acid(-), and substance P(+, plus other peptides) are found in small cortical neurons presumed to function as local circuit cells or in corticocortical connections. Glutamate(+) is present in cortical efferent fibers that project to the spinal cord. Glutaminergic corticospinal fibers and terminals are found in all spinal levels but are especially concentrated in cervical and lumbosacral enlargements. Lower motor neurons are influenced by corticospinal fibers either directly or indirectly via interneurons. Acetylcholine and calcitonin gene related peptide are present in these large motor cells and in their endings in skeletal muscle.

Clinical Correlations: *Myasthenia gravis*, a disease characterized by moderate to profound weakness of skeletal muscles, is caused by circulating antibodies that react with postsynaptic nicotinic acetylcholine receptors. Injury to corticospinal fibers on one side of the cervical spinal cord (as in the *Brown-Sequard syndrome*) results in weakness (*hemiparesis*) or paralysis (*hemiplegia*) of the ipsilateral arm and leg. In addition, and with time, these patients exhibit features of an *upper motor neuron lesion* (*hyperreflexia, spasticity*, loss of superficial abdominal reflexes, and the *Babinski sign*). Rostral to the pyramidal decussation, vascular lesions in the medulla (*medial medullary syndrome*), pons (*Millard-Gubler* or *Foville's syndromes*), or midbrain (*Weber's syndrome*) all produce *alternating hemiplegia's*. These present as a contralateral hemiplegia of the arm and leg coupled with an ipsilateral paralysis of the tongue (medulla), facial muscles or lateral rectus muscle (pons), and most eye movements (midbrain); sensory deficits can also be part of these syndromes. Lesions in the internal capsule (*lacunar strokes*) produce contralateral hemiparesis sometimes coupled with various cranial nerve signs due to corticobulbar involvement. Bilateral weakness, indicative of corticospinal involvement, is also present in *amyotrophic lateral sclerosis*.

Abbreviations

ACSp	Anterior Corticospinal Tract		**RNu**	Red Nucleus
ALS	Anterolateral System		**SN**	Substantia Nigra
APL	Anterior Paracentral Lobule		**TecSp**	Tectospinal Tract
BP	Basilar Pons		**VesNu**	Vestibular Nuclei
CBul	Corticobulbar Fibers			
CC	Crus Cerebri			
CSp	Corticospinal Fibers			
IC	Internal Capsule			
IO	Inferior Olivary Nucleus			
LCSp	Lateral Corticospinal Tract			
ML	Medial Lemniscus			
MLF	Medial Longitudinal Fasciculus			
PrCGy	Precentral Gyrus			
Py	Pyramid			
RB	Restiform Body			

Somatotopy of **CSp** Fibers

A position of fibers coursing to upper extremity regions of spinal cord

L position of fibers coursing to lower extremity regions of spinal cord

T position of fibers coursing to thoracic regions of spinal cord

Review of Blood Supply to Corticospinal Fibers

Structures	Arteries
Posterior Limb of **IC**	lateral striate branches of middle cerebral (see Fig. 5–38)
Crus Cerebri in Midbrain	paramedian and short circumferential branches of basilar and posterior communicating (see Fig. 5–27)
CSp in **BP**	paramedian branches of basilar (see Fig. 5–21)
Py in Medulla	anterior spinal (see Fig. 5–14)
LCSp in Spinal Cord	penetrating branches of arterial vasocorona (leg fibers), branches of central artery (arm fibers) (see Fig. 5–6)

Corticospinal Tracts

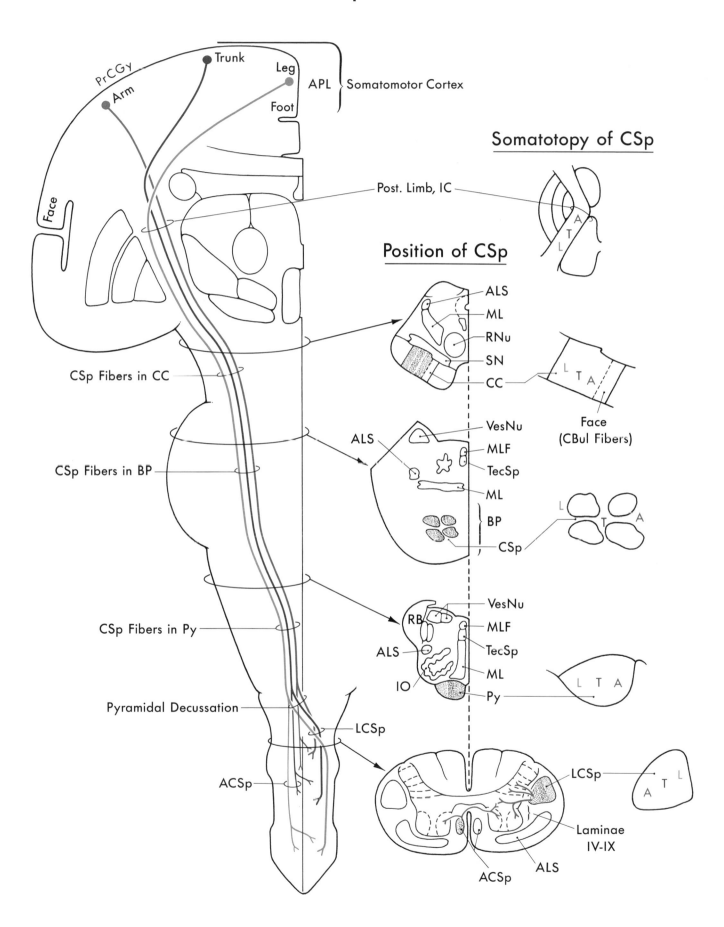

Somatomotor Cortex

Somatotopy of CSp

Position of CSp

Post. Limb, IC

Face (CBul Fibers)

Corticobulbar Fibers

7–11   The origin, course, and distribution of corticobulbar fibers to brainstem motor nuclei. These fibers influence, either directly or through neurons in the immediately adjacent reticular formation, the motor nuclei of oculomotor, trochlear, trigeminal, abducens, facial, glossopharyngeal and vagus (both via nucleus ambiguus), spinal accessory, and hypoglossal nerves. Corticobulbar fibers occupy the genu and, sometimes, the adjacent rostral portion of the posterior limb of the internal capsule. In addition to their origin from the precentral gyrus (somatomotor cortex, area 4), corticobulbar fibers also arise from the postcentral gyrus (somatosensory cortex, areas 3, 1, 2) and from the frontal eye field (area 8). Corticobulbar fibers that influence the oculomotor, trochlear, and abducens nuclei arise primarily from the frontal eye field (area 8) and the supplemental eye field (area 6). The posterior eye field (area 7) influences eye movement through the superior colliculus. Although not illustrated here, it should be noted that descending cortical fibers also project to the sensory nuclei of some cranial nerves and to other sensory relay nuclei in the brainstem, such as those of the dorsal column system.

Neurotransmitters: Glutamate(+) is found in many corticofugal axons that directly innervate cranial nerve motor nuclei and in those fibers that terminate near (indirect), but not in, the various motor nuclei.

Clinical Correlations: Lesions involving the motor cortex (as in cerebral artery occlusion) or the internal capsule (as in *lacunar strokes* or occlusion of lenticulostriate branches of M_1 give rise to a contralateral *hemiplegia* of the arm and leg coupled with certain cranial nerve signs. Strictly cortical lesions may produce a transient *gaze palsy* due to damage to cortical gaze areas. In addition to a contralateral *hemiplegia* due to corticospinal involvement, the most common cranial nerve findings in capsular lesions are (1) deviation of the tongue to the side of the weakness when protruded and (2) paralysis of facial muscles on the contralateral lower half of the face (central facial palsy). This reflects the fact that corticobulbar fibers to genioglossus motor neurons and to facial motor nerves serving the lower face are primarily crossed. In rare cases there may be an ipsilateral deviation of the uvula on attempted phonation and/or a drooping of the shoulder (trapezius) and weakness of the sternocleidomastoid muscle ipsilateral to the infarcted hemisphere. In contrast to the *alternating hemiparesis* seen in some brainstem lesions, hemisphere lesions result in spinal and cranial nerve deficits that are both contralateral to the cerebral injury.

Abbreviations

AbdNu	Abducens Nucleus
AccNu	Accessory Nucleus (Spinal Accessory Nu.)
F	Face Area of Internal Capsule
FacNu	Facial Nucleus
HyNu	Hypoglossal Nucleus
IC	Internal Capsule
NuAm	Nucleus Ambiguus
OcNu	Oculomotor Nucleus
TriMoNu	Trigeminal Motor Nucleus
TroNu	Trochlear Nucleus

Review of Blood Supply to Cranial Nerve Motor Nuclei

Structures	Arteries
OcNu and **EWNu**	paramedian branches of basilar bifurcation and medial branches of posterior cerebral and posterior communicating (see Fig. 5–27)
TriMoNu	long circumferential branches of basilar (see Fig. 5–21)
AbdNu and **FacNu**	long circumferential branches of basilar (see Fig. 5–21)
NuAm	posterior inferior cerebellar (see Fig. 5–14)
HyNu	anterior spinal (see Fig. 5–14)

Corticobulbar Fibers

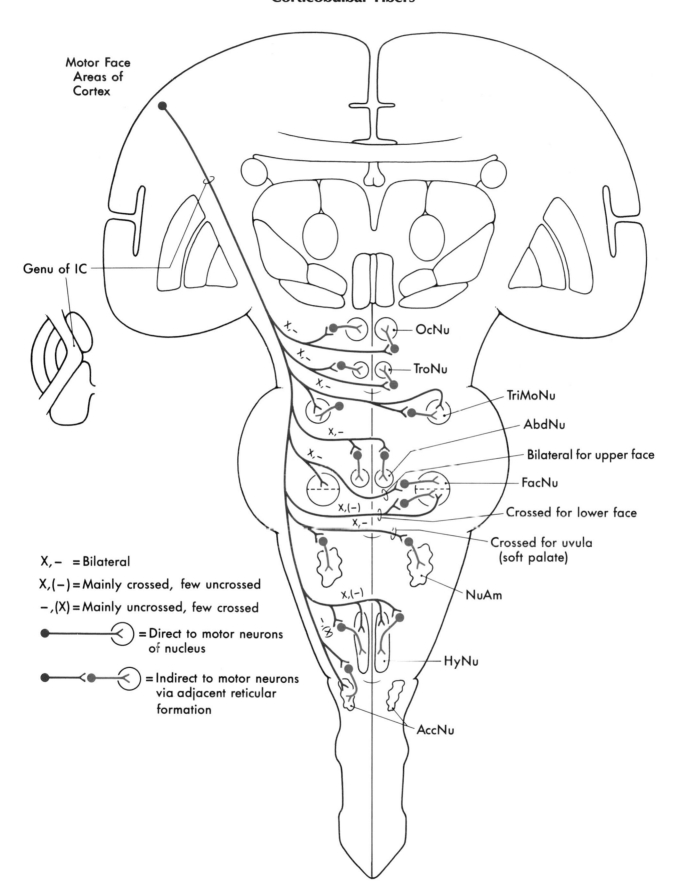

Motor Face Areas of Cortex

Genu of IC

OcNu

TroNu

TriMoNu

AbdNu

Bilateral for upper face

FacNu

Crossed for lower face

Crossed for uvula (soft palate)

NuAm

HyNu

AccNu

X, − = Bilateral

X, (−) = Mainly crossed, few uncrossed

−, (X) = Mainly uncrossed, few crossed

= Direct to motor neurons of nucleus

= Indirect to motor neurons via adjacent reticular formation

Tectospinal and Reticulospinal Tracts

7–12 The origin, course, position in representative cross-sections of brainstem and spinal cord, and general distribution of tectospinal and reticulospinal tracts. Tectospinal fibers originate from deeper layers of the superior colliculus, cross in the dorsal tegmental decussation, and distribute to cervical cord levels. While several regions of cerebral cortex (e.g., frontal, parietal, temporal) project to the tectum, the most highly organized corticotectal projections arise from the visual cortex. Pontine reticulospinal fibers (medial reticulospinal) tend to be uncrossed, while those from the medulla (lateral reticulospinal) are bilateral but with a pronounced ipsilateral preponderance. Corticoreticular fibers are bilateral with a slight contralateral preponderance and originate from several cortical areas.

Neurotransmitters: Corticotectal projections, especially those from the visual cortex, utilize glutamate(+). This substance is also present in most corticoreticular fibers. Some neurons of the gigantocellular reticular nucleus that send their axons to the spinal cord, as reticulospinal projections, contain enkephalin(-) and substance P(+). Enkephalinergic reticulospinal fibers may be part of the descending system that modulates pain transmission at the spinal level. Many reticulospinal fibers influence the activity of lower motor neurons.

Clinical Correlations: Isolated lesions of only tectospinal and reticulospinal fibers are essentially never seen. Tectospinal fibers project to upper cervical levels where they influence reflex movement of the head and neck. Such movements may be diminished in patients with damage to these fibers. Medial (pontine) reticulospinal fibers are excitatory to extensor motor neurons and to neurons innervating axial musculature; some of these fibers may also inhibit flexor motor neurons. In contrast, lateral (medullary) reticulospinal fibers are primarily inhibitory to extensor motor neurons and to neurons innervating muscles of the neck and back; these fibers may also excite flexor motor neurons via interneurons. Reticulospinal (and vestibulospinal) fibers contribute to the *spasticity* that develops in patients with lesions of corticospinal fibers. These reticulospinal and vestibulospinal also contribute to the tonic extension of the arms and legs seen in *decerebrate rigidity* when spinal motor neurons are released from descending cortical control.

Abbreviations

ALS	Anterolateral System	**Py**	Pyramid
BP	Basilar Pons	**RB**	Restiform Body
CC	Crus Cerebri	**RetNu**	Reticular Nuclei
CRet	Corticoreticular Fibers	**RetSp**	Reticulospinal Tract(s)
CTec	Corticotectal Fibers	**RNu**	Red Nucleus
DTegDec	Dorsal Tegmental Decussation (Tectospinal Fibers)	**RuSp**	Rubrospinal Tract
		SC	Superior Colliculus
GigRetNu	Gigantocellular Reticular Nucleus	**SN**	Substantia Nigra
IO	Inferior Olivary Nucleus	**SpTec**	Spinotectal Tract
LCSp	Lateral Corticospinal Tract	**SpVNu**	Spinal (or Inferior) Vestibular Nucleus
ML	Medial Lemniscus	**TecSp**	Tectospinal Tract
MLF	Medial Longitudinal Fasciculus	**VTegDec**	Ventral Tegmental Decussation (Rubrospinal Fibers)
MVNu	Medial Vestibular Nucleus		
OcNu	Oculomotor Nucleus		

Review of Blood Supply to **SC,** Reticular Formation of Pons and Medulla, and **TecSp** and **RetSp** Tracts in Cord

Structures	Arteries
Sc	long circumferential branches (quadrigeminal branch) of posterior cerebral plus some from superior cerebellar and posterior choroidal (see Fig. 5–27)
Pontine Reticular Formation	long circumferential branches of basilar plus branches of superior cerebellar in rostral pons (see Fig. 5–21)
Medullary Reticular Formation	branches of vertebral plus paramedian branches of basilar at medulla-pons junction (see Fig. 5–14)
TecSp and **RetSp** Tracts	branches of central artery (TecSp and Medullary RetSp); penetrating branches of arterial vasocorona (Pontine RetSp) (see Figs. 5–14, 5–6)

Tectospinal and Reticulospinal Tracts

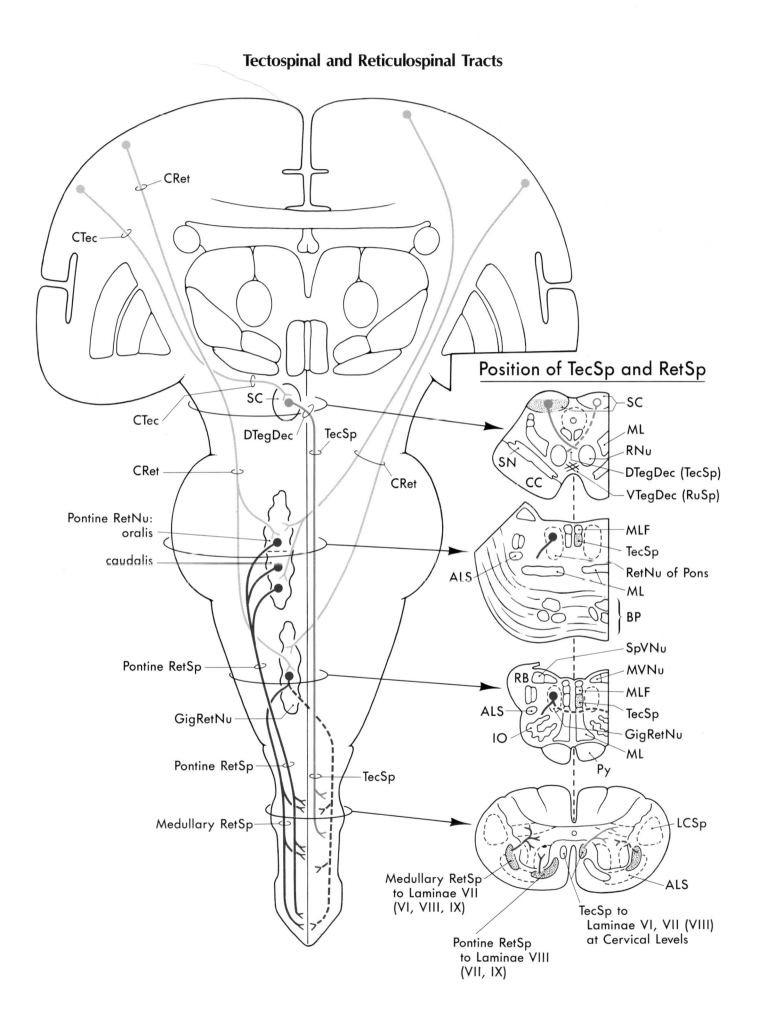

Position of TecSp and RetSp

CRet

CTec

CTec

SC

DTegDec

TecSp

CRet

CRet

Pontine RetNu:
oralis

caudalis

ALS

Pontine RetSp

GigRetNu

Pontine RetSp

Medullary RetSp

TecSp

SC

ML

RNu

DTegDec (TecSp)

VTegDec (RuSp)

SN

CC

MLF

TecSp

RetNu of Pons

ML

BP

SpVNu

MVNu

MLF

TecSp

GigRetNu

ML

Py

RB

ALS

IO

LCSp

ALS

Medullary RetSp
to Laminae VII
(VI, VIII, IX)

Pontine RetSp
to Laminae VIII
(VII, IX)

TecSp to
Laminae VI, VII (VIII)
at Cervical Levels

Rubrospinal and Vestibulospinal Tracts

7–13 The origin, course, and position in representative cross-sections of brainstem and spinal cord, and general distribution of rubrospinal and vestibulospinal tracts. Rubrospinal fibers cross in the ventral tegmental decussation and distribute to all spinal levels. Cells in dorsomedial regions of the red nucleus receive input from arm areas of the motor cortex and project to cervical cord, while those in ventrolateral areas of the nucleus receive fibers from leg cortex and project to lumbosacral levels. The red nucleus also projects, via the central tegmental tract, to the ipsilateral inferior olivary complex (rubro-olivary fibers). Medial and lateral vestibular nuclei give rise to the medial and lateral vestibulospinal tracts, respectively. The former tract is primarily ipsilateral, projects to upper spinal levels, and is considered a component of the medial longitudinal fasciculus in the cord. The latter tract is ipsilateral and somatotopically organized; fibers to lumbosacral levels originate from dorsal and caudal regions of the lateral nucleus, while those to cervical levels arise from its rostral and more ventral areas.

Neurotransmitters: Glutamate(+) is present in corticorubral fibers. Some lateral vestibulospinal fibers contain aspartate(+), while glycine(-) is present in a portion of the medial vestibulospinal projection. There are numerous gamma-aminobutyric acid(-)-containing fibers in the vestibular complex; these represent the endings of cerebellar corticovestibular fibers.

Clinical Correlations: Isolated injury to rubrospinal and vestibulospinal fibers is not seen in humans. Deficits in fine distal limb movements seen in monkeys following rubrospinal lesions may be present in humans. However, these deficits are overshadowed by the *hemiplegia* associated with injury to the adjacent corticospinal fibers. The contralateral tremor seen in patients with *Claude's syndrome* (a lesion of the medial midbrain) is partially related to damage to the red nucleus. Medial vestibulospinal fibers primarily inhibit neurons innervating extensors and neurons serving muscles of the back and neck. Lateral vestibulospinal fibers may inhibit some flexor motor neurons, but they mainly facilitate spinal reflexes via their excitatory influence on neurons innervating extensors. Vestibulospinal (and reticulospinal) fibers contribute to the *spasticity* seen in patients with damage to corticospinal fibers or to the tonic extension of the arms and legs in patients with *decerebrate rigidity*.

Abbreviations

CC	Crus Cerebri		**MVNu**	Medial Vestibular Nucleus
CorRu	Corticorubral Fibers		**OcNu**	Oculomotor Nucleus
DTegDec	Dorsal Tegmental Decussation (Tectospinal Fibers)		**Py**	Pyramid
FacNu	Facial Nucleus		**RNu**	Red Nucleus
IO	Inferior Olivary Nucleus		**RuSp**	Rubrospinal Tract
LCSp	Lateral Corticospinal Tract		**SC**	Superior Colliculus
LRNu	Lateral Reticular Nucleus		**SN**	Substantia Nigra
LVNu	Lateral Vestibular Nucleus		**SVNu**	Superior Vestibular Nucleus
LVesSp	Lateral Vestibulospinal Tract		**SpVNu**	Spinal (or Inferior) Vestibular Nucleus
ML	Medial Lemniscus		**TecSp**	Tectospinal Tract
MLF	Medial Longitudinal Fasciculus		**VesSp**	Vestibulospinal Tracts
MVesSp	Medial Vestibulospinal Tract		**VTegDec**	Ventral Tegmental Decussation (Rubrospinal Fibers)

Review of Blood Supply to **RNu**, Vestibular Nuclei, **MFL** and **RuSp**, and Vestibulospinal Tracts in Cords

Structures	Arteries
RNu	medial branches of posterior cerebral and posterior communicating plus some from short circumferential branches of posterior cerebral (see Fig. 5–27)
Vestibular Nuclei	posterior inferior cerebellar in medulla (see Fig. 5–14) and long circumferential branches in pons (see Fig. 5–21)
MLF	long circumferential branches of basilar in pons (see Fig. 5–21) and anterior spinal in medulla (see Fig. 5–14)
MVesSp	branches of central artery (see Figs. 5–6; 5–14)
LVesSp and **RuSp**	penetrating branches of arterial vasocorona plus terminal branches of central artery (see Fig. 5–6)

Rubrospinal and Vestibulospinal Tracts

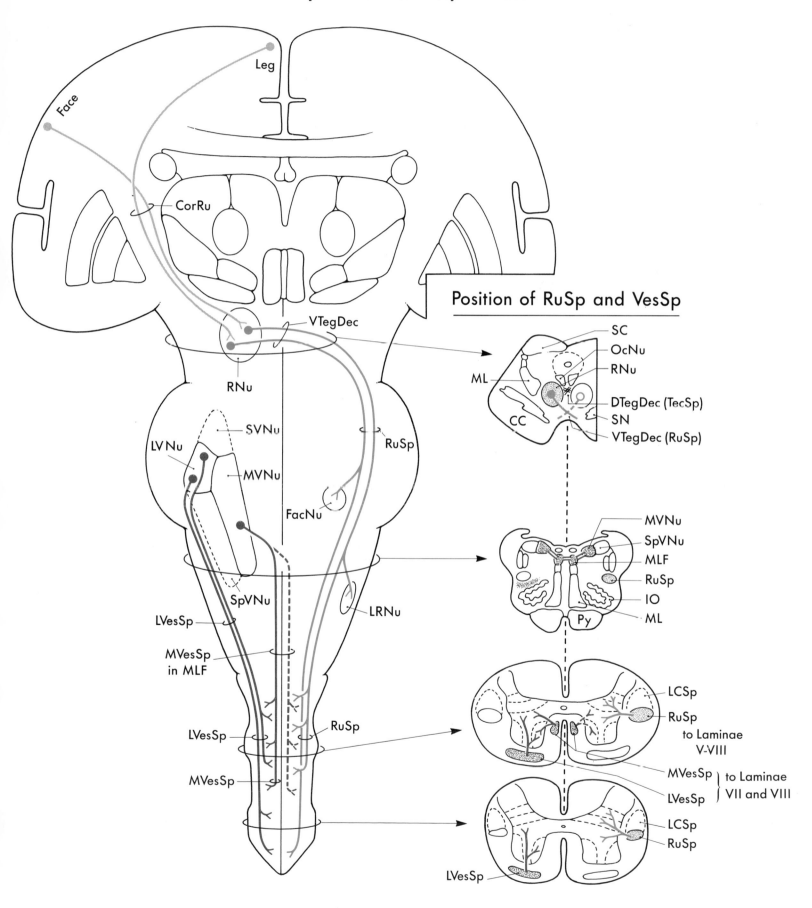

Position of RuSp and VesSp

7–14 Blank master drawing for motor pathways. This illustration is provided for self-evaluation of motor pathway understanding, for the instructor to expand on motor pathways not covered in the atlas, or both.

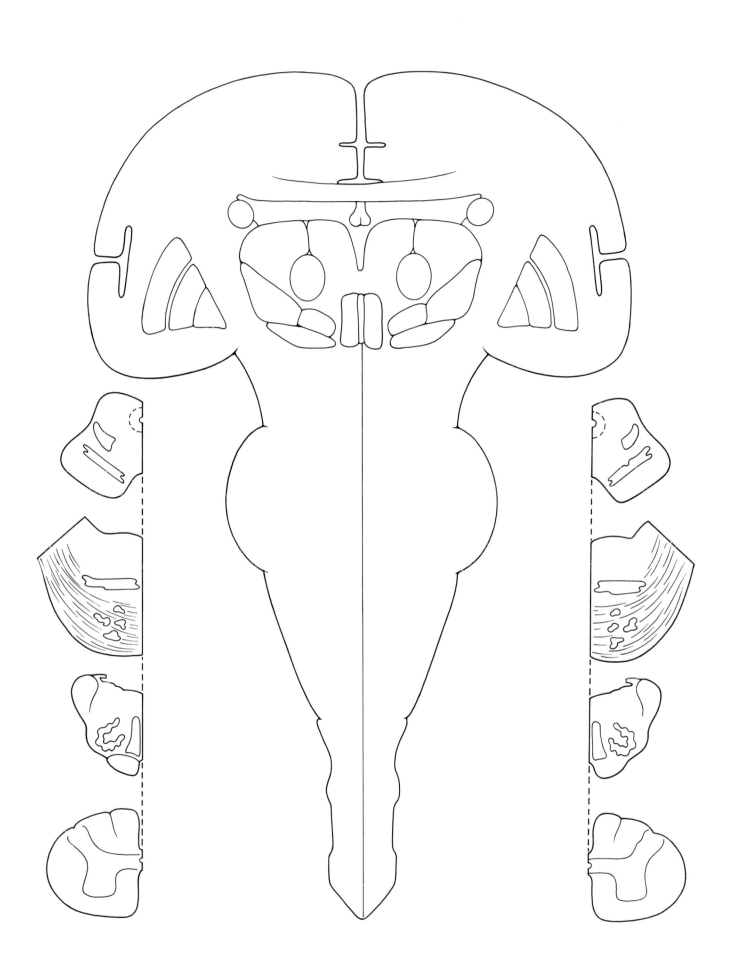

Cranial Nerve Efferents (III, IV, VI, XI-AccNu, XII)

7–15 The origin and peripheral distribution of GSE fibers from the oculomotor, trochlear, abducens, spinal accessory, and hypoglossal nuclei. Also shown are GVE fibers arising from the Edinger-Westphal nucleus and the distribution of postganglionic fibers from the ciliary ganglion. Internuclear abducens neurons project, via the MLF, to contralateral oculomotor neurons that innervate the medial rectus muscle (internuclear ophthalmoplegia pathway). Some authors specify the functional component of neurons in the accessory nucleus as special visceral efferent, some specify it as somatic efferent, and some are noncommittal. Since, in humans, the trapezius and sternocleidomastoid muscles originate from cervical somites located caudal to the last pharyngeal arch, the functional component is designated here as GSE.

Neurotransmitters: Acetylcholine (and probably calcitonin gene-related peptide, CGRP) is found in the motor neurons of cranial nerve nuclei and in their peripheral endings. This substance is also found in cells of the Edinger-Westphal nucleus and the ciliary ganglion.

Clinical Correlations: In patients with *myasthenia gravis*, a disease caused by antibodies to postsynaptic nicotinic acetylcholine receptors on skeletal muscles, ocular movement disorders are common. Tongue and neck movements may also be impaired. Lesions of the IIIrd nerve (as in *Weber's syndrome* or *carotid cavernous aneurysms*) may result in (1) *ptosis*, (2) lateral and downward deviation of the eye, and, (3) *diplopia* (except on lateral gaze). In addition, the pupil may be unaffected (pupillary sparing) or dilated and fixed. Damage to the MLF (as in *multiple sclerosis* or small vessel occlusion) between the VIth and IIIrd nuclei results in *internuclear ophthalmoplegia*. A lesion of the IVth nerve produces *diplopia* on downward and inward gaze (tilting the head may give some relief) and the eye is slightly elevated when looking straight ahead. *Diabetes mellitus*, trauma, or *pontine gliomas* are some causes of VIth nerve dysfunction. In these patients the affected eye is slightly adducted, and *diplopia* is pronounced on attempted gaze to the lesioned side. The XIth nerve may be damaged centrally (as in *syringobulbia* or *amyotrophic lateral sclerosis*) or at the jugular foramen with resultant paralysis of the ipsilateral sternocleidomastoid and upper parts of the trapezius muscle. Central injury to the XIIth nucleus or fibers (as in the *medial medullary syndrome* or in *syringobulbia*) or to its peripheral part (as in *polyneuropathy* or tumors) results in deviation of the tongue toward the lesioned side when protruded.

Abbreviations

AbdNr	Abducens Nerve		**RNu**	Red Nucleus
AbdNu	Abducens Nucleus		**SC**	Superior Colliculus
AccNu	Accessory Nucleus (Spinal Accessory Nu.)		**SCP,Dec**	Superior Cerebellar Peduncle, Decussation
BP	Basilar Pons		**SN**	Substantia Nigra
CC	Crus Cerebri		**SpAccNr**	Spinal Accessory Nerve
DVagNu	Dorsal Motor Nucleus of Vagus		**TecSp**	Tectospinal Tract
EWNu	Edinger-Westphal Nucleus		**TroDec**	Trochlear Decussation
FacCol	Facial Colliculus		**TroNr**	Trochlear Nerve
HyNr	Hypoglossal Nerve		**TroNu**	Trochlear Nucleus
HyNu	Hypoglossal Nucleus			
IO	Inferior Olivary Nucleus			
ML	Medial Lemniscus			
MLF	Medial Longitudinal Fasciculus			
OcNr	Oculomotor Nerve			
OcNu	Oculomotor Nucleus			
Py	Pyramid			

Ganglion

1 ciliary

Review of Blood Supply to **OcNu, TroNu, AbdNu** and **HyNu,** and the Internal Course of their Fibers

Structures	Arteries
OcNu and Fibers	medial branches of posterior cerebral and posterior communicating (see Fig. 5–27)
TroNu	paramedian branches of basilar bifurcation (see Fig. 5–27)
AbdNu	long circumferential branches of basilar (see Fig. 5–21)
Abducens Fibers in **BP**	paramedian branches of basilar (see Fig. 5–21)
HyNu and Fibers	anterior spinal (see Fig. 5–14)

Cranial Nerve Efferents (III, IV, VI, XI-AccNu, XII)

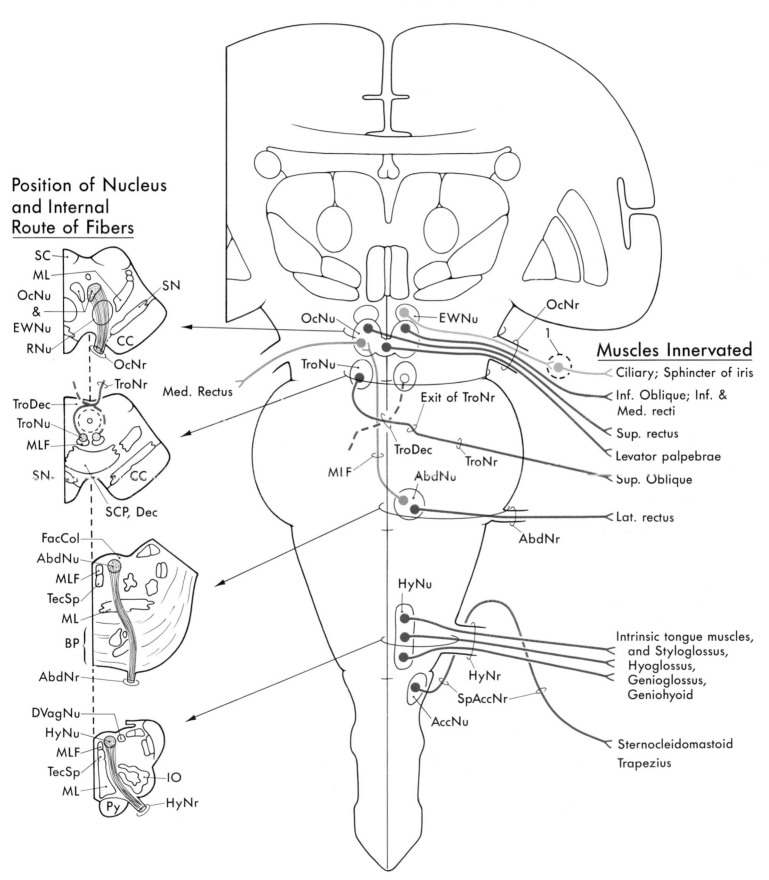

Position of Nucleus
and Internal
Route of Fibers

SC
ML
OcNu
&
EWNu
RNu
SN
CC
OcNr

TroDec
TroNu
MLF
SN
SCP, Dec
TroNr
CC

FacCol
AbdNu
MLF
TecSp
ML
BP
AbdNr

DVagNu
HyNu
MLF
TecSp
ML
Py
IO
HyNr

OcNu
EWNu
OcNr
1
TroNu
Med. Rectus
Exit of TroNr
TroDec
TroNr
MLF
AbdNu
AbdNr

HyNu
HyNr
SpAccNr
AccNu

Muscles Innervated

Ciliary; Sphincter of iris
Inf. Oblique; Inf. & Med. recti
Sup. rectus
Levator palpebrae
Sup. Oblique
Lat. rectus

Intrinsic tongue muscles, and Styloglossus, Hyoglossus, Genioglossus, Geniohyoid

Sternocleidomastoid
Trapezius

Cranial Nerve Efferents (V, VII, IX, X)

7–16   The origin and peripheral distribution of fibers arising from the SVE motor nuclei of the trigeminal, facial, and glossopharyngeal and vagus (via the nucleus ambiguus) nerves. Also shown are the origin of GVE preganglionic parasympathetic fibers from the superior (to facial nerve) and inferior (to glossopharyngeal nerve) salivatory nuclei and from the dorsal motor vagal nucleus. Their respective ganglia are indicated as well as the structures innervated by postganglionic fibers arising from each. The SVE functional component specifies cranial nerve motor nuclei that innervate head muscles that arose, embryologically, from pharyngeal arches. Muscles innervated by the trigeminal nerve come from the 1st arch, those served by the facial nerve from the 2nd arch; the stylopharyngeal muscle originates from the 3rd arch and is innervated by the glossopharyngeal nerve, and the muscles derived from the 4th arch are served by the vagus nerve.

Neurotransmitters: The transmitter found in the cells of cranial nerve motor nuclei, and in their peripheral endings, is acetylcholine; CGRP is also co-localized in these motor neurons. This substance is also present in pre- and post-ganglionic parasympathetic neurons.

Clinical Correlations: Patients with *myasthenia gravis* have difficulty with facial movements, their jaw may hang open because of muscle weakness, and they may have *dysphagia* and *dysarthria*. Le-

sions of the Vth nerve (as in *meningiomas* or trauma) result in (1) loss of pain, temperature, and touch on the ipsilateral face and in the oral and nasal cavities, (2) *paralysis* of ipsilateral masticatory muscles (jaw deviates to the lesioned side when closed), and (3) loss of the afferent limb of the *corneal reflex. Trigeminal neuralgia (tic douloureux)* is an intense, sudden, intermittent pain emanating from the area of the cheek, oral cavity, or adjacent parts of the nose (distribution of V_2 or V_3). Tumors (such as *chordomas* or *acoustic neuroma)*, trauma, or *meningitis* may damage the VIIth nerve, resulting in (1) an ipsilateral *facial* (or *Bell's) palsy*, (2) loss of taste from the ipsilateral two-thirds of the tongue, and (3) decreased secretion from the ipsilateral lacrimal, nasal, and sublingual and submandibular glands. Injury distal to the chorda tympani produces only an ipsilateral *facial palsy*. Because of their common origin from NuAm, adjacent exit from the medulla, and passage through the jugular foramen, the IXth and Xth nerves may be damaged together (as in *amyotrophic lateral sclerosis* or in *syringobulbia).* The results are *dysarthria, dysphagia, dyspnea,* loss of taste from the ipsilateral caudal tongue, and loss of the *gag reflex,* but no significant autonomic deficits. Bilateral lesions of the Xth nerve are life-threatening because of the resultant total paralysis (and closure) of the vocal folds.

Abbreviations

AbdNu	Abducens Nucleus	**SpTTr**	Spinal Trigeminal Tract
ALS	Anterolateral System	**SSNu**	Superior Salivatory Nucleus
BP	Basilar Pons	**TecSp**	Tectospinal Tract
CSNu	Chief Sensory Nucleus	**TriMoNu**	Trigeminal Motor Nucleus
DVagNu	Dorsal Motor Nucleus of Vagus	**TriNr**	Trigeminal Nerve
		VagNr	Vagus Nerve
FacNr	Facial Nerve		
FacNu	Facial Nucleus		
GlNr	Glossopharyngeal Nerve		
HyNu	Hypoglossal Nucleus		
ISNu	Inferior Salivatory Nucleus		
MesNu	Mesencephalic Nucleus		
ML	Medial Lemniscus		
MLF	Medial Longitudinal Fasciculus		
NuAm	Nucleus Ambiguus		
SpTNu	Spinal Trigeminal Nucleus		

Ganglia

1 pterygopalatine
2 submandibular
3 otic
4 terminal and/or intramural

Review of Blood Supply to **TriMoNu, FacNu, DMNu** and **NuAm,** and the Internal Course of their Fibers

Structures	Arteries
TriMoNu and Trigeminal Root	long circumferential branches of basilar (see Fig. 5–21)
FacNu and Internal Genu	long circumferential branches of basilar (see Fig. 5–21)
DMNu and **NuAm**	branches of vertebral and posterior inferior cerebellar (see Fig. 5–14)

Cranial Nerve Efferents (V, VII, IX, X)

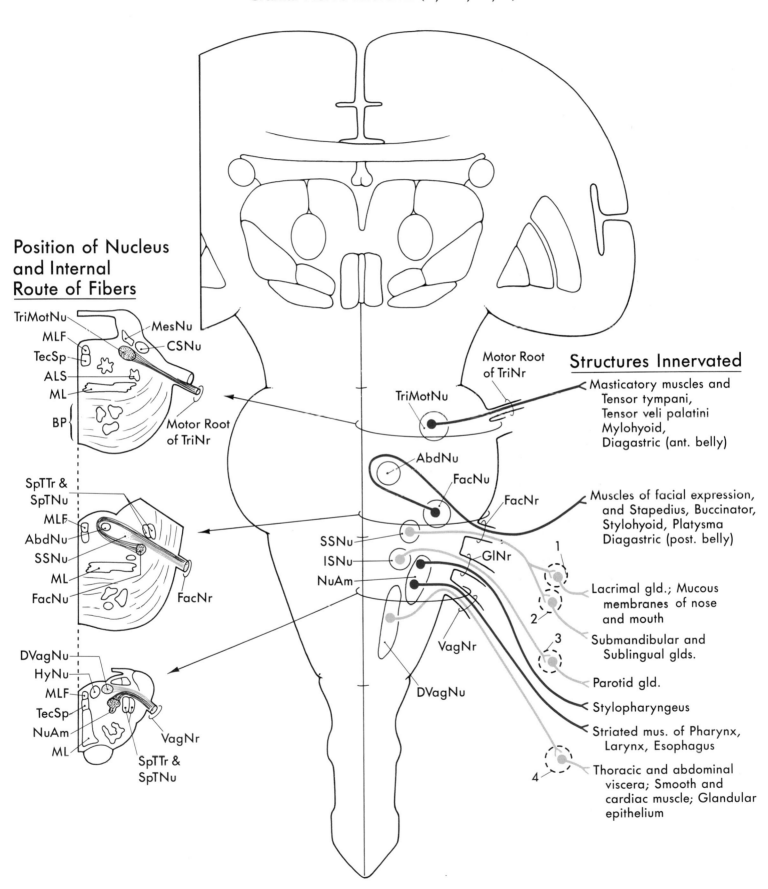

Position of Nucleus and Internal Route of Fibers

TriMotNu
MLF
TecSp
ALS
ML
BP
MesNu
CSNu
Motor Root of TriNr

SpTTr & SpTNu
MLF
AbdNu
SSNu
ML
FacNu
FacNr

DVagNu
HyNu
MLF
TecSp
NuAm
ML
VagNr
SpTTr & SpTNu

Motor Root of TriNr
TriMotNu
AbdNu
FacNu
FacNr
SSNu
ISNu
NuAm
GlNr
VagNr
DVagNu

Structures Innervated

Masticatory muscles and Tensor tympani, Tensor veli palatini Mylohyoid, Diagastric (ant. belly)

Muscles of facial expression, and Stapedius, Buccinator, Stylohyoid, Platysma Diagastric (post. belly)

1

Lacrimal gld.; Mucous membranes of nose and mouth

2

Submandibular and Sublingual glds.

3

Parotid gld.

Stylopharyngeus

Striated mus. of Pharynx, Larynx, Esophagus

4

Thoracic and abdominal viscera; Smooth and cardiac muscle; Glandular epithelium

Spinocerebellar Tracts

7–17 The origin, course, and distribution pattern of fibers to the cerebellar cortex and nuclei from the spinal cord (dorsal and ventral spinocerebellar tracts, rostral spinocerebellar fibers) and from the external cuneate nucleus (cuneocerebellar fibers). Also illustrated is the somatotopy of those fibers originating from the spinal cord. These fibers enter the cerebellum via the restiform body, the larger portion of the inferior cerebellar peduncle, or in relationship to the superior cerebellar peduncle. After entering the cerebellum, collaterals are given off to the cerebellar nuclei while the parent axons of spino- and cuneo-cerebellar fibers pass on to the cortex, where they end as mossy fibers. Although not shown here, there are important ascending spinal projections to the medial and dorsal accessory nuclei of the inferior olivary complex (spino-olivary fibers).

Neurotransmitters: Glutamate(+) is found in some spinocerebellar fibers, in their mossy fiber terminals in the cerebellar cortex, and in their collateral branches that innervate the cerebellar nuclei.

Clinical Correlations: Lesions, or tumors, that selectively damage only spinocerebellar fibers are rarely, if ever, seen in humans. The *ataxia* one might expect to see in patients with a spinal cord hemisection (as in the *Brown-Sequard syndrome*) is masked by the *hemiplegia* resulting from the concomitant damage to lateral corticospinal (and other) fibers. However, in *Friedreich's ataxia (hereditary spinal ataxia)* there is degeneration of both major spinocerebellar tracts plus the corticospinal tracts and dorsal columns. The axial and appendicular *ataxia* seen in these patients correlates with this spinocerebellar degeneration.

Abbreviations

ALS	Anterolateral System	**MesNu**	Mesencephalic Nucleus
AMV	Anterior Medullary Velum	**ML**	Medial Lemniscus
Cbl	Cerebellum	**Py**	Pyramid
CblNu	Cerebellar Nuclei	**RB**	Restiform Body
CCblF	Cuneocerebellar Fibers	**RSCF**	Rostral Spinocerebellar Fibers
CSNu	Chief Sensory Nucleus	**RuSp**	Rubrospinal Tract
DNuC	Dorsal Nucleus of Clarke	**S**	Sacral Representation
DRG	Dorsal Root Ganglion	**SBC**	Spinal Border Cells
DSCT	Dorsal Spinocerebellar Tract	**SCP**	Superior Cerebellar Peduncle
ECNu	External (Lateral) Cuneate Nucleus	**SpTNu**	Spinal Trigeminal Nucleus
FNL	Flocculonodular Lobe	**SpTTr**	Spinal Trigeminal Tract
ICP	Inferior Cerebellar Peduncle	**T**	Thoracic Representation
IZ	Intermediate Zone	**TriMoNu**	Trigeminal Motor Nucleus
JRB	Juxtarestiform Body	**VesNu**	Vestibular Nuclei
L	Lumbar Representation	**VSCT**	Ventral Spinocerebellar Tract

Review of Blood Supply to Spinal Cord Gray Matter, Spinocerebellar Tracts, **RB**, and **SCP**

Structures	Arteries
Spinal Cord Gray	branches of central artery (see Fig. 5–6)
DSCT and **VSCT** in Cord	penetrating branches of arterial vasocorona (see Fig. 5–6)
RB	posterior inferior cerebellar (see Fig. 5–14)
SCP	long circumferential branches of basilar and superior cerebellar (see Fig. 5–21)
Cerebellum	posterior and anterior inferior cerebellar and superior cerebellar

Spinocerebellar Tracts

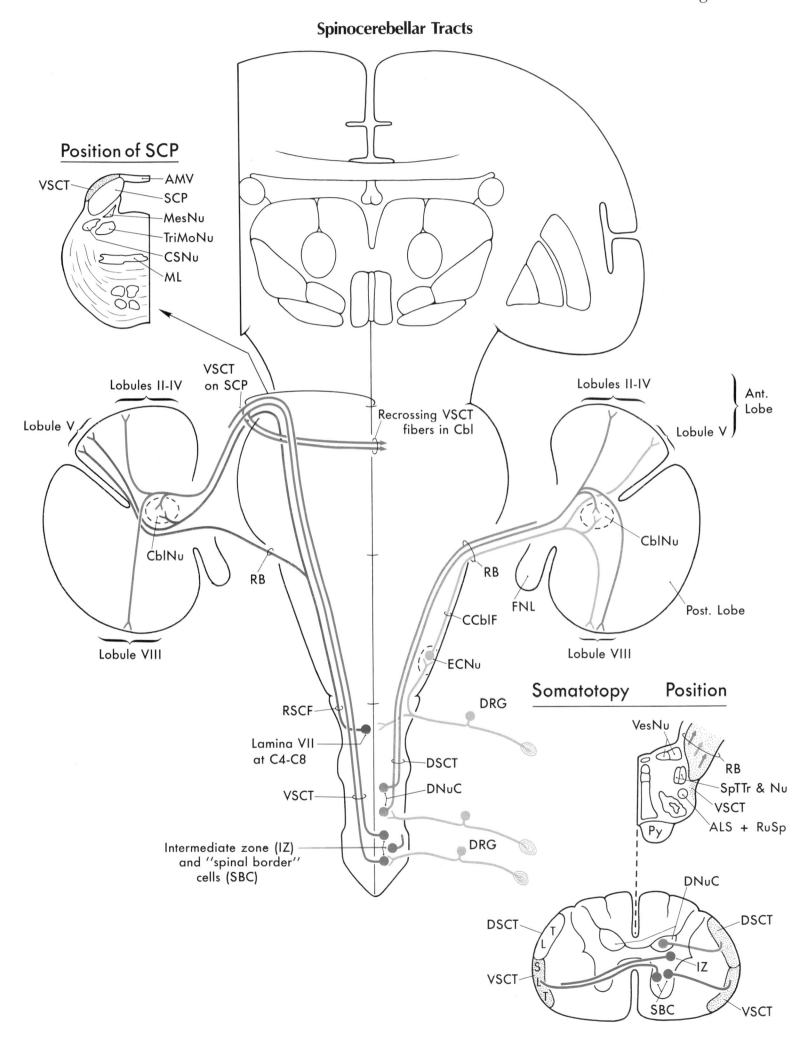

Position of SCP

VSCT
AMV
SCP
MesNu
TriMoNu
CSNu
ML

VSCT on SCP

Recrossing VSCT fibers in Cbl

Lobules II-IV
Lobule V
CblNu
RB
Lobule VIII

Lobules II-IV
Lobule V
} Ant. Lobe
CblNu
RB
FNL
CCblF
ECNu
DRG
Post. Lobe
Lobule VIII

RSCF
Lamina VII at C4-C8
VSCT
Intermediate zone (IZ) and "spinal border" cells (SBC)

DSCT
DNuC
DRG

Somatotopy   Position

VesNu
RB
SpTTr & Nu
VSCT
ALS + RuSp
Py

DNuC
DSCT
DSCT
L
T
L
S
L
T
IZ
VSCT
SBC
VSCT

Ponto-, Reticulo-, Olivo-, Ceruleo-, Hypothalamo-, and Raphe-cerebellar Fibers

7–18 Afferent fibers to the cerebellum from selected brainstem areas and the organization of corticopontine fibers in the internal capsule and crus cerebri. The cerebellar peduncles are also indicated. Pontocerebellar axons are mainly crossed, reticulocerebellar fibers may be bilateral (from Ret- TegNu) or mainly uncrossed (from LRNu and PRNu), and olivocerebellar fibers are exclusively crossed. Raphe-, hypothalamo-, and ceruleo-cerebellar fibers are, to varying degrees, bilateral projections. Although all afferent fibers to the cerebellum give rise to collaterals to the cerebellar nuclei, those from pontocerebellar axons are modest. Olivocerebellar axons end as climbing fibers, reticulo- and ponto-cerebellar fibers as mossy fibers, and hypothalamo- and ceruleo-cerebellar axons end in all cortical layers.

Neurotransmitters: Glutamate(+) is found in corticopontine projections and in most pontocerebellar fibers. Aspartate(+) and corticotropin-releasing factor(+) are present in many olivocerebellar fibers.

Ceruleocerebellar fibers contain nonradrenalin, histamine is found in hypothalamocerebellar fibers, and some reticulocerebellar fibers contain enkephalin. Serotonergic fibers to the cerebellum arise from neurons found in medial areas of the reticular formation (open cell in Fig. 7-18) and, most likely, from some cells in the adjacent raphe nuclei.

Clinical Correlations: Common symptoms seen in patients with lesions involving nuclei and tracts that project to the cerebellum are *ataxia* (of trunk or limbs), an *ataxic gait, dysarthria, dysphagia,* and disorders of eye movement. These deficits are seen in some hereditary diseases (such as *olivopontocerebellar degeneration, ataxia telangiectasia,* or *hereditary cerebellar ataxia*), in tumors (brainstem gliomas), in vascular diseases (*lateral pontine syndrome*), or in other conditions such as *alcoholic cerebellar degeneration* or pontine hemorrhages.

Abbreviations

AntLb	Anterior Limb of Internal Capsule	**PO**	Principal (Inferior) Olivary Nucleus
CblNu	Cerebellar Nuclei	**PPon**	Parietopontine Fibers
CerCblF	Ceruleocerebellar Fibers	**PRNu**	Paramedian Reticular Nuclei
CPonF	Cerebropontine Fibers	**Py**	Pyramid
CSp	Corticospinal Fibers	**RB**	Restiform Body
DAO	Dorsal Accessory Olivary Nucleus	**RCblF**	Reticulocerebellar Fibers
FPon	Frontopontine Fibers	**RetLenLb**	Retrolenticular Limb of Internal Capsule
Hyth	Hypothalamus		
HythCblF	Hypothalamocerebellar Fibers	**RNu**	Red Nucleus
IC	Internal Capsule	**RetTegNu**	Reticulotegmental Nucleus
IO	Inferior Olivary Nucleus	**SCP**	Superior Cerebellar Peduncle
LoCer	(Nucleus) Locus Ceruleus	**SubLenLb**	Sublenticular Limb of Internal Capsule
LRNu	Lateral Reticular Nucleus	**SN**	Substantia Nigra
MAO	Medial Accessory Olivary Nucleus	**TPon**	Temporopontine Fibers
MCP	Middle Cerebellar Peduncle		
ML	Medial Lemniscus		
NuRa	Raphe Nuclei		
OCblF	Olivocerebellar Fibers		
OPon	Occipitopontine Fibers		
PCblF	Pontocerebellar Fibers		
PostLb	Posterior Limb of Internal Capsule		
PonNu	Pontine Nuclei		

Number Key

1 Nucleus Raphe, Pontis
2 Nucleus Raphe, Magnus
3 Raphecerebellar Fibers

Review of Blood Supply to Precerebellar Relay Nuclei in Pons and Medulla, **MCP,** and **RB**

Structures	Arteries
Pontine Tegmentum	long circumferential branches of basilar plus some from superior cerebellar (see Fig. 5–21)
Basilar Pons	paramedian and short circumferential branches of basilar (see Fig. 5–21)
Medulla **RetF** and **IO**	branches of vertebral and posterior inferior cerebellar (see Fig. 5–14)
MCP	long circumferential branches of basilar and branches of anterior inferior and superior cerebellar (see Fig. 5–21)
RB	posterior inferior cerebellar (see Fig. 5–14)

Ponto-, Reticulo-, Olivo-, Ceruleo-, Hypothalamo-, and Raphecerebellar Fibers

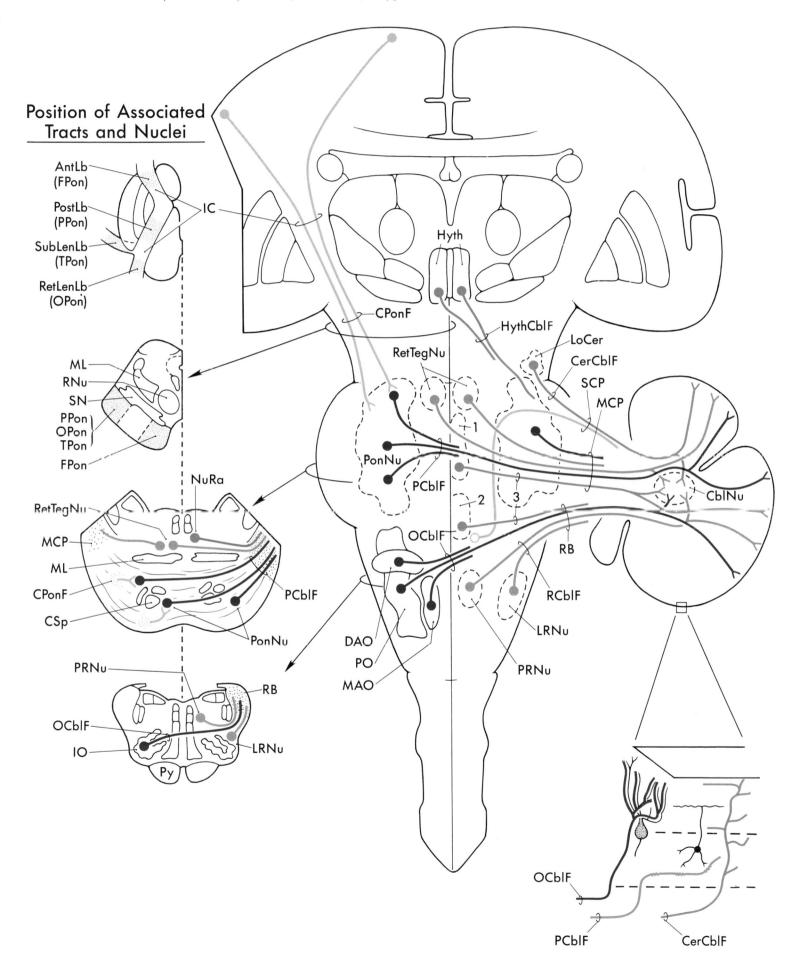

Position of Associated Tracts and Nuclei

Corticonuclear, Nucleocortical, and Corticovestibular Fibers

7–19 Corticonuclear fibers arise from all regions of the cortex and terminate in an orderly (mediolateral and rostrocaudal) sequence in the cerebellar nuclei. Corticovestibular fibers originate from the vermis and flocculonodular lobe, exit the cerebellum via the juxtarestiform body, and end in the vestibular nuclei. These projections are ipsilateral and arise from Purkinje cells. Nucleocortical processes originate from cerebellar nuclear neurons and pass to the overlying cortex in a pattern that basically reciprocates that of the corticonuclear projection; they end as mossy fibers. Some nucleocortical fibers are collaterals of cerebellar efferent axons. The cerebellar cortex may influence the activity of lower motor neurons through, for example, the cerebellovestibular-vestibulospinal route.

Neurotransmitters: Gamma-aminobutyric acid (GABA)(-) is found in many Purkinje cells and is the principal transmitter substance present in cerebellar corticonuclear and corticovestibular projections. However, taurine(-) and motilin(-) are also found in some Purkinje cells. GABAergic terminals are numerous in the cerebellar nuclei and vestibular complex. Some of the glutamate-containing mossy fibers in the cerebellar cortex represent the endings of nucleocortical fibers that originate from cells in the cerebellar nuclei.

Clinical Correlations: Numerous disease entities can result in cerebellar dysfunction including virus infections (*echovirus*), hereditary diseases (see Fig. 7–18), trauma, tumors (*glioma, medulloblastoma*), occlusion of cerebellar arteries (cerebellar stroke), *arteriovenous malformation* of cerebellar vessels, development errors (such as the *Dandy-Walker syndrome* or *Arnold-Chiari deformity*), or the intake of toxins. In general, damage to only the cortex results in little or no dysfunction unless the lesion is quite large or causes increases in intracranial pressure. However, lesions involving both the cortex and nuclei, or only the nuclei, will produce obvious cerebellar signs.

Lesions involving midline structures (vermal cortex, fastigial nuclei) and/or the flocculonodular lobe result in *truncal ataxia* (*titubation* or *tremor*), *nystagmus*, and head tilting. These patients may also have a wide-based (*cerebellar*) *gait*. Damage to the intermediate and lateral cortices and the globose, emboliform and dentate nuclei result in *dysarthria, dysmetria* (*hypometria, hypermetria*), *dysdiadochokinesia, tremor* (*static, kinetic, intention*), *rebound phenomenon*, unsteady and wide-based (*cerebellar*) *gait*, and *nystagmus*. Cerebellar damage in these lateral areas causes movement disorders on the side of the lesion with ataxia and gait problems on that side; the patient may tend to fall toward the side of the lesion. This is because the cerebellar nuclei project to the contralateral thalamus, which projects to the motor cortex on the same side, which projects to the contralateral side of the spinal cord via the corticospinal tract. Other circuits (cerebellorubal-rubrospinal) and feedback loops (cerebelloolivary-olivocerebellar) follow similar routes. Consequently, the motor expression of unilateral cerebellar damage is toward the lesioned side because of these doubly-crossed pathways.

Abbreviations

CorNu	Corticonuclear Fibers	**MVesSp**	Medial Vestibulospinal Tract
CorVes	Corticovestibular Fibers	**MVNu**	Medial Vestibular Nucleus
Flo	Flocculus	**NL, par**	Lateral Cerebellar Nucleus, Parvocellular Region
IC	Intermediate Cortex	**NM, par**	Medial Cerebellar Nucleus, Parvocellular Region
JRB	Juxtarestiform Body		
LC	Lateral Cortex	**NuCor**	Nucleocortical Fibers
LVesSp	Lateral Vestibulospinal Tract	**SpVNu**	Spinal (Inferior) Vestibular Nucleus
LVNu	Lateral Vestibular Nucleus	**SVNu**	Superior Vestibular Nucleus
MLF	Medial Longitudinal Fasciculus	**VC**	Vermal Cortex

Review of Blood Supply to Cerebellum and Vestibular Nuclei

Structures	Arteries
Cerebellar Cortex	branches of posterior and anterior inferior cerebellar and superior cerebellar
Cerebellar Nuclei	anterior inferior cerebellar and superior cerebellar
Vestibular Nuclei	posterior inferior cerebellar in medulla, long circumferential branches of basilar in pons

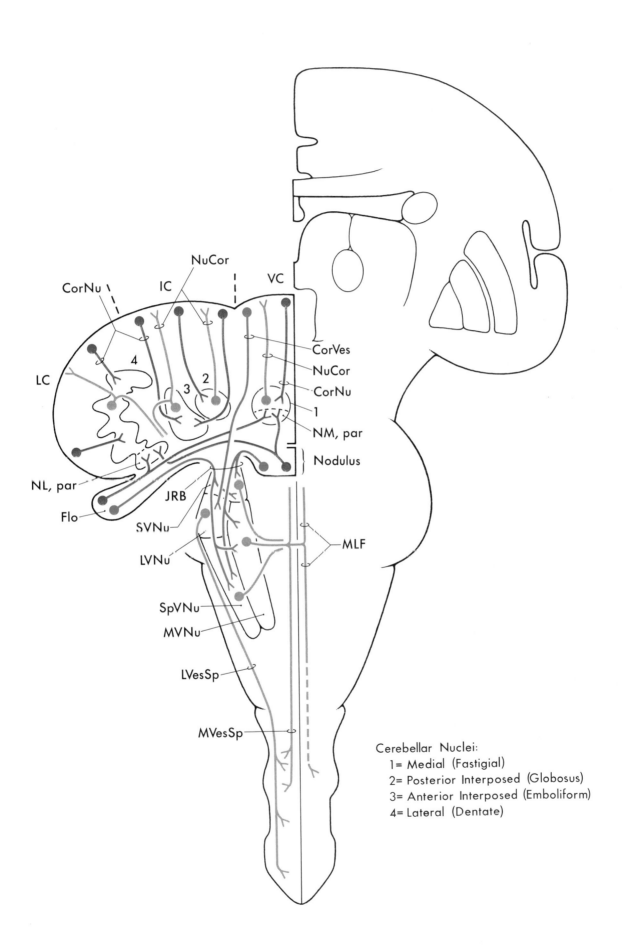

CorNu
NuCor
IC
VC
CorVes
NuCor
CorNu
1
NM, par
Nodulus
LC
4
2
3
NL, par
Flo
JRB
SVNu
LVNu
MLF
SpVNu
MVNu
LVesSp
MVesSp

Cerebellar Nuclei:
1= Medial (Fastigial)
2= Posterior Interposed (Globosus)
3= Anterior Interposed (Emboliform)
4= Lateral (Dentate)

Cerebellar Efferent Fibers

7–20   The origin, course, topography, and general distribution of fibers arising in the cerebellar nuclei. Cerebellofugal fibers project to several thalamic areas (VL and VA), to intralaminar relay nuclei in addition to the centromedian, and to a number of midbrain, pontine, and medullary targets. Most of the latter nuclei project back to the cerebellum (e.g., reticulocerebellar, pontocerebellar), some in a highly organized manner. For example, cerebello-olivary fibers from the dentate nucleus (DNu) project to the principal olivary nucleus (PO), and neurons of the PO send their axons back to the lateral cerebellar cortex, with collaterals going to the DNu. The cerebellar nuclei can influence motor activity through, as examples, the follow-ing routes: (1) cerebellorubral-rubrospinal, (2) cerebelloreticular-re-ticulospinal, (3) cerebellothalamic-thalamocortical-corticospinal, and others.

Neurotransmitters: Many cells in the cerebellar nuclei contain glutamate(+), aspartate(+), or gamma-aminobutyric acid(-). Gluta-mate and aspartate are found in cerebellorubral and cerebellothalamic fibers, while some GABA-containing cells give rise to cerebellopon-tine and cerebello-olivary fibers. Cerebelloreticular projections may also contain GABA.

Clinical Correlations: Deficits related to lesions of the cerebellar nuclei are described in Figure 7–19.

Abbreviations

ALS	Anterolateral System
AMV	Anterior Medullary Velum
BP	Basilar Pons
CblOl	Cerebello-olivary Fibers
CblTh	Cerebellothalamic Fibers
CblRu	Cerebellorubral Fibers
CC	Crus Cerebri
CeGy	Central Gray (Periaqueductal Gray)
CM	Centromedian Nucleus of Thalamus
CSp	Corticospinal Fibers
DAO	Dorsal Accessory Olive
DNu	Dentate Nucleus (Lateral Cerebellar Nucleus)
ENu	Emboliform Nucleus (Anterior Interposed Cerebellar Nucleus)
EWNu	Edinger-Westphal Nucleus
FNu	Fastigial Nucleus (Medial Cerebellar Nucleus)
GNu	Globose Nucleus (Posterior Interposed Cerebellar Nucleus)
IC	Inferior Colliculus
INu	Interstitial Nucleus
LRNu	Lateral Reticular Nucleus
LVNu	Lateral Vestibular Nucleus
MAO	Medial Accessory Olive
ML	Medial Lemniscus
MLF	Medial Longitudinal Fasciculus
MVNu	Medial Vestibular Nucleus
NuDark	Nucleus of Darkschewitsch
OcNu	Oculomotor Nucleus
PO	Principal Olivary Nucleus
PonNu	Pontine Nuclei

RetForm	Reticular Formation
RNu	Red Nucleus
RuSp	Rubrospinal Tract
SC	Superior Colliculus
SCP	Superior Cerebellar Peduncle
SCP, Dec	Superior Cerebellar Peduncle, Decussation
SN	Substantia Nigra
SpVNu	Spinal Vestibular Nucleus
SVNu	Superior Vestibular Nucleus
ThCor	Thalamocortical Fibers
ThFas	Thalamic Fasciculus
TriMoNu	Trigeminal Motor Nucleus
VL	Ventral Lateral Nucleus of Thalamus
VPL	Ventral Posterolateral Nucleus of Thalamus
VSCT	Ventral Spinocerebellar Tract
ZI	Zona Incerta

Number Key

1   ascending projections to superior colliculus, and possibly ventral lateral and ventromedial thalamic nuclei

2   descending crossed fibers from superior cerebellar peduncle

3   uncinate fasciculus (of Russell)

4   juxtarestiform body to vestibular nuclei

5   reticular formation

Review of Blood Supply to Cerebellar Nuclei and their Principal Efferent Pathways

Structures	Arteries
Cerebellar Nuclei	anterior inferior cerebellar and superior cerebellar
SCP	long circumferential branches of basilar and superior cer-ebellar (see Fig. 5–21)
Midbrain Tegmentum **(RNu, CblTh, CblRu, OcNu)**	paramedian branches of basilar bifurcation, short cir-cumferential branches of posterior cerebral, branches of superior cerebellar (see Fig. 5–27)
VPL, CM, VL, VA	thalamogeniculate branches of posterior cerebral, thala-moperforating branches of the posteromedial group of posterior cerebral (see Fig. 5–38)
IC	lateral striate branches of middle cerebral (see Fig. 5–38)

Cerebellar Efferent Fibers

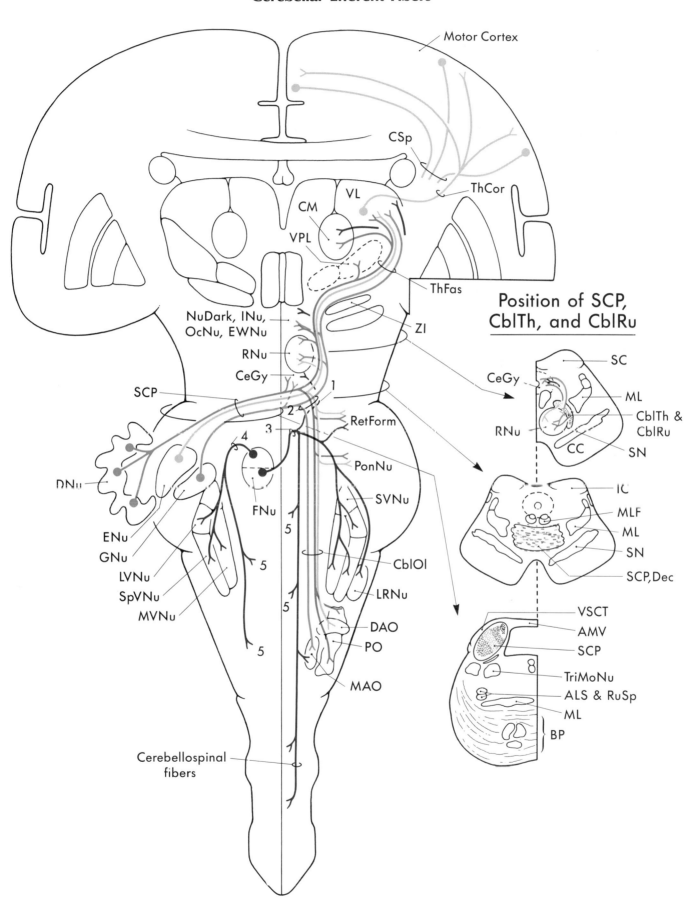

Motor Cortex

CSp

VL

CM

VPL

ThCor

ThFas

NuDark, INu,
OcNu, EWNu

ZI

RNu

CeGy

SCP

RetForm

1

2

DNu

4

3

PonNu

FNu

SVNu

ENu

GNu

LVNu

SpVNu

MVNu

5

5

5

5

CblOl

LRNu

DAO

PO

MAO

Cerebellospinal
fibers

Position of SCP,
CblTh, and CblRu

CeGy

SC

ML

RNu

CblTh &
CblRu

CC

SN

IC

MLF

ML

SN

SCP,Dec

VSCT

AMV

SCP

TriMoNu

ALS & RuSp

ML

BP

7–21 Blank master drawing for pathways projecting to the cerebellar cortex, and for efferent projections of cerebellar nuclei. This illustration is provided for self-evaluation of understanding of pathways to the cerebellar cortex and from the cerebellar nuclei, for the instructor to expand on cerebellar afferent/efferent pathways not covered in the atlas, or both.

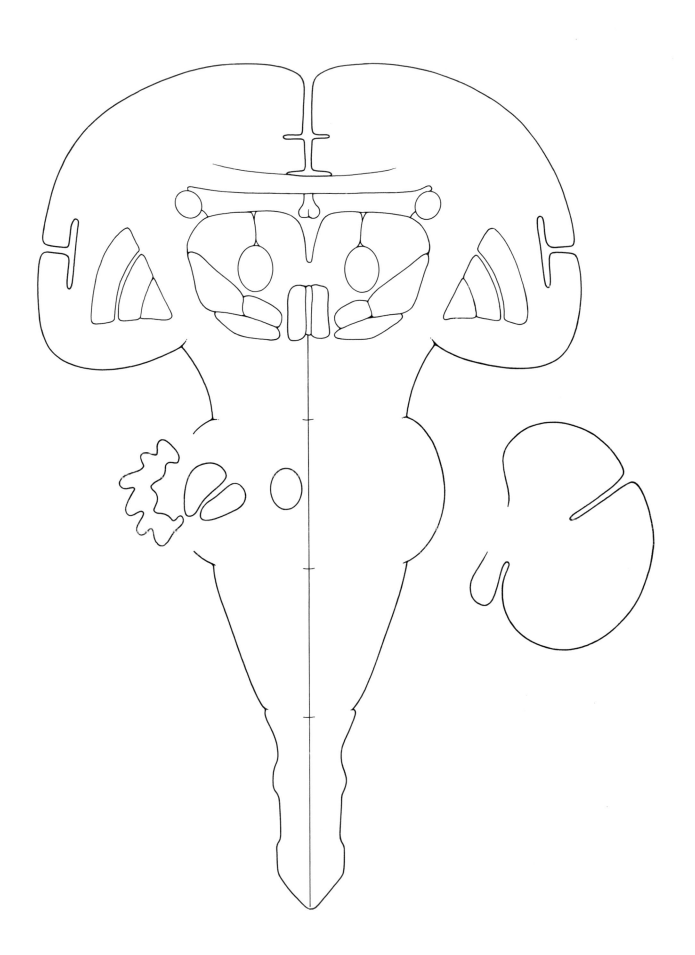

Striatal Connections

7–22　The origin, course, and distribution of afferent fibers to, and efferent projections from, the neostriatum. These projections are extensive, complex, and in large part topographically organized; only their general patterns are summarized here. Afferents to the caudate and putamen originate from the cerebral cortex (corticostriate fibers), from several of the intralaminar thalamic nuclei (thalamostriate), from the substantia nigra-pars compacta (nigrostriate), and from some of the raphe nuclei. Neostriatal cells send axons into the globus pallidus (paleostriatum) as striopallidal fibers and into the substantia nigra-pars reticulata as a strionigral projection.

Neurotransmitters: Glutamate(+) is found in corticostriate fibers, and serotonin is found in raphestriatal fibers from the nucleus raphe dorsalis. Four neuroactive substances are associated with striatal efferent fibers, these being gamma-aminobutyric acid (GABA)(-), dynorphin, enkephalin(-), and substance P(+). Enkephalinergic and GABAergic striopallidal projections are numerous to the lateral pallidum (origin of pallidosubthalamic fibers), while dynorphin-containing terminals are more concentrated in its medial segment (source of pallidothalamic fibers). Enkephalin and GABA are also present in strionigral projections to the pars reticulata. Since substance P and GABA are found in striopallidal *and* strionigral fibers, some of the former may be collaterals of the latter. Dopamine is present in nigrostriatal projection neurons and in their terminals in the neostriatum.

Clinical Correlations: Degenerative changes in, and eventual loss of, neurons in the caudate and putamen may be seen as a complication of rheumatic fever (as in *Sydenham's chorea*) or in patients with the dominately inherited disorder, *Huntington's disease. Choreiform* movements of limb, facial, and oral musculature with varying degrees of weakness and *dystonia* are characteristic. Huntington's patients frequently try to mask the abnormal movements by attempting to incorporate them into an intended/purposeful movement. *Dementia,* presumably due to cell loss in the cerebral cortex, is also seen in Huntington's disease. A reduction of substance P terminals in the nigra and of enkephalinergic endings in the globus pallidus is seen in the brains of Huntington's patients. In *Wilson's disease (hepatolenticular degeneration)* there is a genetic error in the ability to metabolize copper with the resultant accumulation of this metal in the basal ganglia and frontal cortex. These patients show *athetoid* movements, rigidity and contractures, and a resting *tremor*. A unique movement of the hand and/or arm in these patients is called a wing-beating tremor (*asterixis*). Copper can also be seen in the cornea (*Kayser-Fleischer ring*) in these patients. In *Parkinson's disease* there is a progressive loss of dopaminergic cells in the substantia nigra-pars compacta, of their terminals in the caudate and putamen, and of their dendrites that extend into the substantia nigra-pars reticulata. Patients with Parkinson's disease characteristically show a *resting tremor* (pill-rolling), *rigidity* (*cog wheel* or *lead pipe*), and *bradykinesia* or *hypokinesia*. These patients have a distinct stooped flexed posture and a *festinating gait*. Parkinson's disease and Huntington's disease are progressive neurodegenerative disorders.

Abbreviations

CaNu	Caudate Nucleus	**SNpc**	Substantia Nigra, pars compacta
CorSt	Corticostriate Fibers	**SNpr**	Substantia Nigra, pars reticulata
GP	Globus Pallidus	**StNig**	Striatonigral Fibers
NigSt	Nigrostriatal Fibers	**StPal**	Striatopallidal Fibers
Put	Putamen	**SThNu**	Subthalamic Nucleus
RaNu	Raphe Nuclei	**ThSt**	Thalamostriatal Fibers
RaSt	Raphestriatal Fibers	**ZI**	Zona Incerta

Review of Blood Supply to Caudate, Putamen, **Sn, CC,** and **IC**

Structures	Arteries
Caudate, Putamen and **IC**	lateral striate branches of middle cerebral (see Fig. 5–38)
SN and **CC**	paramedian branches of basilar bifurcation, short circumferential branches of posterior cerebral and some from superior cerebellar (see Fig. 5–27)

Striatal Connections

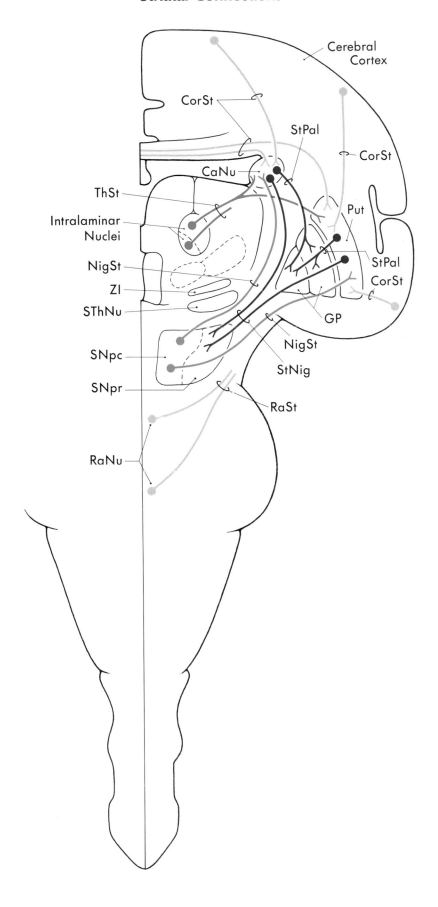

Pallidal Efferents and Nigral Connections

7–23 The origin, course, and distribution of efferent projections of the globus pallidus (upper illustration), and connections of the substantia nigra (lower drawing) that were not shown in relation to the pallidum or in Figure 7–22. The ansa lenticularis (broken line) arches around the internal capsule and passes caudally to join in the formation of the thalamic fasciculus. Pallidosubthalamic fibers originate primarily from the lateral pallidal segment, while pallidothalamic projections, via the ansa lenticularis and lenticular fasciculus, arise mainly from its medial segment. The substantia nigra has extensive connections, the clinically most important being the dopaminergic nigrostriatal fibers. The globus pallidus influences motor activity by way of pallidothalamic-thalamocortical-corticospinal (and corticobulbar) pathways.

Neurotransmitters: Gamma-aminobutyric acid(-)-containing cells in the globus pallidus give rise to pallidonigral projections, which end primarily in the substantia nigra-pars reticulata. Although GABA is also found in some subthalamopallidal axons, this latter projection contains many glutaminergic(+) fibers. Dopamine-, GABA(-)-, and glycine(-)-containing cells are present in the substantia nigra. Of these, dopamine is found in pars compacta neurons, which give rise to nigrostriatal, nigroamygdaloid, and several other projections; GABA in pars reticulata cells, which give rise to nigrocollicular and nigrothalamic fibers; and glycine in some local circuit nigral neurons. Glutamate(+) is found in corticonigral fibers, and serotonin(-) is associated with raphenigral fibers; these latter fibers originate primarily from the nucleus raphe dorsalis.

The dopaminergic projection to the frontal cortex, shown here as arising only from SNpc, originates from this cell group as well as from the immediately adjacent ventral tegmental area. Excessive activity in neurons comprising this projection may play a partial role in schizophrenia.

Clinical Correlations: Movement disorders associated with lesions in the neostriatum and substantia nigra are reviewed in Figure 7–22. Hemorrhage into, or the occlusion of vessels serving, the subthalamic nucleus will result in violent flailing movements of the extremities, a condition called *hemiballismus.* Hemiballistic movements are seen contralateral to the lesion. Lesions confined to the globus pallidus, as in hemorrhage of lenticulostriate arteries, may result in *hypokinesia* and *rigidity* without tremor.

Abbreviations

AmyNig	Amygdalonigral Fibers	**PedPonNu**	Pedunculopontine Nucleus
AmyNu	Amygdaloid Nucleus (Complex)	**Put**	Putamen
AnLent	Ansa Lenticularis	**RaNu**	Raphe Nuclei
CaNu	Caudate Nucleus	**SC**	Superior Colliculus
CM	Centromedian Nucleus of Thalamus	**SNpc**	Substantia Nigra, pars compacta
CorNig	Corticonigral Fibers	**SNpr**	Substantia Nigra, pars reticulata
CSp	Corticospinal Fibers	**SThFas**	Subthalamic Fasciculus
GP	Globus Pallidus	**SThNig**	Subthalamonigral Fibers
LenFas	Lenticular Fasciculus (H$_{(2)}$)	**SThNu**	Subthalamic Nucleus
NigAmy	Nigroamygdaloid Fibers	**ThCor**	Thalamocortical Fibers
NigCol	Nigrocollicular Fibers	**ThFas**	Thalamic Fasciculus (H$_{(1)}$)
NigTec	Nigrotectal Fibers	**VA**	Ventral Anterior Nucleus of Thalamus
NigSTh	Nigrosubthalamic Fibers	**VL**	Ventral Lateral Nucleus of Thalamus
NigTh	Nigrothalamic Fibers	**VM**	Ventromedial Nucleus of Thalamus
PalNig	Pallidonigral Fibers	**ZI**	Zona Incerta

Review of Blood Supply to Palladum, Subthalamic Area, and **SN**

Structures	Arteries
GP	lateral striate branches of middle cerebral and branches of anterior choroidal (see Fig. 5–38)
SThNu	posteromedial branches of posterior cerebral and posterior communicating (see Fig. 5–38)
SN	branches of basilar bifurcation, medial branches of posterior cerebral and posterior communicating, short circumferential branches of posterior cerebral (see Fig. 5–27)

Pallidal Efferents and Nigral Connections

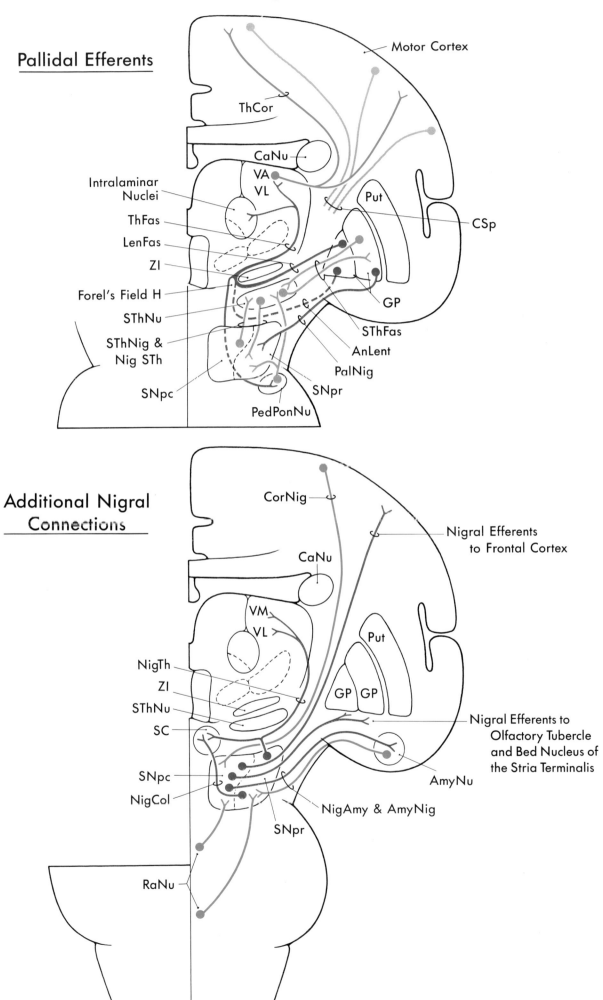

7–24 Blank master drawing for connections of the basal ganglia. This illustration is provided for self-evaluation of understanding of basal ganglia connections, for the instructor to expand on basal ganglia pathways not covered in this atlas, or both.

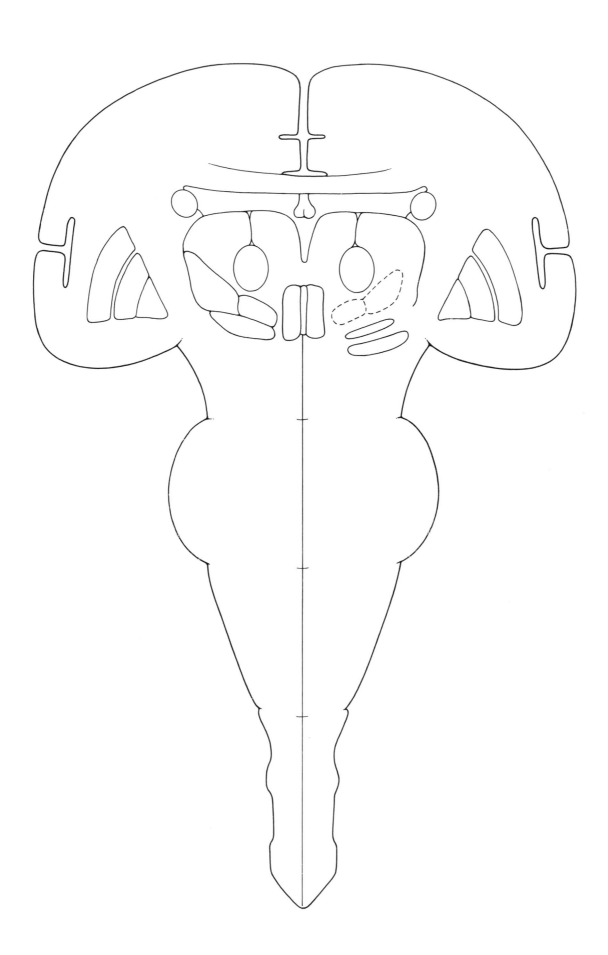

Pupillary/Accommodation Pathways

7–25 The origin, course, and distribution of fibers involved in the pathway for the pupillary light reflex. In addition, the pathway for sympathetic innervation of the dilator muscle of the iris is also depicted. The pathway from the midbrain reticular formation to the intermediolateral cell column may also have a multisynaptic component with relay stations in the pontine and medullary reticular formations. Postganglionic sympathetic fibers to the head originate from the superior cervical ganglion. Although not shown, descending projections to the intermediolateral cell column also originate from various hypothalamic areas and nuclei, some of which receive retinal input.

Neurotransmitters: Acetylcholine is the transmitter found in the pre- and post-ganglionic autonomic fibers shown in this illustration. In addition, N-acetylaspartylglutamate is present in some retinal ganglion cells (retinogeniculate projections).

Clinical Correlations: Total or partial blindness in one or both eyes may result from a variety of causes (such as *gliomas, meningiomas, strokes, aneurysms*, infections, and demyelinating diseases); such lesions may occur at any locus along the visual pathway. Lesions of the optic nerve result in *blindness* and loss of the *pupillary light reflex* (direct response) in the involved eye. A *pituitary adenoma* may damage the crossing fibers in the optic chiasm (producing a *bitemporal hemianopsia*) or the uncrossed fibers in the right (or left) side of the optic chiasm. These lateral lesions produce a *right* (or *left*) *nasal hemianopsia*). Optic (geniculocalcarine) radiations (see Figs. 7–26 and 7–27) may pass directly caudal to the upper lip (cuneus) of the calcarine sulcus or follow an arching route (*Meyer's*, or *Meyer-Archambault, loop*) through the temporal lobe to the lower bank (lingual gyrus) of the calcarine sulcus. Temporal lobe lesions involving Meyer's loop, or involving fibers entering the lingual gyrus, can produce a *homonymous superior quadrantanopia*. A *homonymous inferior quadrantanopia* is seen in patients with damage to upper (parietal) parts of the geniculocalcarine radiations or to these fibers as they enter the cuneus. Damage to the visual cortex adjacent to the calcarine sulcus (distal posterior cerebral artery occlusion) results in a *right* (or *left*) *homonymous hemianopsia*. With the exception of macular sparing, this deficit is the same as that seen in optic tract lesions. Vascular lesions (as in the *lateral medullary syndrome*), tumors (such as *brainstem gliomas*) or *syringobulbia* may interrupt the descending projections from hypothalamus and midbrain to the intermediolateral cell column at upper thoracic levels. This will produce *Horner's syndrome* (*ptosis, miosis, enophthalmos, anhidrosis*) on the ipsilateral side.

Abbreviations

CC	Crus Cerebri	**PoCom**	Posterior Commissure
CilGang	Ciliary Ganglion	**PrTecNu**	Pretectal Nucleus
EWNu	Edinger-Westphal Nucleus	**PulNu**	Pulvinar Nuclear Complex
ILCC	Intermediolateral Horn (Cell Column)	**RetF**	Reticular Formation
LGB	Lateral Geniculate Body (Nucleus)	**RNu**	Red Nucleus
MGB	Medial Geniculate Body (Nucleus)	**SC**	Superior Colliculus
ML	Medial Lemniscus	**SC,Br**	Superior Colliculus, Brachium
OcNr	Oculomotor Nerve	**SCerGang**	Superior Cervical Ganglion
OpCh	Optic Chiasm	**SN**	Substantia Nigra
OpNr	Optic Nerve	**WRCom**	White Ramus Communicans
OpTr	Optic Tract		

Review of Blood Supply to **OpTr, MGB, LGB, Sc,** and Midbrain Tegementum, including **PrTecNu**

Structures	Arteries
OpTr	anterior choroidal (see Fig. 5–38)
MGB, LGB	thalamogeniculate branches of posterior cerebral (see Fig. 5–38)
SC and PrTecNu	long circumferential branches (quadrigeminal) of posterior cerebral, posterior choroidal and some from superior cerebellar (to SC) (see Figs. 5–27; 5–38)
Midbrain Tegmentum	paramedian branches of basilar bifurcation, medial branches of posterior cerebral and posterior communicating, short circumferential branches of posterior cerebral (see Fig. 5–27)

Pupillary/Accommodation Pathways

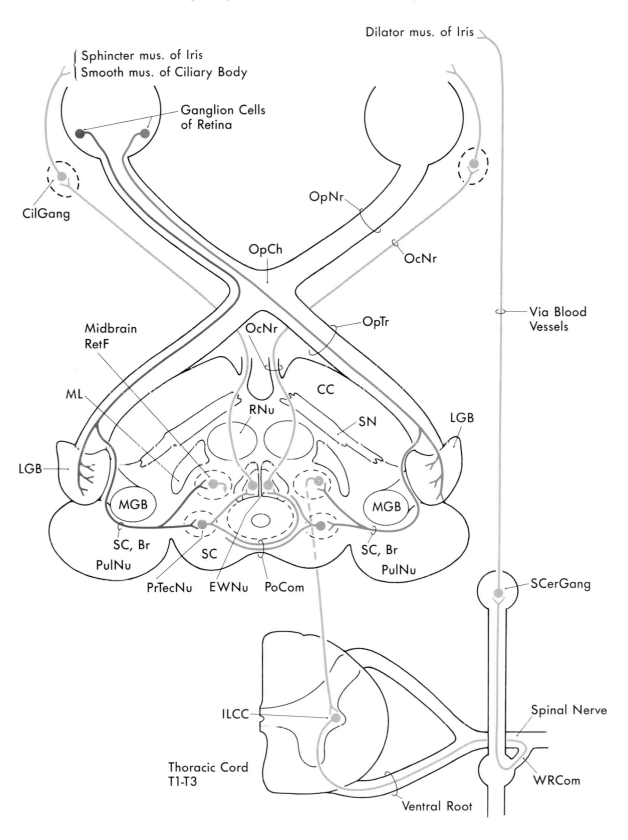

Sphincter mus. of Iris
Smooth mus. of Ciliary Body
Ganglion Cells of Retina
Dilator mus. of Iris
CilGang
OpNr
OcNr
OpCh
Via Blood Vessels
Midbrain RetF
OcNr
OpTr
ML
CC
RNu
SN
LGB
LGB
MGB
MGB
SC, Br
PulNu
SC
SC, Br
PulNu
PrTecNu   EWNu   PoCom
SCerGang
ILCC
Spinal Nerve
WRCom
Thoracic Cord
T1-T3
Ventral Root

Visual Pathways

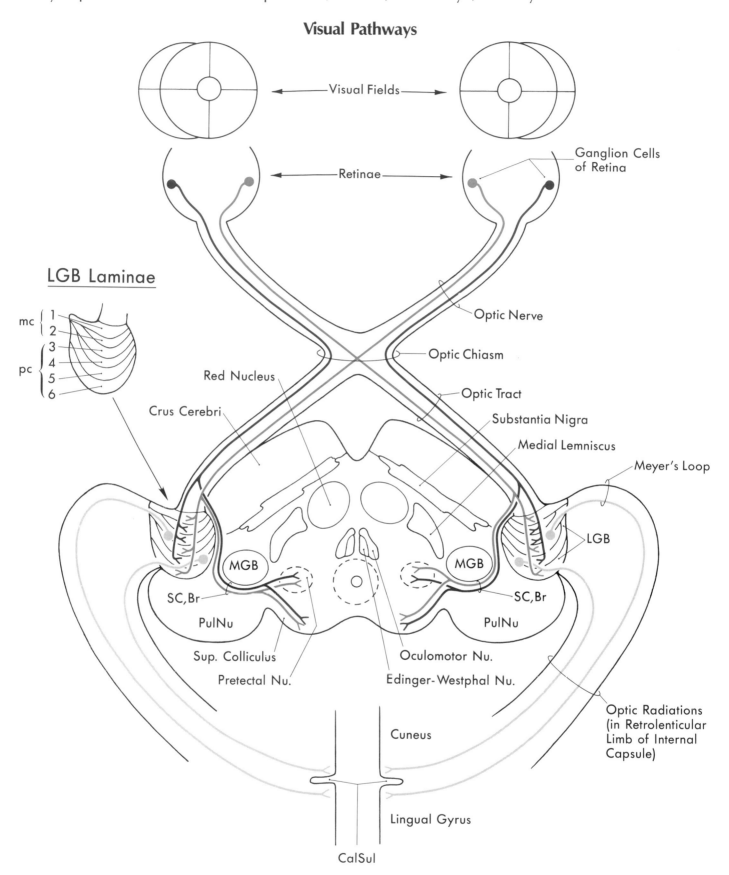

LGB Laminae

Visual Fields

Ganglion Cells of Retina

Retinae

Optic Nerve

Optic Chiasm

Red Nucleus

Optic Tract

Crus Cerebri

Substantia Nigra

Medial Lemniscus

Meyer's Loop

LGB

MGB

MGB

SC,Br

SC,Br

PulNu

PulNu

Sup. Colliculus

Oculomotor Nu.

Pretectal Nu.

Edinger-Westphal Nu.

Optic Radiations (in Retrolenticular Limb of Internal Capsule)

Cuneus

Lingual Gyrus

CalSul

7–26 The origin, course, and distribution of the visual pathway are shown. Uncrossed retinogeniculate fibers terminate in laminae 2, 3, and 5, while crossed fibers end in laminae 1, 4, and 6. Geniculocalcarine fibers arise from laminae 3–6. Retinogeniculate and geniculocalcarine pathways are retinotopically organized (see facing page).

Neurotransmitters: Cholecystokinin(+) is present in some geniculocalcarine fibers. N-acetylaspartylglutamate is found in some retinogeniculate fibers, and in some lateral geniculate and visual cortex neurons. Abbreviations: **CalSul**—Calcarine Sulcus; **LGB**—Lateral Geniculate Body, **mc**—magnocellular, **pc**—parvocellular; **MGB**—Medial Geniculate Body; **PulNu**—Pulvinar Nuclear Complex; **SC,Br**—Superior Colliculus, Brachium.

Clinical Correlations: Deficits seen following lesions of various parts of the visual pathway are described in Figure 7–25 on p. 206.

Visual Pathways

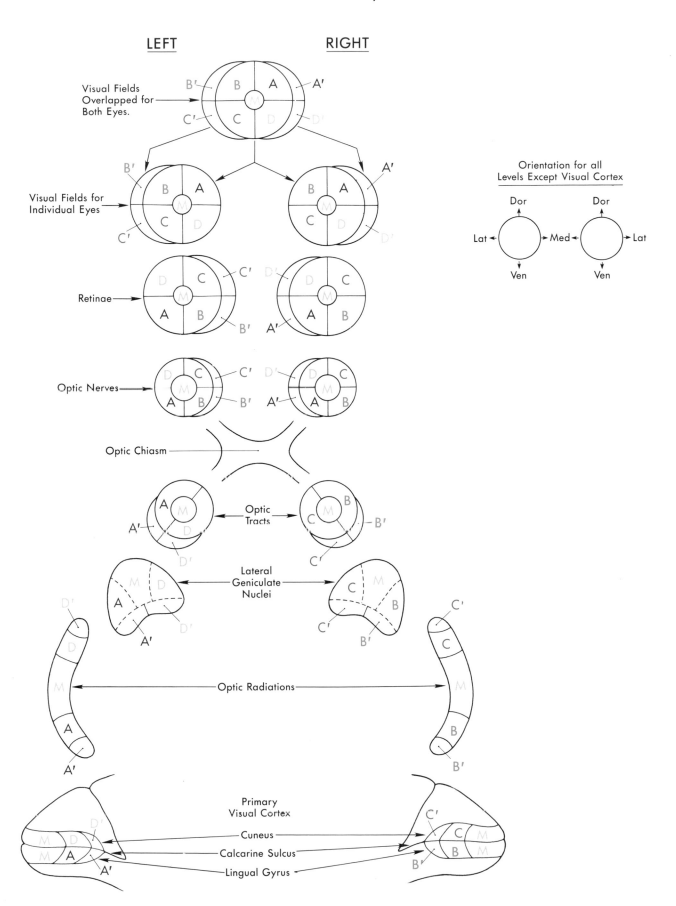

LEFT   **RIGHT**

Visual Fields Overlapped for Both Eyes.

Visual Fields for Individual Eyes

Retinae

Optic Nerves

Optic Chiasm

Optic Tracts

Lateral Geniculate Nuclei

Optic Radiations

Primary Visual Cortex
Cuneus
Calcarine Sulcus
Lingual Gyrus

Orientation for all Levels Except Visual Cortex

Dor   Dor

Lat ← → Med ← → Lat

Ven   Ven

7–27   Semi-diagrammatic representation of the retinographic arrangement of visual and retinal fields, and the subsequent topography of these projections throughout the visual system. Upper-case letters identify the binocular visual fields (A, B, C, D), the macula (M), and the monocular visual fields (A', B', C', D').

Clinical Correlations: Deficits seen following lesions of various parts of the visual pathway are described in Figure 7–25 on p. 206.

7–28   Blank master drawing of visual pathways. This illustration is provided for self-evaluation of visual pathway understanding, for the instructor to expand on aspects of the visual pathways not covered in the atlas, or both.

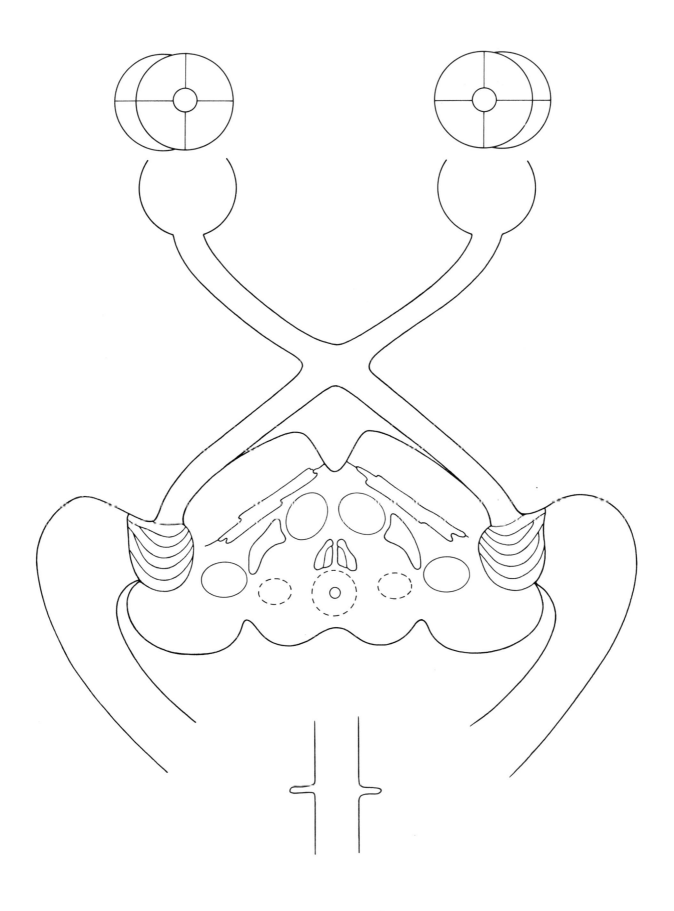

Auditory Pathways

7–29 The origin, course, and distribution of the fibers collectively composing the auditory pathway. Central to the cochlear nerve and dorsal and ventral cochlear nuclei this system is, in a general sense, bilateral and multisynaptic, as input is relayed through brainstem nuclei en route to the auditory cortex. Synapse and crossing (or recrossing) of information can occur at several levels in the neuraxis. The medial geniculate body is the thalamic station for the relay of auditory information to the temporal cortex.

Neurotransmitters: Glutamate(+) and aspartate(+) are found in some spiral ganglion cells and in their central terminations in the cochlear nuclei. Dynorphin- and histamine-containing fibers are also present in the cochlear nuclei; the latter arises from the hypothalamus. A noradrenergic projection to the cochlear nuclei and to the inferior colliculus originates from the nucleus locus ceruleus. Cells in the superior olive that contain cholecystokinin and cells in the nuclei of the lateral lemniscus that contain dynorphin project to the inferior colliculus. Although the olivocochlear bundle is not shown, it is noteworthy that enkephalin is found in some of the cells that contribute to this projection.

Clinical Correlations: Hearing loss may result from trauma (such as fracture of the petrous bone), demyelinating diseases, tumors, certain medications (*streptomycin*), or occlusion of the labyrinthine artery. Damage to the cochlear part of the VIIIth nerve (as in *acoustic neuroma*) results in *tinnitus* and/or *deafness* (partial or total) in the ipsilateral ear. The *Weber test* and *Rinne test* are used to differentiate between neural hearing loss and conduction hearing loss, and to lateralize the deficit. Central lesions (as in gliomas or vascular occlusions) rarely produce unilateral or bilateral hearing losses that can be detected, the possible exception being pontine lesions that damage the trapezoid body and nuclei. Injury to central auditory pathways and/ or primary auditory cortex may diminish auditory acuity, decrease the ability to hear certain tones, or make it difficult to precisely localize sounds in space. Patients with damage to secondary auditory cortex in the temporal lobe experience difficulty in understanding and/ or interpreting sounds (*auditory agnosia*).

Abbreviations

AbdNu	Abducens Nucleus	**MLF**	Medial Longitudinal Fasciculus
ALS	Anterolateral System	**PulNu**	Pulvinar Nuclear Complex
CC	Crus Cerebri	**RB**	Restiform Body
DCNu	Dorsal Cochlear Nucleus	**RetF**	Reticular Formation
FacNu	Facial Nucleus	**SC**	Superior Colliculus
IC	Inferior Colliculus	**SCP,Dec**	Superior Cerebellar Peduncle, Decussation
IC,Br	Inferior Colliculus, Brachium	**SO**	Superior Olive
IC,Com	Inferior Colliculus, Commissure	**SpGang**	Spiral Ganglion
IC,SL	Internal Capsule, Sublenticular Limb	**SpTTr**	Spinal Trigeminal Tract
LGB	Lateral Geniculate Body (Nucleus)	**TrapB**	Trapezoid Body
LL	Lateral Lemniscus	**TrapNu**	Trapezoid Nucleus
LL, Nu	Lateral Lemniscus, Nucleus	**TTGy**	Transverse Temporal Gyrus
MGB	Medial Geniculate Body (Nucleus)	**VCNu**	Ventral Cochlear Nucleus
ML	Medial Lemniscus		

Review of Blood Supply to Cochlear Nuclei, **LL** (and associated structures), Pontine Tegmentum, **IC**, and **MGB**

Structures	Arteries
Cochlear Nuclei	posterior and anterior inferior cerebellar (see Fig. 5–14)
LL, SO in Pons	long circumferential branches of basilar (see Fig. 5–21)
IC	long circumferential branches (quadrigeminal branches) of basilar, superior cerebellar (see Fig. 5–27)
MGB	thalamogeniculate branches of posterior cerebral (see Fig. 5–38)

Auditory Pathways

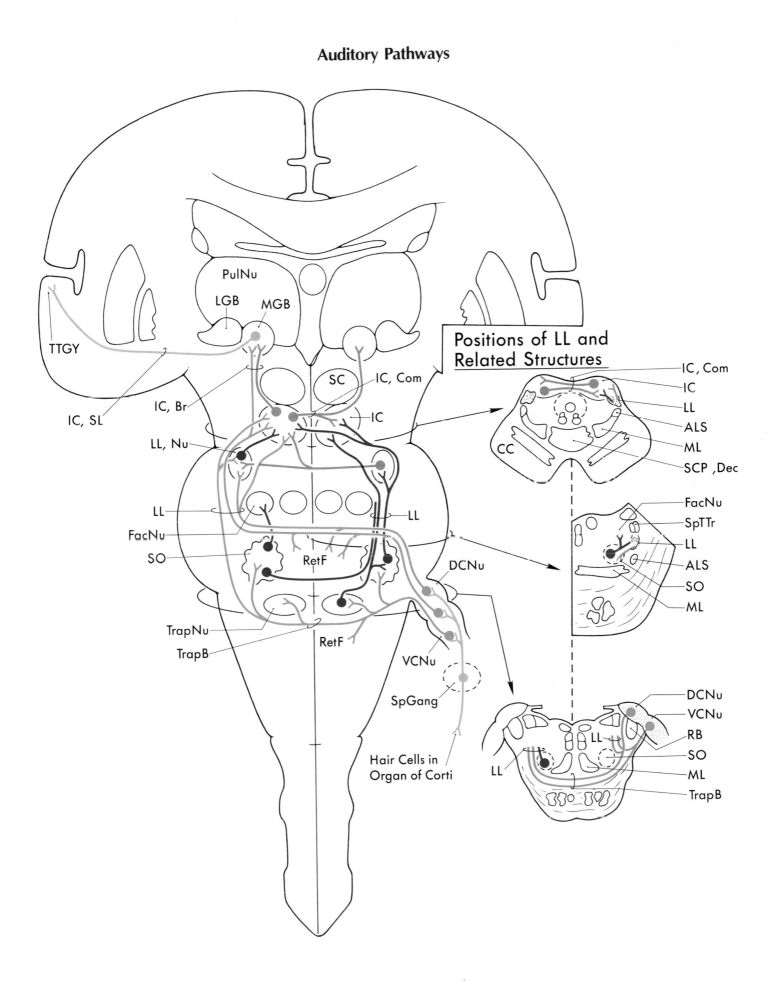

Positions of LL and Related Structures

Hair Cells in Organ of Corti

Vestibular Pathways

7–30   The origin, course, and distribution of the main afferent and efferent connections of the vestibular nuclei (see also Figs. 7–13, 7–19, and 7–20). Primary vestibular afferent fibers may end in the vestibular nuclei or pass to cerebellar structures via the juxtarestiform body. Secondary vestibulocerebellar axons originate from the vestibular nuclei and follow a similar path to the cerebellum. Efferent projections from the vestibular nuclei also course to the spinal cord (see Fig. 7–13) as well as to the motor nuclei of the oculomotor, trochlear, and abducens nerves by way of the MLF. Cerebellar structures most extensively interconnected with the vestibular nuclei include the lateral regions of the vermal cortex of anterior and posterior lobes, the flocculonodular lobe, and the fastigial (medial) cerebellar nucleus.

Neurotransmitters: Gamma-aminobutyric acid(-) is the transmitter associated with many cerebellar corticovestibular fibers and their terminals in the vestibular complex; this substance is also seen in cerebellar corticonuclear axons. The medial vestibular nucleus also has fibers that are dynorphin- and histamine-positive; the latter arise from cells in the hypothalamus.

Clinical Correlations: The vestibular part of the eighth nerve can be damaged by the same insults that affect the cochlear nerve (see Fig. 7–29). Damage to vestibular receptors of the vestibular nerve commonly results in *vertigo*. The patient may feel that his or her body is moving (*subjective vertigo*) or that objects in the environment are moving (*objective vertigo*). They have equilibrium problems, an unsteady (*ataxic*) gait, and a tendency to fall to the lesioned side. Deficits seen in nerve lesions, or in brainstem lesions involving the vestibular nuclei, include *nystagmus*, nausea, and vomiting, along with *vertigo* and gait problems. A *facial palsy* may also appear in concert with VIIIth nerve damage in patients with an *acoustic neuroma*. These vestibular deficits, along with partial or complete deafness, are seen in *Meniere's disease*. Lesions of those parts of the cerebellum with which the vestibular nerve and nuclei are most intimately connected (flocculonodular lobe and fastigial nucleus) result in *nystagmus*, truncal ataxia, ataxic gait, and a propensity to fall to the injured side. The *nystagmus* seen in patients with vestibular lesions and the *internuclear ophthalmoplegia* seen in some patients with *multiple sclerosis* are signs that correlate with the interruption of vestibular projections to the motor nuclei of III, IV and VI via the MLF.

Abbreviations

AbdNu	Abducens Nucleus		**OcNu**	Oculomotor Nucleus
ALS	Anterolateral System		**PAG**	Periaqueductal Gray
BP	Basilar Pons		**Py**	Pyramid
Cbl	Cerebellar		**RB**	Restiform Body
Cbl-CoVes	Cerebellar Corticovestibular Fibers		**RNu**	Red Nucleus
CblNu	Cerebellar Nuclei		**SC**	Superior Colliculus
CC	Crus Cerebri		**SCP,Dec**	Superior Cerebellar Peduncle, Decussation
HyNu	Hypoglossal Nucleus		**SN**	Substantia Nigra
IC	Inferior Colliculus		**SolNu**	Solitary Nucleus
IO	Inferior Olivary Nucleus		**SolTr**	Solitary Tract
JRB	Juxtarestiform Body		**SpTTr**	Spinal Trigeminal Tract
LVesSp	Lateral Vestibulospinal Tract		**SpVNu**	Spinal (or Inferior) Vestibular Nucleus
LVNu	Lateral Vestibular Nucleus		**SVNu**	Superior Vestibular Nucleus
MesNu	Mesencephalic Nucleus		**TecSp**	Tectospinal Tract
ML	Medial Lemniscus		**TroNu**	Trochlear Nucleus
MLF	Medial Longitudinal Fasciculus		**VesGang**	Vestibular Ganglion
MVesSp	Medial Vestibulospinal Tract		**VesCbl,Prim**	Vestibulocerebellar Fibers, Primary
MVNu	Medial Vestibular Nucleus		**VesCbl,Sec**	Vestibulocerebellar Fibers, Secondary

Review of Blood Supply to Vestibular Nuclei, **TroNu**, and **OcNu**

Structures	Arteries
Vestibular Nuclei	posterior inferior cerebellar in medulla (see Fig. 5–14), long circumferential branches of basilar in pons (see Fig. 5–21)
TroNu and **OcNu**	paramedian branches of basilar bifurcation, medial branches of posterior cerebral and posterior communicating, short circumferential branches of posterior cerebral (see Fig. 5–27)

Vestibular Pathways

Position of Vestibular Nuclei MLF and Related Structures

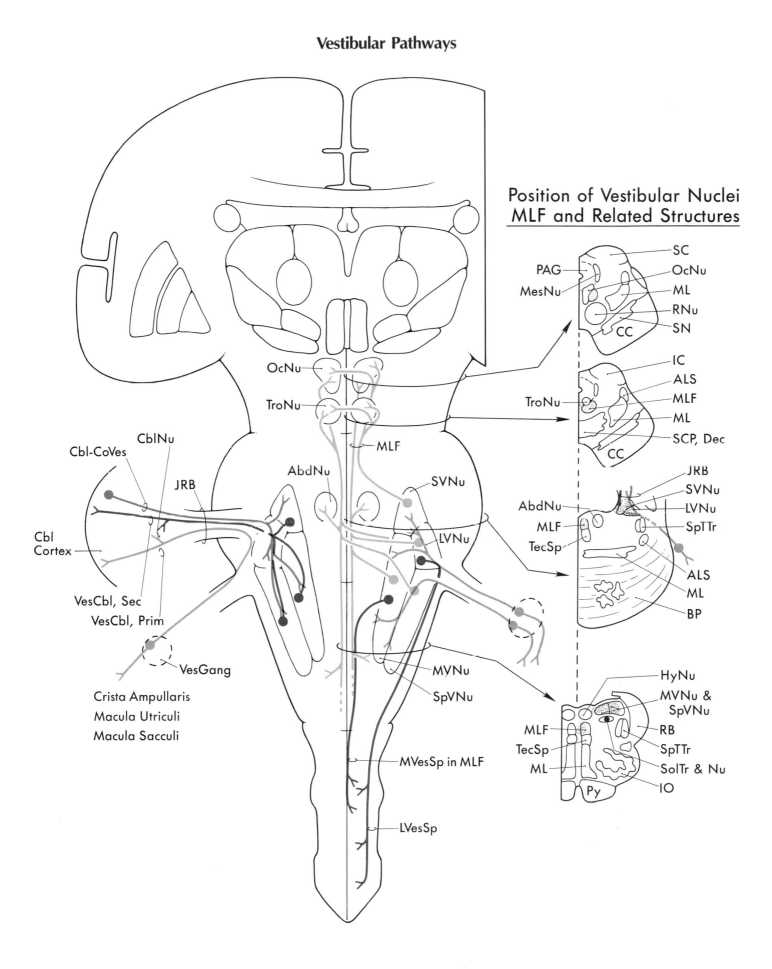

OcNu

TroNu

MLF

CblNu

Cbl-CoVes

JRB

AbdNu

SVNu

Cbl
Cortex

LVNu

VesCbl, Sec

VesCbl, Prim

VesGang

Crista Ampullaris
Macula Utriculi
Macula Sacculi

MVNu

SpVNu

MVesSp in MLF

LVesSp

SC
PAG
OcNu
MesNu
ML
RNu
SN
CC

IC
ALS
TroNu
MLF
ML
SCP, Dec
CC

JRB
SVNu
AbdNu
LVNu
MLF
SpTTr
TecSp
ALS
ML
BP

HyNu
MVNu &
SpVNu
MLF
RB
TecSp
SpTTr
ML
SolTr & Nu
Py
IO

7–31 Blank master drawing for auditory or vestibular pathways. This illustration is provided for self-evaluation of auditory or vestibular pathway understanding, for the instructor to expand on aspects of these pathways not covered in the atlas, or both.

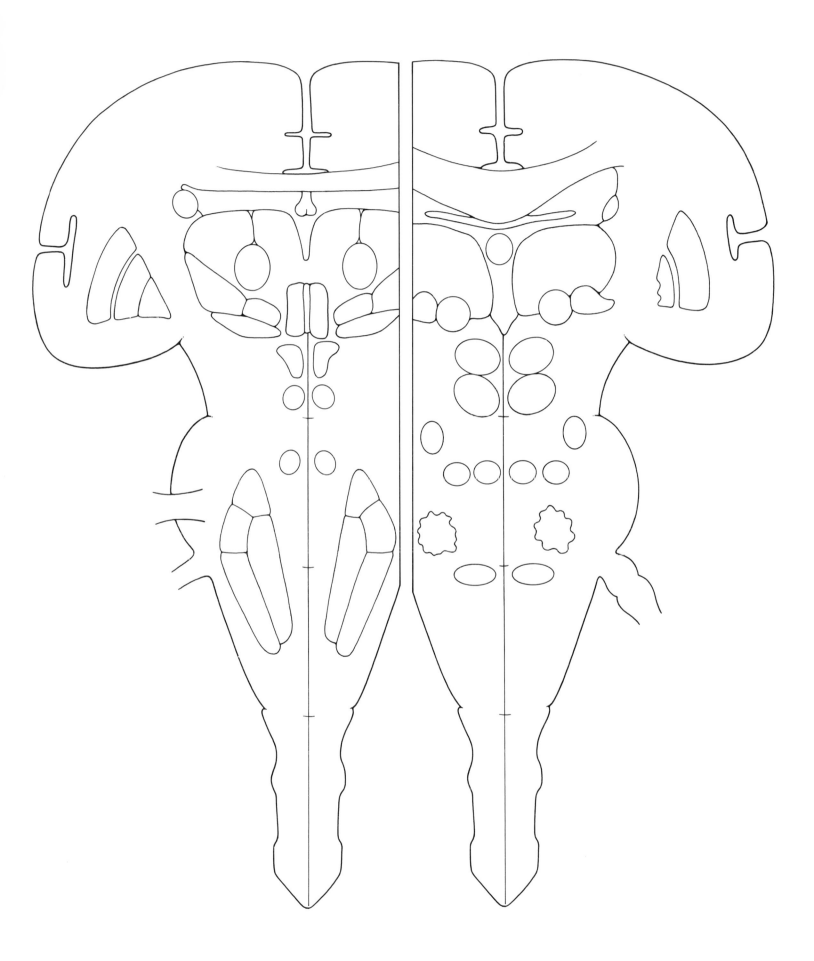

Hippocampal Connections

7–32 Selected afferent and efferent connections of the hippocampus (upper) and the mammillary body (lower) with emphasis on the circuit of Papez. The hippocampus receives input from, and projects to, diencephalic nuclei (especially the mammillary body via the postcommissural fornix), the septal region, and amygdala. The hippocampus receives cortical input from the superior and middle frontal gyri, superior temporal and cingulate gyri, precuneus, lateral occipital cortex, occipitotemporal gyri, and subcallosal cortical areas. The mammillary body is connected with the dorsal and ventral tegmental nuclei, anterior thalamic nucleus (via the mammillothalamic tract), septal nuclei, and, through the mammillotegmental tract, tegmental pontine and reticulotegmental nuclei.

Neurotransmitters: Glutamate(+)-containing cells in the subiculum and Ammon's horn project to the mammillary body, other hypothalamic centers, and the lateral septal nucleus through the fornix. Cholecystokinin(+) and somatostatin(-) are also found in hippocampal cells that project to septal nuclei and hypothalamic structures. The septal nuclei and the nucleus of the diagonal band give rise to cholinergic afferents to the hippocampus that travel in the fornix. In addition, a gamma-aminobutyric acid(-) septohippocampal projection originates from the medial septal nucleus. Enkephalin and glutamate-containing hippocampal afferent fibers arise from the adjacent entorhinal cortex; the locus ceruleus gives origin to noradrenergic fibers to the dentate gyrus, Ammon's horn, and subiculum; and serotoninergic fibers arise from the rostral raphe nuclei.

Clinical Correlations: Dysfunction associated with damage to the hippocampus is seen in patients with trauma to the temporal lobe, as a sequel to alcoholism, and as a result of neurodegenerative changes seen in the dementing diseases (such as *Alzheimer's disease* and *Pick's disease*). Bilateral injury to the hippocampus results in loss of recent memory (remote memory is unaffected), impaired ability to remember recent (new) events, and difficulty in acquiring new information. Also, memory that depends on visual, tactile or auditory discrimination is noticeably affected. In *Korsakoff's syndrome (amnestic confabulatory syndrome)* there is memory loss, dementia, amnesia, and a tendency to give confabulated responses. In addition to lesions in the hippocampus in these patients, the mammillary bodies and dorsomedial nucleus of the thalamus are noticeably affected. The Korsakoff's syndrome seen in chronic alcoholics is largely due to thiamine deficiency and can be treated with therapeutic doses of this vitamin.

Abbreviations

AC	Anterior Commissure		**LT**	Lamina Terminalis
AmHrn	Ammon's Horn		**MB**	Mammillary Body
Amy	Amygdaloid Nucleus (Complex)		**MedFCtx**	Medial Frontal Cortex
AntNu	Anterior Nucleus of Thalamus		**MedTh**	Medial Thalamus
CC, G	Corpus Callosum, Genu		**MTegTr**	Mammillotegmental Tract
CC,Spl	Corpus Callosum, Splenium		**MTTr**	Mammillothalamic Tract
Cing	Cingulum		**NuAccSep**	Nucleus Accumbens Septi
CingGy	Cingulate Gyrus		**OpCh**	Optic Chiasm
CorHip	Corticohippocampal Fibers		**Pi**	Pineal
DenGy	Dentate Gyrus		**RSplCtx**	Retrosplenial Cortex
EnCtx	Entorhinal Cortex		**SepNu**	Septal Nuclei
For	Fornix		**SMNu**	Supramammillary Nucleus
GyRec	Gyrus Rectus		**Sub**	Subiculum
Hip	Hippocampus		**TegNu**	Tegmental Nuclei
Hyth	Hypothalamus		**VmNu**	Ventromedial Hypothalamic Nucleus
IC,G	Internal Capsule, Genu			

Review of Blood Supply to **Hip, MB, Hyth and CingGy**

Structures	Arteries
Hip	Anterior choroidal (see Fig. 5–38)
MB, Hyth	branches of circle of Willis (see Fig. 2–21)
AntNu	thalamoperforating (see Fig. 5–38)
CingGy	branches of anterior cerebral

Hippocampal Connections

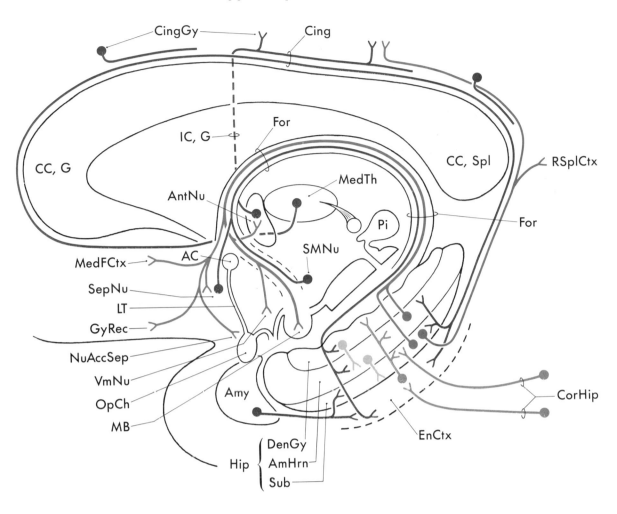

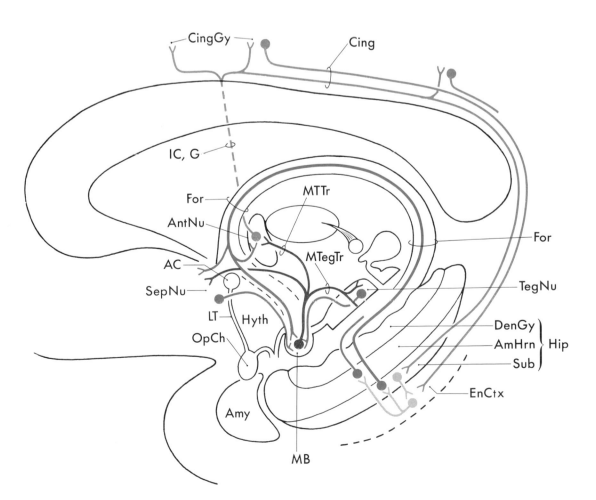

Amygdaloid Connections

7–33 The origin, course, and distribution of selected afferent and efferent connections of the amygdaloid nuclear complex in sagittal (upper) and coronal (lower) planes. The amygdala receives input from, and projects to, brainstem and forebrain centers via the stria terminalis and the ventral amygdalofugal pathway. Corticoamygdaloid and amygdalocortical fibers interconnect the basal and lateral amygdaloid nuclei with select cortical areas.

Neurotransmitters: Cells in the amygdaloid complex contain vasoactive intestinal polypeptide (VIP, +), neurotensin (NT), somatostatin (SOM,-), enkephalin (ENK,-), and substance P (SP, +). These neurons project, via the stria terminalis or the ventral amygdalofugal path, to the septal nuclei (VIP, NT), the bed nucleus of the stria terminalis (NT, ENK, SP), the hypothalamus (VIP, SOM, SP), the nucleus accumbens septi, and the caudate and putamen (NT). Serotonergic amygdaloid fibers originate from the nucleus raphe dorsalis and the superior central nucleus, dopaminergic axons from the ventral tegmental area and the substantia nigra-pars compacta, and noradrenalin-containing fibers from the locus ceruleus. Glutamate(+) is found in olfactory projections to the prepiriform cortex and the amygdaloid complex. Acetylcholine is present in afferents to the amygdala from

the substantia innominata, as well as from the septal area. In patients with Alzheimer's disease and the associated dementia there is a marked loss of acetylcholine-containing neurons in the basal nucleus of the substantia innominata, in the cortex, and in the hippocampus.

Clinical Correlations: Dysfunctions related to damage to the amygdaloid complex are seen in patients with trauma to the temporal lobe, herpes simplex, *encephalitis*, bilateral temporal lobe surgery to treat intractable epileptic activity, and in some CNS degenerative disorders (such as *Alzheimer's disease* and *Pick's disease*). The behavioral changes seen in individuals with amygdala lesions collectively form the *Kluver-Bucy syndrome*. In humans these changes/deficits are (1) *hyperorality*, (2) *visual, tactile,* and *auditory agnosia*, (3) *placidity*, (4) *hyperphagia* or other dietary manifestations, (5) an intense desire to explore the immediate environment (*hypermetamorphosis*), and (6) what is commonly called hypersexuality. These changes in sexual attitudes are usually in the form of comments, suggestions, and attempts to make a sexual contact rather than in actual intercourse or masturbation. These patients may also show *aphasia, dementia,* and *amnesia*.

Abbreviations

AC	Anterior Commissure	**NuRa,m**	Nucleus Raphe, Magnus
Amy	Amygdaloid Nuclear Complex	**NuRa,o**	Nucleus Raphe, Obscurus
AmyCor	Amygdalocortical Fibers	**NuRa,p**	Nucleus Raphe, Pallidus
AmyFugPath	Amygdalofugal Pathway	**NuStTer**	Nucleus of the Stria Terminalis
AntHyth	Anterior Hypothalamus	**OlfB**	Olfactory Bulb
Ba-LatNu	Basal and Lateral Nuclei	**OpCh**	Optic Chiasm
CaNu	Caudate Nucleus	**PAG**	Periaqueductal Gray
Cen-MedNu	Central, Cortical and Medial Nuclei	**PBrNu**	Parabrachial Nuclei
CorAmy	Corticoamygdaloid Fibers	**PfNu**	Parafascicular Nucleus
DVagNu	Dorsal Motor Vagal Nucleus	**Pi**	Pineal
EnCtx	Entorhinal Cortex	**POpNu**	Preoptic Nucleus
For	Fornix	**PPriCtx**	Prepiriform Cortex
GP	Globus Pallidus	**Put**	Putamen
Hyth	Hypothalamus	**SepNu**	Septal Nuclei
LT	Lamina Terminalis	**SNpc**	Substantia Nigra, pars compacta
LHAr	Lateral Hypothalamic Area	**SolNu**	Solitary Nucleus
LocCer	(Nucleus) Locus Ceruleus	**StTer**	Stria Terminalis
MedThNu	Medial Thalamic Nuclei	**Sub**	Subiculum
MGB	Medial Geniculate Body	**SubIn**	Substantia Innominata
MidTh	Midline Thalamic Areas	**VenTegAr**	Ventral Tegmental Area
NuAccSep	Nucleus Accumbens Septi	**VmNu**	Ventromedial Hypothalamic Nucleus
NuCen,s	Nucleus Centralis, Superior		
NuRa,d	Nucleus Raphe, Dorsalis		

Review of Blood Supply to **Amy** and Related Centers

Structures	Arteries
Amy	anterior choroidal (see Fig. 5–38)
Hyth	branches of circle of Willis (see Fig. 5–38)
Brainstem	see Figs. 5–14, 5–21, 5–27)
Thalamus	thalamoperforating, thalamogeniculate (see Fig. 5–38)

Amygdaloid Connections

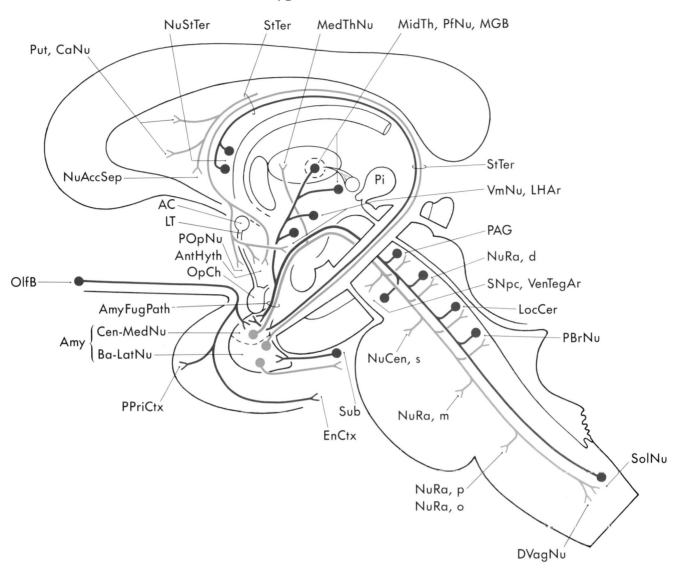

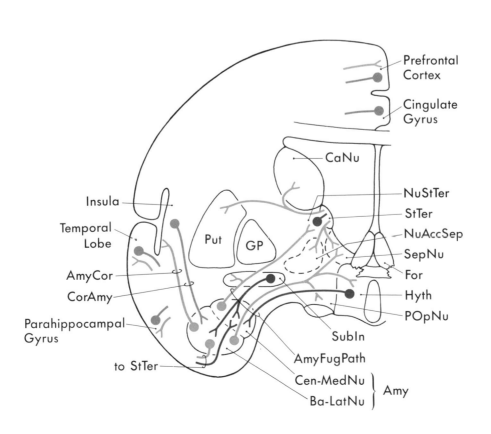

7–34 Blank master drawing for limbic pathways. This illustration is provided for self-evaluation of limbic pathways or connections, for the instructor to expand on aspects of these pathways not covered in the atlas, or both.

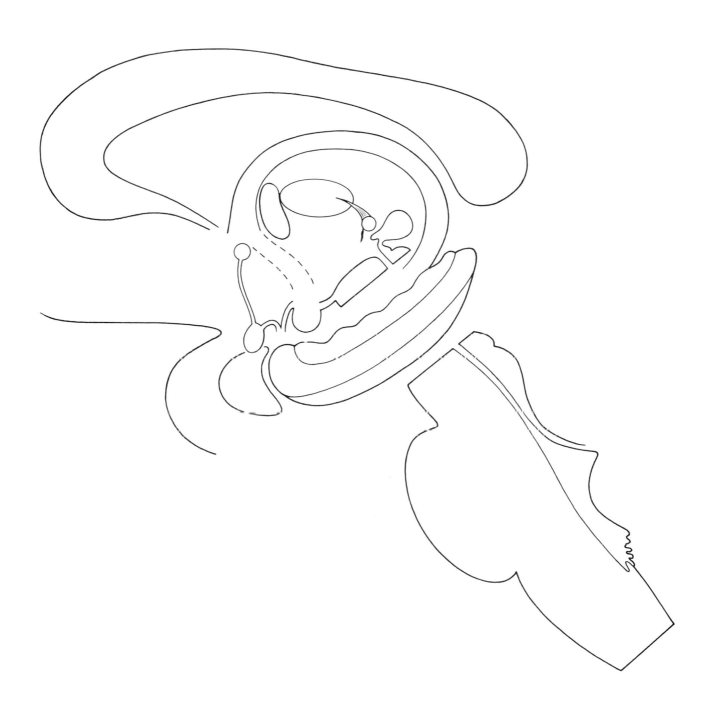

Chapter 8

Anatomical-Clinical Correlations:

Cerebral Angiogram and MRA

Brain Slice-CT Scan—MRI Correlation

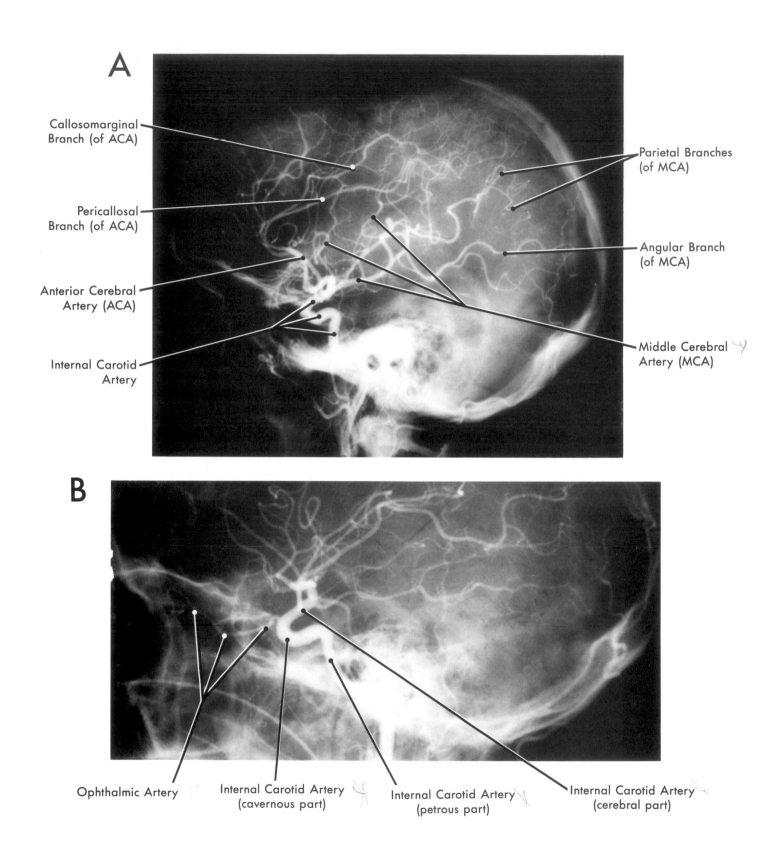

A

Callosomarginal
Branch (of ACA)

Pericallosal
Branch (of ACA)

Anterior Cerebral
Artery (ACA)

Internal Carotid
Artery

Parietal Branches
(of MCA)

Angular Branch
(of MCA)

Middle Cerebral
Artery (MCA)

B

Ophthalmic Artery

Internal Carotid Artery
(cavernous part)

Internal Carotid Artery
(petrous part)

Internal Carotid Artery
(cerebral part)

8–1   Internal carotid angiogram (left lateral projection, arterial phase) showing the general patterns of the internal carotid, middle, and anterior cerebral arteries (**A,B**) and an image with especially good filling of the ophthalmic artery (**B** arrows). The ophthalmic artery leaves the cerebral part of the internal carotid and enters the orbit via the optic canal. Its terminal branches will anastomose with superficial vessels around the orbit. Compare with Figures 2-10 and 2-23.

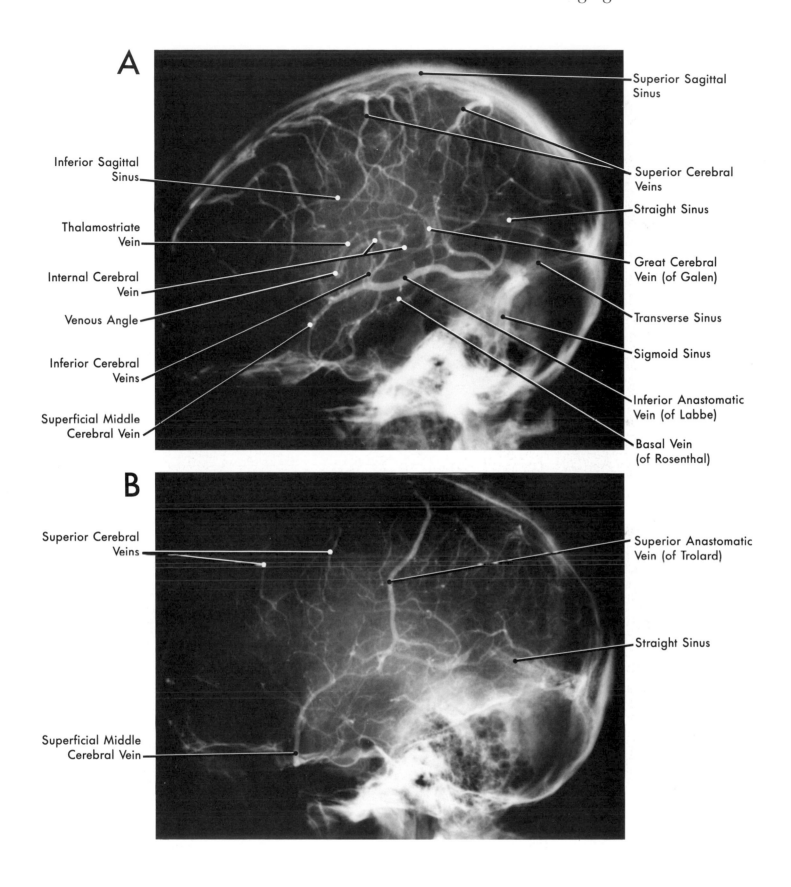

A

Inferior Sagittal Sinus

Thalamostriate Vein

Internal Cerebral Vein

Venous Angle

Inferior Cerebral Veins

Superficial Middle Cerebral Vein

Superior Sagittal Sinus

Superior Cerebral Veins

Straight Sinus

Great Cerebral Vein (of Galen)

Transverse Sinus

Sigmoid Sinus

Inferior Anastomatic Vein (of Labbe)

Basal Vein (of Rosenthal)

B

Superior Cerebral Veins

Superficial Middle Cerebral Vein

Superior Anastomatic Vein (of Trolard)

Straight Sinus

8–2 Two internal carotid angiograms (left lateral projection, venous phase). Superficial and deep venous structures are clear in **A**, while **B** shows a particularly obvious vein of Trolard. Compare these images with the drawings of veins and sinuses in Figures 2–11 and 2–24.

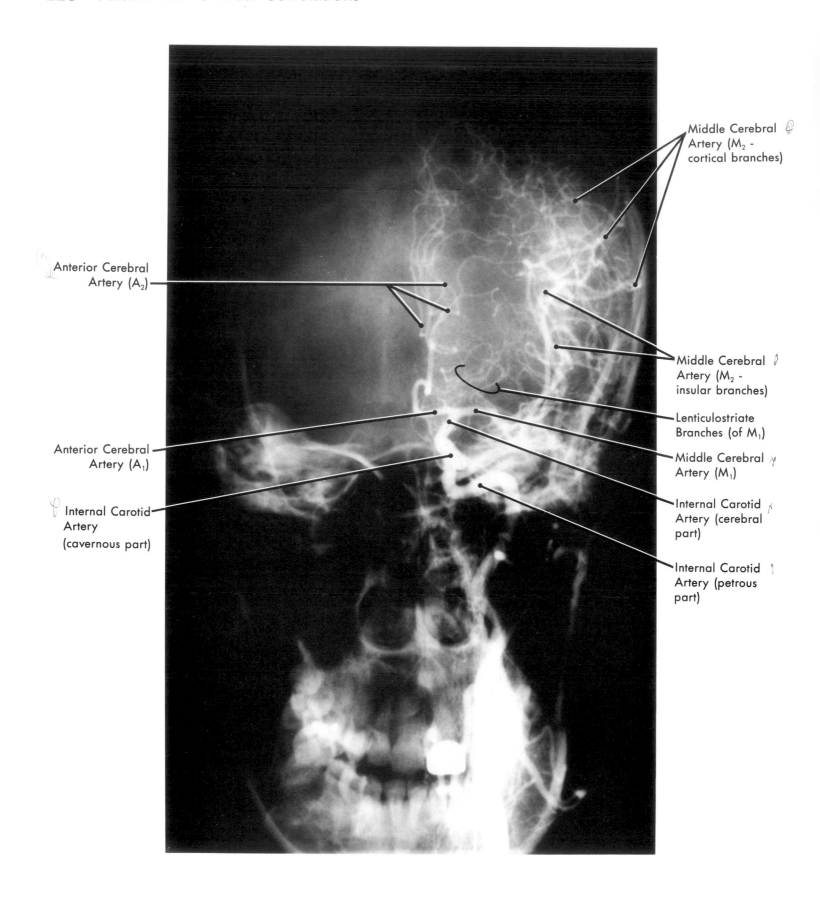

Middle Cerebral Artery (M$_2$ - cortical branches)

Anterior Cerebral Artery (A$_2$)

Middle Cerebral Artery (M$_2$ - insular branches)

Anterior Cerebral Artery (A$_1$)

Lenticulostriate Branches (of M$_1$)

Middle Cerebral Artery (M$_1$)

Internal Carotid Artery (cavernous part)

Internal Carotid Artery (cerebral part)

Internal Carotid Artery (petrous part)

8–3   Internal carotid angiogram (right anterior-posterior projection, arterial phase). Note general distribution patterns of anterior and middle cerebral arteries and the location of lenticulostriate branches. The A$_1$ segment of the anterior cerebral artery is located between the internal carotid bifurcation and the anterior communicating artery; the A$_2$ segment is distal to the anterior communicator. The M$_1$ segment of the middle cerebral is located between the internal carotid bifurcation and the point at which this vessel branches into superior and inferior trunks on the insular cortex. Distally these insular and cortical branches are parts of the M$_2$ segment.

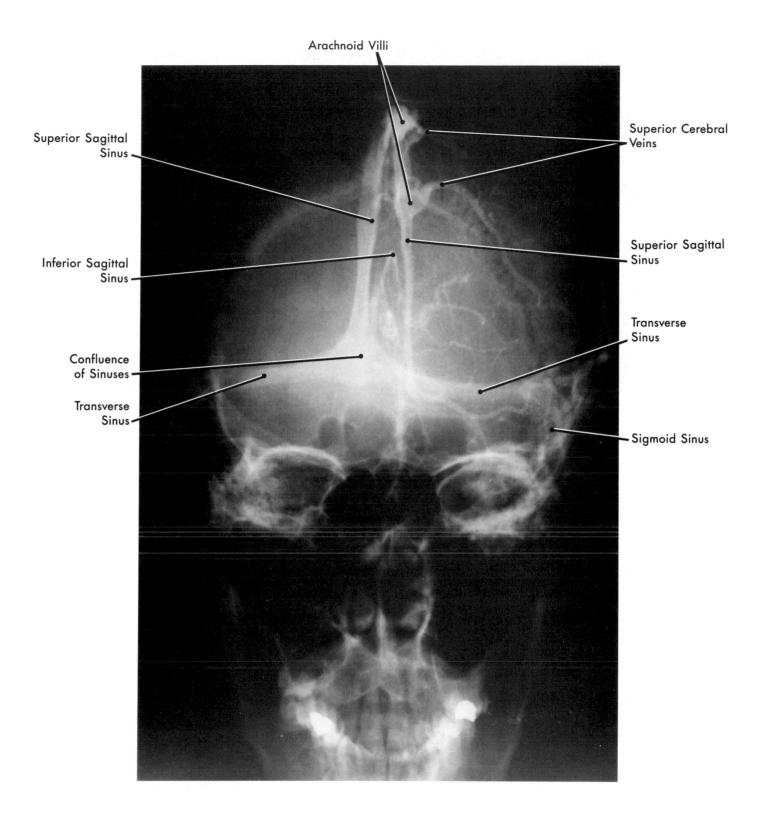

Arachnoid Villi

Superior Sagittal
Sinus

Superior Cerebral
Veins

Inferior Sagittal
Sinus

Superior Sagittal
Sinus

Transverse
Sinus

Confluence
of Sinuses

Transverse
Sinus

Sigmoid Sinus

8–4 Internal carotid angiogram (right anterior-posterior projection, venous phase). The patient's head is tilted slightly; this shows
the arching shapes of the superior and inferior sagittal sinuses to full
advantage. Note the other venous structures in this image and compare
with the arterial phase shown in Figure 8–3.

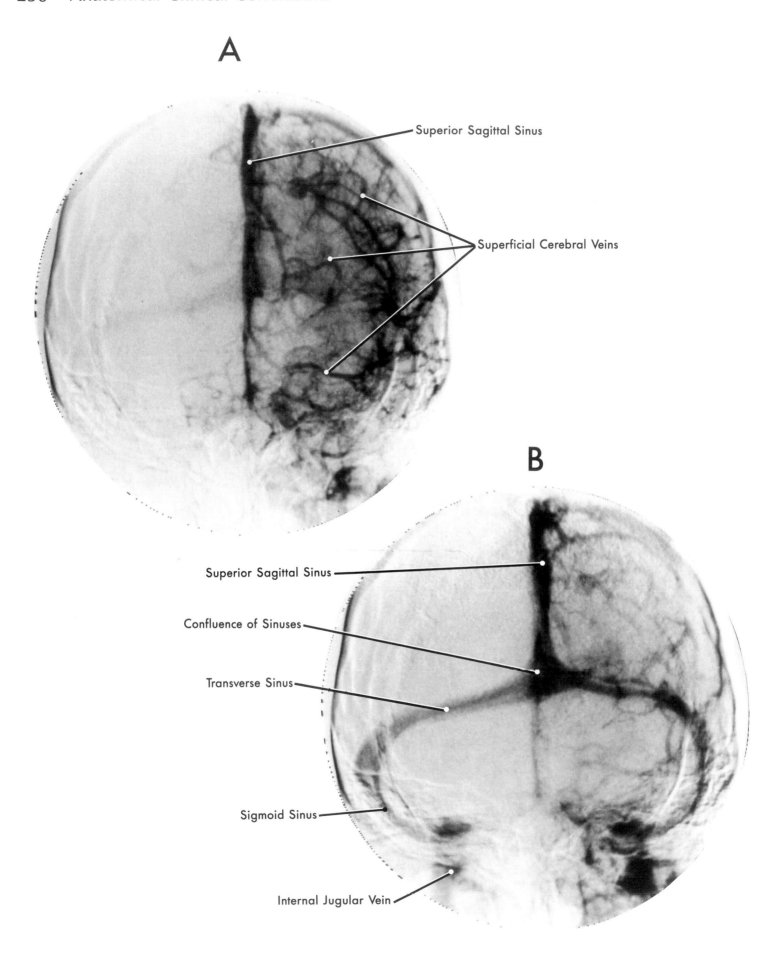

A

Superior Sagittal Sinus

Superficial Cerebral Veins

B

Superior Sagittal Sinus

Confluence of Sinuses

Transverse Sinus

Sigmoid Sinus

Internal Jugular Vein

8–5 Digital subtraction image of an internal carotid angiogram (anterior-posterior projection, venous phase). Image **A** is early in the venous phase (greater filling of cortical veins), while image **B** is later in the venous phase (greater filling of the sinuses and jugular vein). Both images are of the same patient.

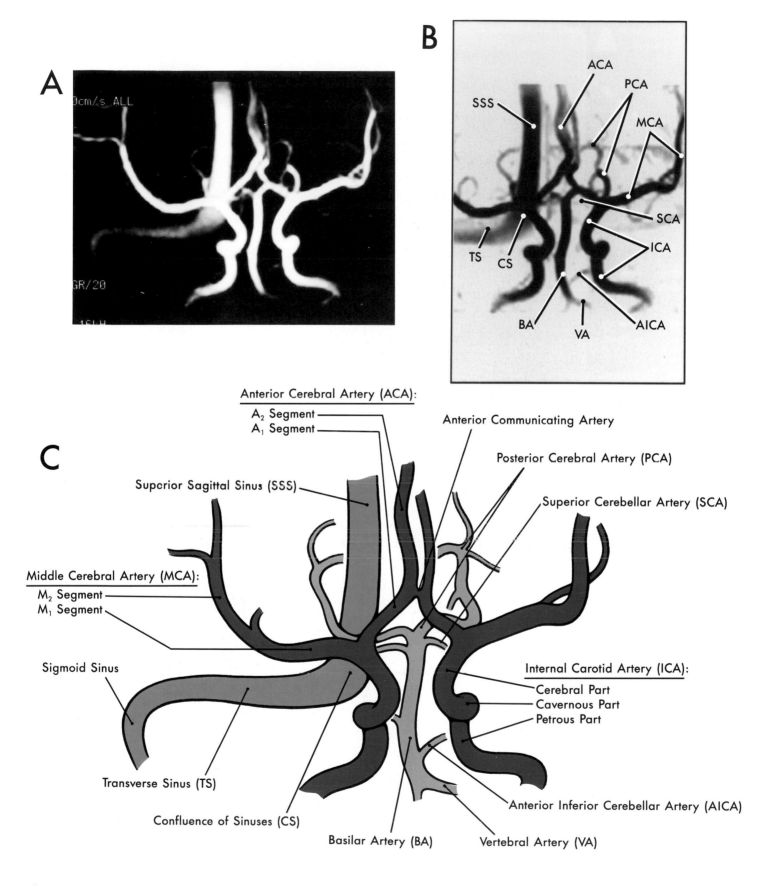

A

B

ACA
PCA
SSS
MCA
SCA
ICA
TS   CS
BA   VA   AICA

C

Anterior Cerebral Artery (ACA):
A₂ Segment
A₁ Segment

Anterior Communicating Artery

Superior Sagittal Sinus (SSS)

Posterior Cerebral Artery (PCA)

Superior Cerebellar Artery (SCA)

Middle Cerebral Artery (MCA):
M₂ Segment
M₁ Segment

Sigmoid Sinus

Internal Carotid Artery (ICA):
Cerebral Part
Cavernous Part
Petrous Part

Transverse Sinus (TS)

Anterior Inferior Cerebellar Artery (AICA)

Confluence of Sinuses (CS)

Basilar Artery (BA)   Vertebral Artery (VA)

8–6   Magnetic resonance angiography (MRA) is a noninvasive method for imaging cerebral arteries, veins, and sinuses simultaneously. A 3-D phase contrast MRA (**A**) and an inverted video image window (**B**) of the same view show major vessels and sinuses from anterior to posterior. **C** shows the relative position of the major vessels and dural sinuses as imaged in A and B.

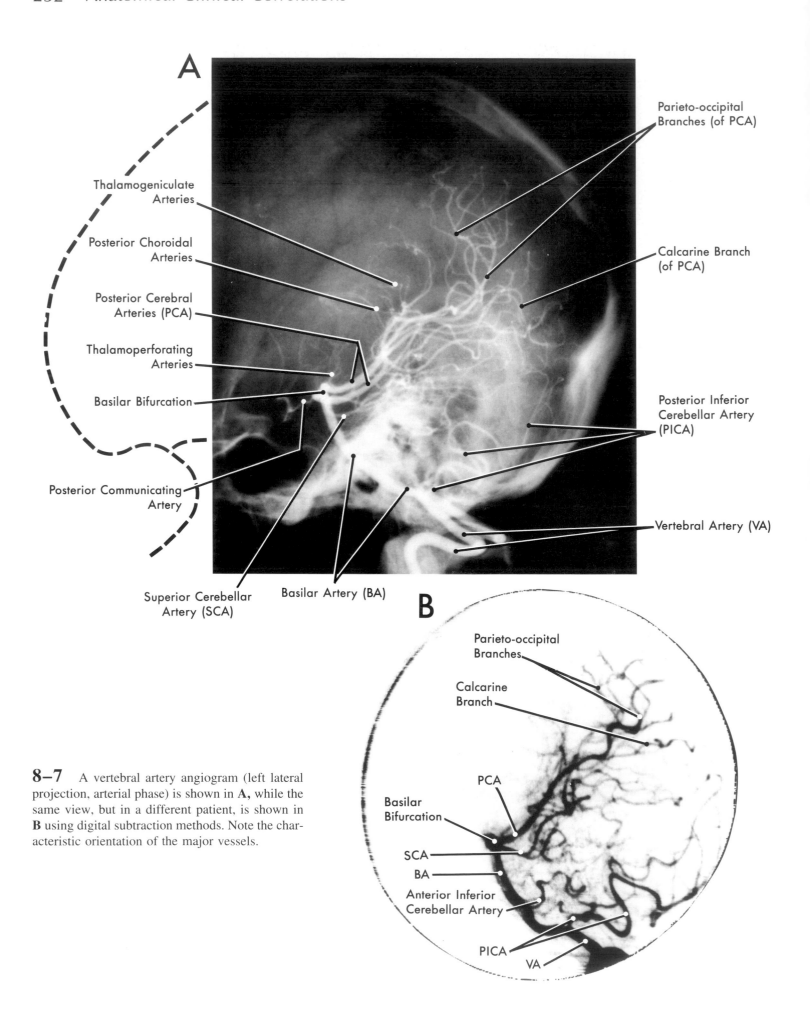

A

Parieto-occipital
Branches (of PCA)

Thalamogeniculate
Arteries

Posterior Choroidal
Arteries

Calcarine Branch
(of PCA)

Posterior Cerebral
Arteries (PCA)

Thalamoperforating
Arteries

Basilar Bifurcation

Posterior Inferior
Cerebellar Artery
(PICA)

Posterior Communicating
Artery

Vertebral Artery (VA)

Superior Cerebellar
Artery (SCA)

Basilar Artery (BA)

B

Parieto-occipital
Branches

Calcarine
Branch

PCA

Basilar
Bifurcation

SCA

BA

Anterior Inferior
Cerebellar Artery

PICA

VA

8–7 A vertebral artery angiogram (left lateral projection, arterial phase) is shown in **A,** while the same view, but in a different patient, is shown in **B** using digital subtraction methods. Note the characteristic orientation of the major vessels.

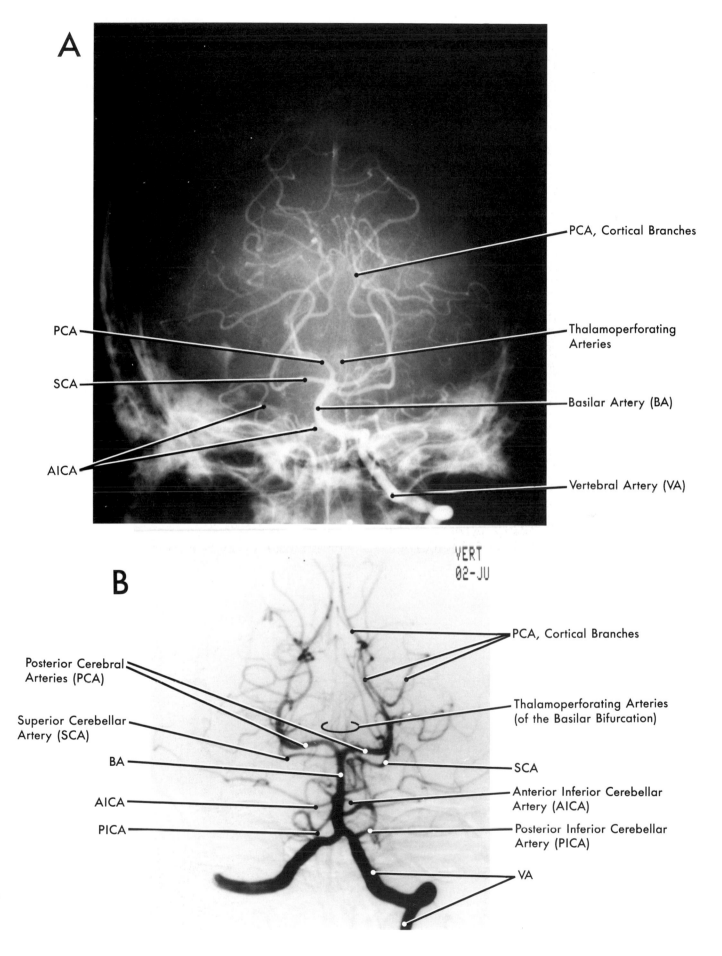

A

PCA, Cortical Branches

PCA

Thalamoperforating
Arteries

SCA

Basilar Artery (BA)

AICA

Vertebral Artery (VA)

B

VERT
02-JU

PCA, Cortical Branches

Posterior Cerebral
Arteries (PCA)

Thalamoperforating Arteries
(of the Basilar Bifurcation)

Superior Cerebellar
Artery (SCA)

SCA

BA

Anterior Inferior Cerebellar
Artery (AICA)

AICA

PICA

Posterior Inferior Cerebellar
Artery (PICA)

VA

8–8   A vertebral artery angiogram (anterior-posterior projection, arterial phase) is shown in **A,** while the same view, but in a different patient, is shown in **B** using digital subtraction methods. Even though the injection is into the left vertebral, there is bilateral filling of the vertebral arteries and of branches of the basilar artery.

Anterior cerebral Artery:
A₂ Segment
A₁ Segment

Middle Cerebral Artery (MCA):
M₁ Segment
M₂ Segment

MCA, Insular Branches

Posterior Cerebral Artery (PCA)

Basilar Artery (BA)

MCA, Cortical Branches

Internal Cerebral Vein

PCA, Temporal Branch

Superior Petrosal Sinus

Lateral Ventricular Vein

Great Cerebral Vein (of Galen)

Transverse Sinus (TS)

Straight Sinus (SS)

TS

Superior Sagittal Sinus

Great Cerebral Vein

Anterior Cerebral Artery (A₂)

MCA, M₂ Segment

SS

Internal Carotid Artery

TS

BA

PCA

Posterior Communicating Artery

Superior Cerebellar Artery

8–9 MRA images arteries, veins, and sinuses simultaneously based on the movement of fluid in these structures. These are inverted video images of 3-D phase contrast MRA images as viewed from the dorsal to ventral (**A**) and from the lateral (**B**) aspects. Compare these images with arteries and veins as depicted in Figures 2–16, 2–17, 2–24, and 2–25.

Brain Slide-CT Scan—MRI Correlation

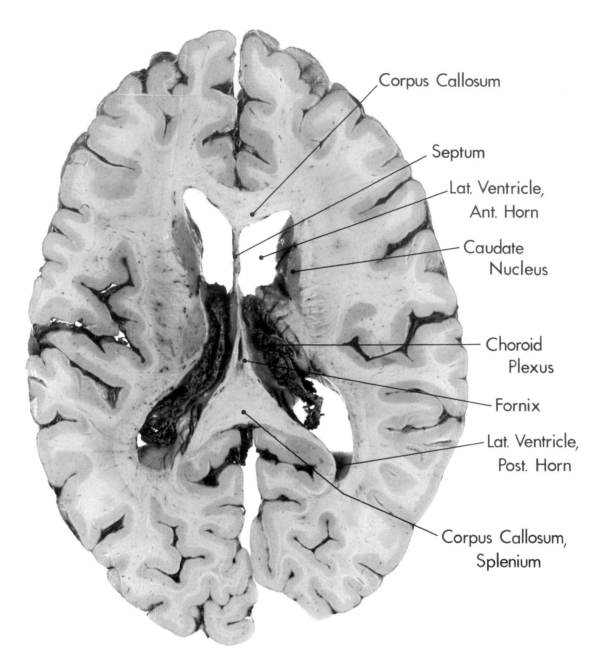

Corpus Callosum

Septum

Lat. Ventricle,
Ant. Horn

Caudate
Nucleus

Choroid
Plexus

Fornix

Lat. Ventricle,
Post. Horn

Corpus Callosum,
Splenium

8–10   Dorsal surface of a axial (horizontal) slice of brain just ventral to the *corpus callosum* (for greater detail see Fig. 4–16 on page 62). Structures that can be easily identified in a corresponding CT or MRI scan of a normal brain (Figs. 8–11, 8–12, facing page) are labeled.

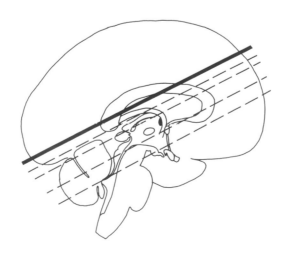

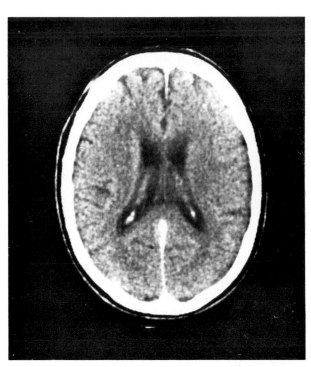

8–11   CT scan of normal brain at a level corresponding to the slice shown in Figure 8–10 (facing page). Identify the internal structures visible in this scan by comparing it with Figure 8–10.

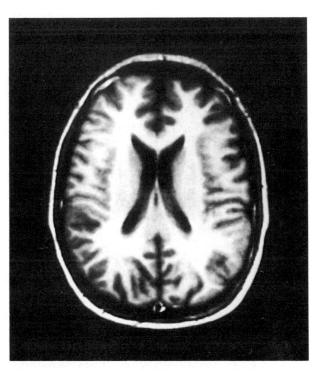

8–12   MRI scan (T1 image) of normal brain at a level corresponding to the slice shown in Figure 8–10 (facing page). Identify the structures visible in this image by comparing it with Figure 8–10.

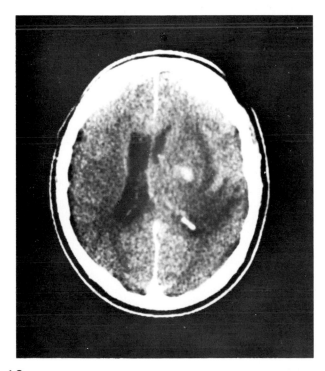

8–13   CT scan of abnormal brain (lymphoma) corresponding to the level of normal brain shown in Figure 8–11 (above). With the exception of some recognizable features of the ventricular system, note that all morphological relationships are disrupted on the right.

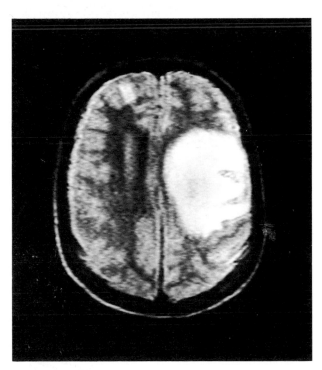

8–14   MRI scan (T2 image) of abnormal brain (metastatic lung carcinoma) corresponding to the level of normal brain shown in Figure 8–12 (above). Note the prominent appearance of the lesion and the disruption of normal morphological relationships on the right.

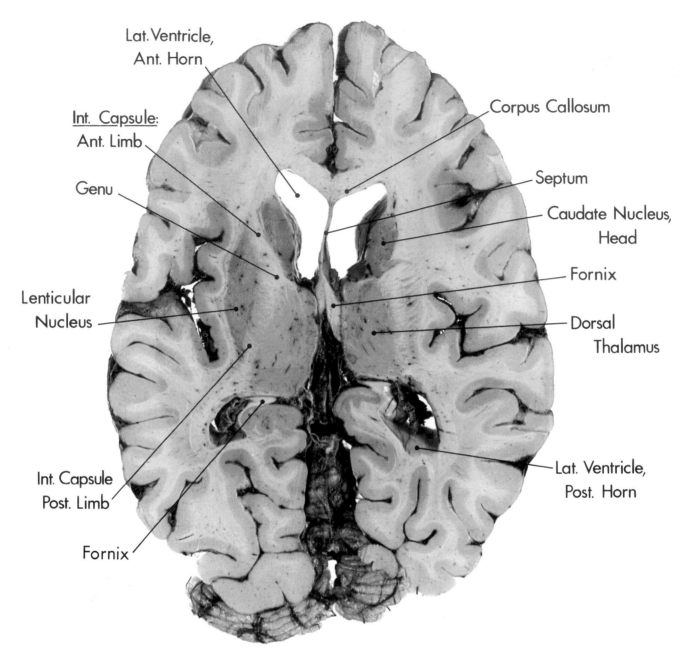

Lat. Ventricle, Ant. Horn

Int. Capsule: Ant. Limb

Genu

Lenticular Nucleus

Int. Capsule Post. Limb

Fornix

Corpus Callosum

Septum

Caudate Nucleus, Head

Fornix

Dorsal Thalamus

Lat. Ventricle, Post. Horn

8–15   Dorsal surface of a axial (horizontal) slice of brain through the *dorsal thalamus* and *caudate and lenticular nuclei* just dorsal to the third ventricle (for greater detail see Fig. 4-17 on page 63). Structures that can be easily identified in a CT or MRI scan of normal brain at corresponding levels (Figs. 8–16, 8–17, facing page) are labeled.

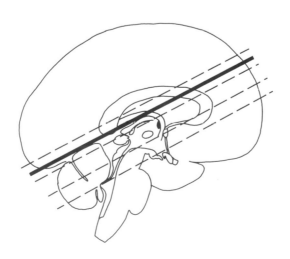

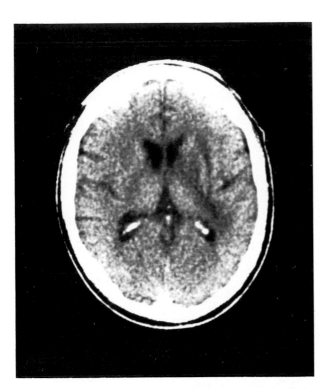

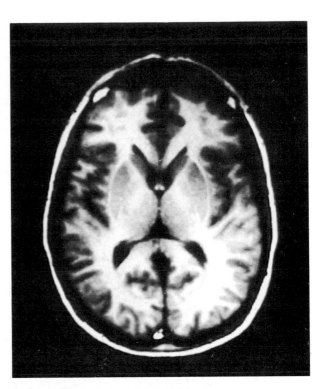

8–16 CT scan of normal brain at a level corresponding to the slice shown in Figure 8–15 (facing page). Identify the internal structures visible in this scan by comparing it with Figure 8–15.

8–17 MRI scan (T1 image) of normal brain at a level corresponding to the slice shown in Figure 8–15 (facing page). Identify the structures visible in this image by comparing it with Figure 8–15.

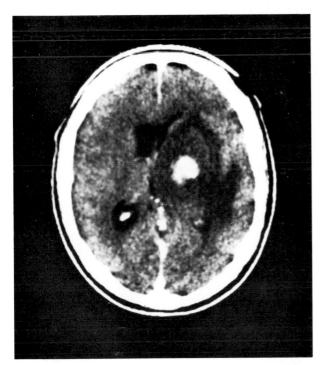

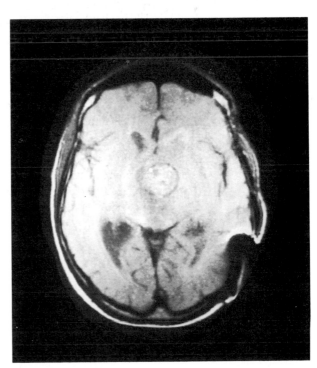

8–18 CT scan of abnormal brain (lymphoma) corresponding to the level of normal brain shown in Figure 8–16 (above). Note that most morphological relationships on the right are disrupted, although portions of the caudate and lenticular nuclei can be identified. On the left, the thalamus, caudate and lenticular nuclei, and main portions of the internal capsule are visible.

8–19 MRI scan (T2 image) of abnormal brain (grade 3 diencephalic glioma) corresponding to the level of normal brain shown in Figure 8–17 (above). The third ventricle is displaced to the left, and the anterior horn of the lateral ventricle is almost completely obliterated on the right and partially deformed on the left. The anatomical relationships of the thalamus and the caudate and lenticular nuclei are totally disrupted, mainly on the right.

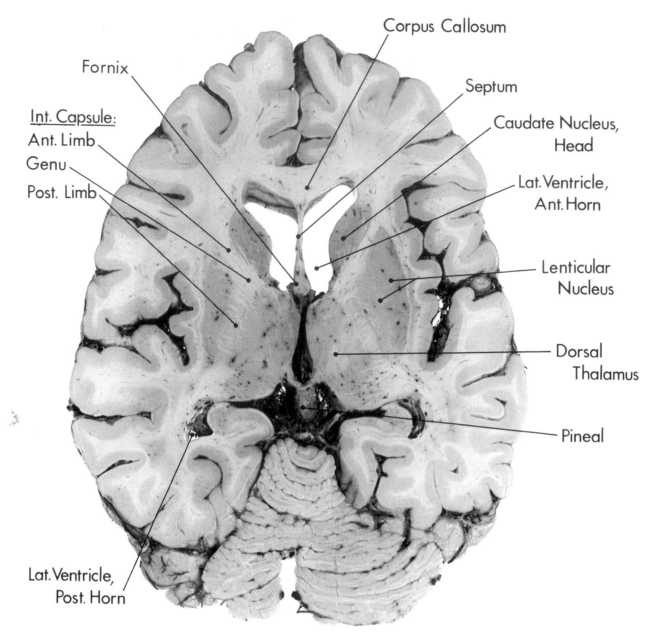

Fornix

Int. Capsule:
Ant. Limb
Genu
Post. Limb

Corpus Callosum

Septum

Caudate Nucleus,
Head

Lat. Ventricle,
Ant. Horn

Lenticular
Nucleus

Dorsal
Thalamus

Pineal

Lat. Ventricle,
Post. Horn

8–20   Ventral surface of a axial (horizontal) slice of brain through the *dorsal thalamus, head of the caudate nucleus,* and *pineal* (for greater detail see Fig. 4–18 on page 64). Structures that can be easily identified in a CT or MRI scan of normal brain at corresponding levels (Figs. 8–21, 8–22, facing page) are labeled.

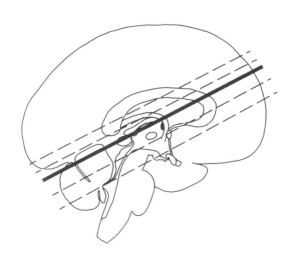

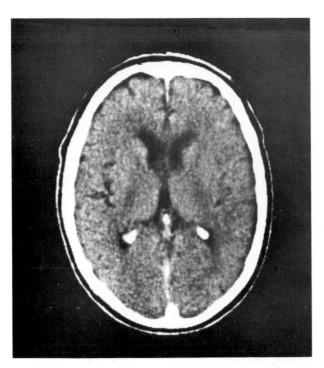

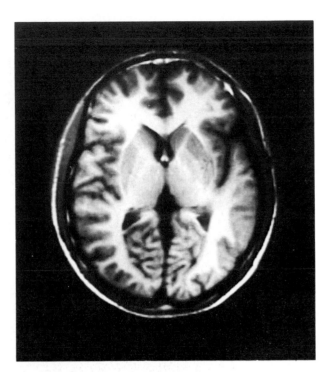

8–21 CT scan of normal brain at a level corresponding to the slice shown in Figure 8–20 (facing page). Identify the internal structures visible in this scan by comparing it with Figure 8–20.

8–22 MRI scan (T1 image) of normal brain at a level corresponding to the slice shown in Figure 8–20 (facing page). Identify the structures visible in this image by comparing it with Figure 8–20. Note the differentiation of the putamen from the globus pallidus.

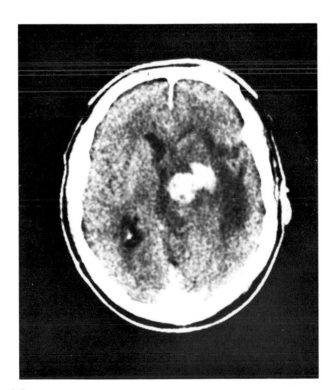

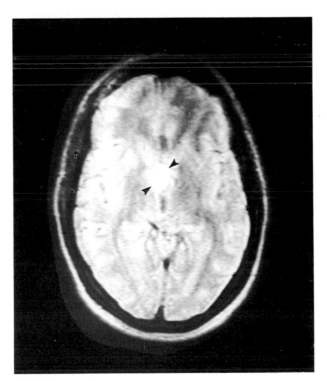

8–23 CT scan of abnormal brain (lymphoma) corresponding to the level of normal brain shown in Figure 8–21 (above). Note that all normal morphological relationships are disrupted on the right. The head of the caudate nucleus is pushed into, and partially obliterates, the anterior horn of the lateral ventricle, and the lymphoma impinges over the midline displacing the third ventricle. On the left, parts of thalamus, internal capsule, and caudate and lenticular nuclei can be identified.

8–24 MRI scan (T2 image) of abnormal brain (suprasellar craniopharyngioma) corresponding to the level of normal brain shown in Figure 8–22 (above). The lesion (arrows) is located in the midline and has disrupted anatomical relationships in the area. Note that the space of the third ventricle is partially obliterated.

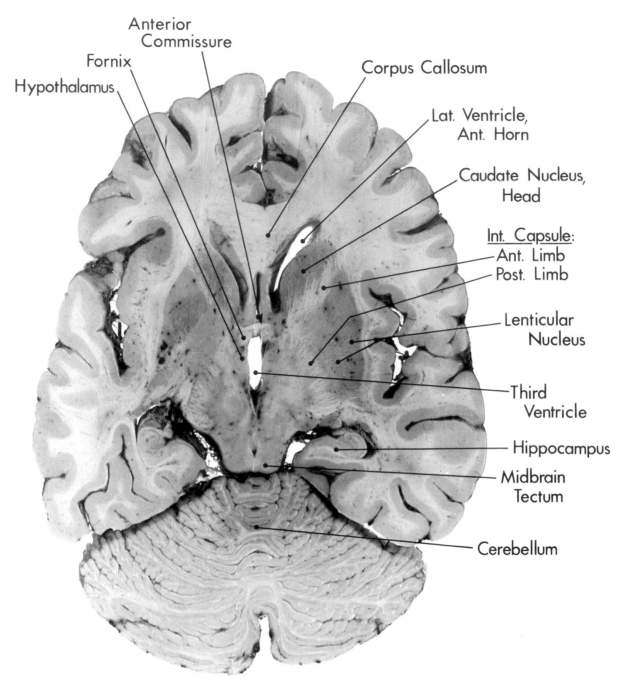

Hypothalamus

Fornix

Anterior Commissure

Corpus Callosum

Lat. Ventricle, Ant. Horn

Caudate Nucleus, Head

Int. Capsule:
Ant. Limb
Post. Limb

Lenticular Nucleus

Third Ventricle

Hippocampus

Midbrain Tectum

Cerebellum

8–25   Dorsal surface of a axial (horizontal) slice of brain through the *anterior commissure*, basal areas of the *rostral forebrain*, and the *midbrain tectum* (for greater detail see Fig. 4-20 on page 66). Structures that can be easily identified in a CT or MRI scan of normal brain at corresponding levels (Figs. 8–26, 8–27, facing page) are labeled.

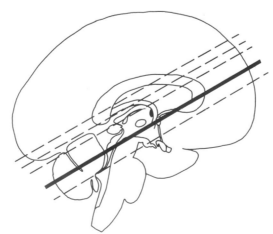

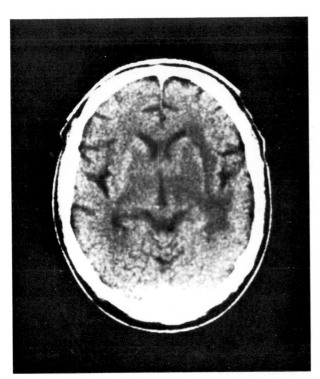

8–26   CT scan of normal brain at a level corresponding to that shown in Figure 8–25 (facing page). Identify the internal structures visible in this scan by comparing it with Figure 8–25. The appearance of the cerebellum is masked by portions of the overlying tentorium cerebelli.

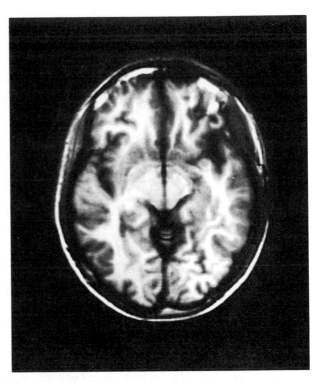

8–27   MRI scan (T1 image) of normal brain at a level corresponding approximately to the slice shown in Figure 8–25 (facing page). Identify the structures visible in this image by comparing it with Figure 8–25. Note the differences in appearance of the putamen and globus pallidus.

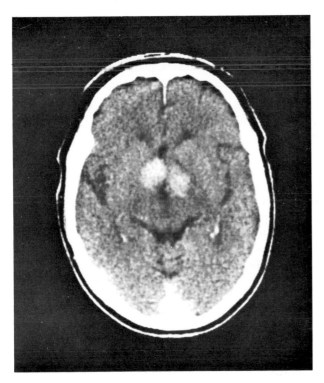

8–28   CT scan of abnormal brain (pituitary adenoma) corresponding to the level of normal brain shown in Figure 8–26 (above). Note that the entire tectal area is clear and that portions of the caudate and lenticular nuclei are recognizable. However, portions of the third ventricle, most of the hypothalamus, and medial areas of the internal capsule are disrupted bilaterally. The appearance of the cerebellum is partially masked by the overlying tentorium cerebelli.

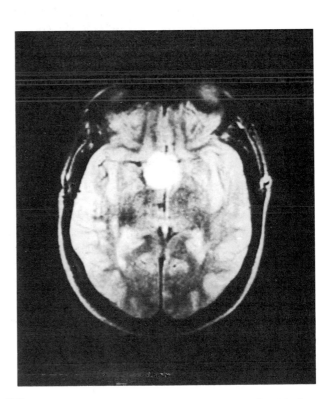

8–29   MRI scan (T2 image) of abnormal brain (pituitary adenoma) corresponding approximately to the level of normal brain shown in Figure 8–27 (above). Note the midline position of the tumor and the bilateral disruption of structures in the immediate area. Caudal portions of the third ventricle are clearly recognizable.

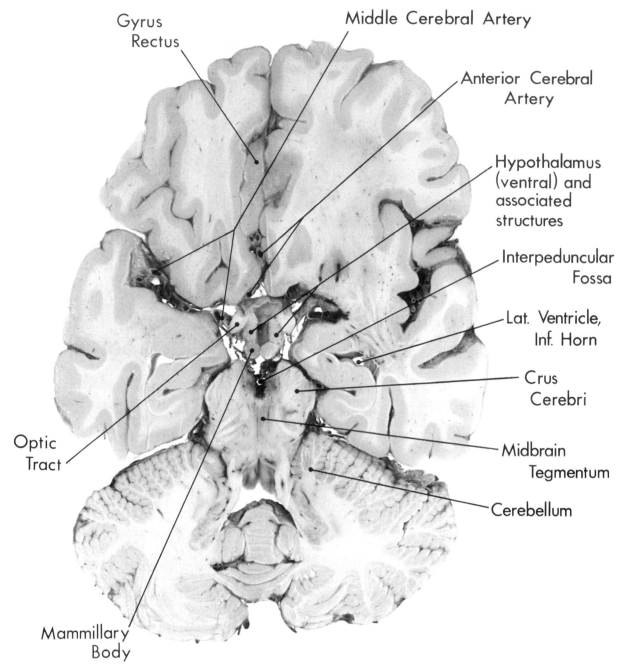

Gyrus Rectus

Middle Cerebral Artery

Anterior Cerebral Artery

Hypothalamus (ventral) and associated structures

Interpeduncular Fossa

Lat. Ventricle, Inf. Horn

Crus Cerebri

Midbrain Tegmentum

Cerebellum

Optic Tract

Mammillary Body

8–30   Dorsal surface of a axial (horizontal) slice of brain through ventral portions of the *hypothalamus* and *midbrain* and through the *superior cerebellar peduncles* and *fourth ventricle* (for greater detail see Fig. 4–22 on page 68). Structures that can be easily identified in a CT or MRI scan of normal brain at corresponding levels (Figs. 8–31, 8–32, facing page) are labeled.

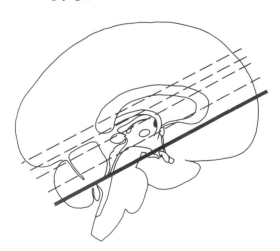

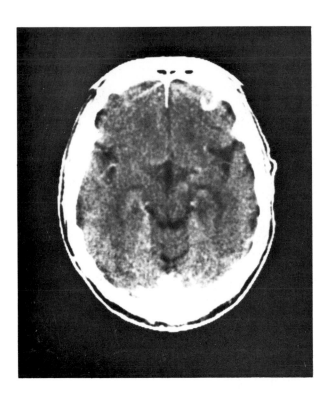

8–31 CT scan of normal brain at a level corresponding to that shown in Figure 8–30 (facing page). Identify the internal structures visible in this scan by comparing it with Figure 8–30.

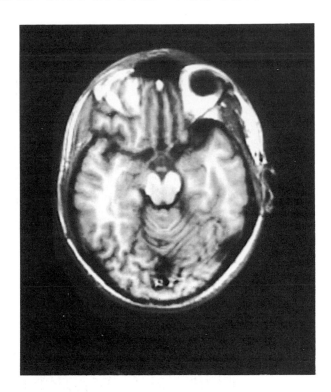

8–32 MRI scan (T1 image) of normal brain at a level corresponding approximately to the slice shown in Figure 8–30 (facing page). Identify the structures visible in this image by comparing it with Figure 8–30. Note the structures in the area of the hypothalamus.

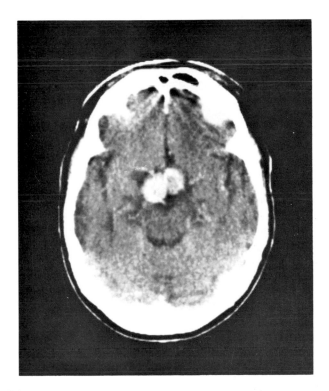

8–33 CT scan of abnormal brain (pituitary adenoma) corresponding to the level of normal brain shown in Figure 8–31 (above). Note that the entire midbrain is clear, including the area of the interpeduncular fossa, while the entire region of hypothalamus is disrupted bilaterally.

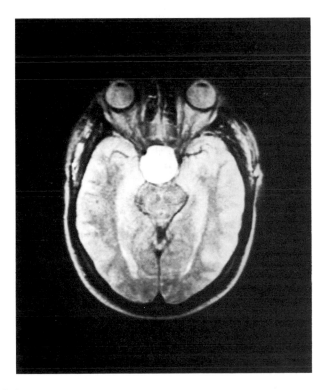

8–34 MRI scan (T2 image) of abnormal brain (pituitary adenoma) corresponding to the level of normal brain shown in Figure 8–32 (above). The tumor has completely disrupted the ventral hypothalamus and structures immediately adjacent to this region (compare with Fig. 8–30, facing page). Although the interpeduncular fossa has been invaded, the general shape of the midbrain is retained. Note the orbit.

Sources and Suggested Readings

Adams, R.D., M. Victor: Principles of Neurology, 5th Edition. McGraw-Hill, Inc., New York, 1993

Afifi, A.K., R.A. Bergman: Basic Neuroscience: A Structural and Functional Approach, 2nd Edition. Urban & Schwarzenberg, Baltimore, 1986

Airaksinen, M.S., P. Panula: The histaminergic system in the guinea pig central nervous system: An immunocytochemical mapping study using an antiserum against histamine. J. Comp. Neurol. 273: 163-186, 1988

Airaksinen, M.S., G. Flugge, E. Fuchs, P. Panula: Histaminergic system in the tree shrew brain. J. Comp. Neurol. 286:289-310, 1989

Anderson, K.D., A. Reiner: Extensive co-occurrence of substance P and dynorphin in striatal projection neurons: An evolutionarily conserved feature of basal ganglia organization. J. Comp. Neurol. 295:339-369, 1990

Angevine, J.B., E.L. Mancall, P.I. Yakovlev: The Human Cerebellum, An Atlas of Gross Topography in Serial Sections. Little, Brown, Boston, 1961

Barr, M.L., J.A. Kiernan: The Human Nervous System. An Anatomic Viewpoint, 6th Edition. J. B. Lippincott Co., Philadelphia, 1993

Beckstead, R.M., J.R. Morse, R, Norgren: The nucleus of the solitary tract in the monkey: Projections to the thalamus and brain stem nuclei. J. Comp. Neurol. 190:259-282, 1980

Bertram, E.G.M., K.L. Moore: An Atlas of the Human Brain and Spinal Cord. Williams & Wilkins, Baltimore, 1982

Bishop, G.A., R.H. Ho, J.S. King: Localization of immunoreactivity in the opossum cerebellum. J. Comp. Neurol. 235:301-321, 1985

Bobillier, P., S. Seguin, F. Petitjean, D. Salvert, M. Touret, M. Jouvert: The raphe nuclei of the cat brain stem: A topographical atlas of their efferent projections as revealed by autoradiography. Brain Res. 113:449-486, 1976

Bossy, J.: Atlas of Neuroanatomy and Special Sense Organs. W.B. Saunders Company, Philadelphia, 1970

Brodal, A.: Neurological Anatomy in Relation to Clinical Medicine, 3rd Edition. Oxford University Press, New York, 1981

Brodal, P.: The Central Nervous System, Structure and Function. Oxford University Press, New York, 1992

Broman, J., A. Blomqvist: Substance P-like immunoreactivity in the lateral cervical nucleus of the owl monkey (Aotus trivirgatus): A comparison with the cat and rat. J. Comp. Neurol. 289:111- 117, 1989

Broman, J., J. Westman, O.P. Ottersen: Spinocervical tract terminals are enriched in glutamate-like immunoreactivity: An anterograde transport-quantitative immunogold study in the cat. Neurosci. Abstr. 15:941, 1989

Brooks, V.B.: The Neural Basis of Motor Control. Oxford University Press, New York, 1986

Brown, A.G.: Organization in The Spinal Cord. Springer-Verlag, Berlin, 1981

Buisseret-Delmas, C., C. Batini, C. Compoint, H. Daniel, D. Menetrey: The GABAergic neurones of the cerebellar nuclei: Projection to the caudal inferior olive and to the bulbar reticular formation. In: P. Strata (ed.), The Olivocerebellar System in Motor Control. Exp. Brain Res. Ser. 17:108-110, Springer-Verlag, New York, 1989

Burt, A.M.: Textbook of Neuroanatomy. W. B. Saunders Co., Philadelphia, 1993

Carpenter, M.B., J. Sutin: Human Neuroanatomy, 8th Edition. Williams & Wilkins, Baltimore, 1983

Cassini, P., R.H. Ho, G.F. Martin: The brainstem origin of enkephalin- and substance-P-like immunoreactive axons in the spinal cord of the North American opossum. Brain Behav. Evol. 34:212-222, 1989

Clemente, C.D.: Anatomy: A Regional Atlas of the Human Body, 3rd Edition. Urban & Schwarzenberg, Baltimore, 1987

Collins, R.D.: Illustrated Manual of Neurologic Diagnosis, 2nd Edition. J.B. Lippincott Company, Philadelphia, 1982

Craig, A.D., Jr., S. Sailer, K.-D. Kniffki: Organization of anterogradely labeled spinocervical tract terminations in the lateral cervical nucleus of the cat. J. Comp. Neurol. 263:214-222, 1987

Craig, A.D., Jr., D.N. Tapper: Lateral cervical nucleus in the cat: Functional organization and characteristics. J. Neurophysiol. 41: 1511-1534, 1978

Crosby, E.C., T. Humphrey, E.W. Lauer: Correlative Anatomy of the Nervous System. Macmillan, New York, 1962

Curtis, B.A., S. Jacobson, E.M. Marcus: An Introduction to the Neurosciences. W.B. Saunders Company, Philadelphia, 1972

Daube, J.R., T.J. Regan, B.A. Sandox, B.F. Westmoreland: Medical Neurosciences: An Approach to Anatomy, Pathology and Physiology by Systems and Levels, 2nd Edition. Little, Brown, Boston, 1986

DeArmond. S.J.. M.M. Fusco. M.M. Dewev: Structure of the Human Brain: A Photographic Atlas, 3rd Edition, Oxford University Press, New York, 1989

de Groot, J.: Correlative Neuroanatomy of Computed Tomography and Magnetic Resonance Imaging. Lea & Febiger, Philadelphia, 1984

de Groot, J., J.G. Chusid: Correlative Neuroanatomy, 21st Edition. Appleton & Lange, Norwalk, CT, 1991

Dietrichs, E., D.E. Haines: Interconnections between hypothalamus and cerebellum. Anat. Embryol. 179:207-220, 1989

DeLacalle, S., L.B. Hersh, C.B. Saper: Cholinergic innervation of the human cerebellum. J. Comp. Neurol. 328:364-376, 1993

Dublin, A.B., W.B. Dublin: Atlas of Neuroanatomy with Radiologic Correlation and Pathologic Illustration. Warren H. Green Inc., St. Louis, 1982

England, M.A., J. Wakely: Color Atlas of the Brain & Spinal Cord. Mosby Year Book, St. Louis, 1991

Fischer, H.W., L. Ketonen: Radiographic Neuroanatomy, A Working Atlas. McGraw-Hill, Inc., New York, 1991

FitzGerald, M.J.T.: Neuroanatomy: Basics and Applied. Bailliere Tindall, Philadelphia, 1985

Fix, J.D.: Atlas of the Human Brain and Spinal Cord. Aspen Publishers Inc., Rockville, MD, 1987

Ford, D.H., J. Illari, J.P. Schade: Atlas of the Human Brain, 3rd Edition. Elsevier/North Holland, Amsterdam and New York, 1978

Gasser, R.F.: Personal Communication, 1989

Gasser, R.F.: Atlas of Human Embryos. Harper & Row, New York, 1975

Giesler, G.J., Jr., M. Bjorkeland, Q. Xu, G. Grant: Organization of the spinocervicothalamic pathway in the rat. J. Comp. Neurol. 268: 223-233, 1989

Gilman, S., S.S. Winans: Manter and Gatz's Essentials of Clinical Neuroanatomy and Neurophysiology, 8th Edition. F.A. Davis Company, Philadelphia, 1992

Giuffrida, R., A. Rustioni: Glutamate and aspartate immunoreactivity in corticospinal neurons of rats. J. Comp. Neurol. 288:154-164, 1989

Gluhbegovic, N., T.H. Williams: The Human Brain, A Photographic Guide. Harper & Row, Hagerstown, MD, 1980

Greenberg, D.A., M.J. Aminoff, R.P. Simon: Clinical Neurology, 2nd Edition. Appleton & Lange, Norwalk, 1993

Groenewegen, H.J., H.W. Berendse: Connections of the subthalamic nucleus with ventral striatopallidal parts of the basal ganglia in the rat. J. Comp. Neurol. 294:607-622, 1990

Haines, D.E., E. Dietrichs: On the organization of interconnections between the cerebellum and hypothalamus. In: J.S. King (ed.), New Concepts in Cerebellar Neurobiology, pp.113-149. Alan R. Liss, New York, 1987

Haines, D.E., P.J. May, E. Dietrichs: Neuronal connections between the cerebellar nuclei and hypothalamus in Macaca fascicularis: Cerebello-visceral circuits. J. Comp. Neurol. 299: 106-122, 1990

Hamilton, W.J., H.W. Mossman: Human Embryology, 4th Edition. Williams & Wilkins, Baltimore, 1972

Heimer, L.: The Human Brain and Spinal Cord: Functional Neuroanatomy and Dissection Guide. Springer-Verlag, New York, 1983

Herbert, H., C.B. Saper: Cholecystokinin-, galamin-, and corticotropin-releasing factor-like immunoreactive projections from the nucleus of the solitary tract to the parabrachial nucleus in the rat. J. Comp. Neurol. 293:581-598, 1990

Huang, X-F., I. Törk, and G. Paxinos: Dorsal motor nucleus of the vagus nerve: A cyto- and chemoarchitectonic study in the human. J. Comp. Neurol. 330:158-182, 1993

Jones, S.L., A.R. Light: Serotoninergic medullary raphespinal projection to the lumbar spinal cord in the rat: A retrograde immunohistochemical study. J. Comp. Neurol. 322:599-610, 1992

Kandel, E.R., J.H. Schwartz, T.M. Jessell: Principles of Neural Sciences. 3rd Edition. Appleton & Lange. Norwalk. CT. 1991

Kiernan, J.A.: Introduction to Human Neuroscience. J.B. Lippincott, Philadelphia, 1987

Kirkwood, J.R.: Essentials of Neuroimaging. Churchill Livingstone, New York, 1990

Krammer, E.B., M.F. Lischka, T.P. Egger, M. Reidl, H. Gruber: The motoneuronal organization of the spinal accessory nuclear complex. Adv. Anat. Embryol. Cell Biol. 103:1-62, 1987

Kretschmann, H.-J., W. Weinrich: Cranial Neuroimaging and Clinical Neuroanatomy, Magnetic Resonance Imaging and Computed Tomography, 2nd Edition. Georg Thieme Verlag, New York, 1992

Larsell, O., J. Jansen: The Comparative Anatomy and Histology of the Cerebellum: The Human Cerebellum, Cerebellar Connections

and Cerebellar Cortex. University of Minnesota Press, Minneapolis, 1972

Leah, J., D. Menetrey, J. dePommery: Neuropeptides in long ascending spinal tract cells in the rat: Evidence for parallel processing of ascending information. Neuroscience 24:195-207, 1988

Lechtenberg, R.: Synopsis of Neurology. Lea & Febiger, Philadelphia, 1991

Lehéricy, S., E.C. Hirsch, P. Cervera-Pierot, L.B. Hersh, S. Bakchine, F. Piette, C. Duyckaerts, J.-J. Hauw, F. Javoy-Agid, and Y. Agid: Heterogeneity and selectivity of the degeneration of cholinergic neurons in the basal forebrain of patients with Alzheimer's disease. J. Comp. Neurol. 330:15-31, 1993

Liebman, M.: Neuroanatomy Made Easy and Understandable, 3rd Edition. Aspen Publishers Inc., Rockville, MD, 1986

Ljungdahl, A., T. Hokfelt, G. Nilsson: Distribution of substance P-like immunoreactivity in the central nervous system of the rat   I. Cell bodies and nerve terminals. Neuroscience 3:861-943, 1978

Lilly, R., J.L. Cummings, D.F. Benson, M. Frankel: The human Kluver-Bucy syndrome. Neurology 33:1141-1145, 1983

Lu, G.W.: Spinocervical tract-dorsal column postsynaptic neurons: A double-projection neuronal system. Somatosens. Mot. Res. 6: 445-454, 1989

Lufkin, R., B.D. Flannigan, I.R. Bentson, G.H. Wilson, W. Rauschning, W. Hanafee: Magnetic resonance imaging of the brainstem and cranial nerves. Surgical and Radiologic Anatomy 8:49-66, 1986

Magnusson, K.R., J.R. Clements, A.A. Larson, J.E. Madl, A.J. Beitz: Localization of glutamate in trigeminothalamic projection neurons: A combined retrograde transport-immunohistochemical study. Somatosens. Res. 4:177-190, 1987

Martin, J.H.: Neuroanatomy, Text and Atlas. Elsevier, New York, 1989

Martinez Martinez, P.F.A.: Neuroanatomy: Development and Structure of the Central Nervous System. W.B. Saunders Company, Philadelphia, 1982

Mihailoff, G.A.: Cerebellar nuclear projections from the basilar pontine nuclei and nucleus reticularis tegmenti pontis as demonstrated with PHA-L tracing in the rat. J. Comp. Neurol. 330:130-146, 1993

Miller, R.A., E. Burack: Atlas of the Central Nervous System in Man, 3rd Edition. Williams & Wilkins, Baltimore, 1982

Monaghan, P.L., A.J. Beitz, A.A. Larson, R.A. Altschuler, J.E. Madl, M.A. Mullett: Immunocytochemical localization of glutamate-, glutaminase- and aspartate aminotransferase-like immunoreactivity in the rat deep cerebellar nuclei. Brain Res. 363:364-370, 1986

Montemurro, D.G., J.E. Bruni: The Human Brain in Dissection, 2nd Edition. Oxford University Press, New York, 1988

Nahin, R.L.: Immunocytochemical identification of long ascending, peptidergic lumbar spinal neurons terminating in either the medial or lateral thalamus in the rat. Brain Res. 443:345-349, 1988

Nelson, B.J., E. Mugnaini: Origins of GABAergic inputs to the inferior olive. In: P. Strata (ed.), The Olivocerebellar System in Motor Control. Exp. Brain Res. Ser. 17:86-107, Springer-Verlag, New York, 1989

Newman, D.B., S.K. Hilleary, C.Y. Ginsberg: Nuclear terminations of corticoreticular fiber systems in rats. Brain Behav. Evol. 34: 223-264, 1989

Nicholls, J.G., A.R. Martin, B.G. Wallace: From Neuron to Brain, 3rd Edition. Sinauer Associates, Inc., Sunderland, MA, 1992

Nieuwenhuys, R.: Chemoarchitecture of the Brain. Springer-Verlag, Berlin, 1985

Nieuwenhuys, R., J. Voogd, C. van Huijzen: The Central Nervous System: A Synopsis and Atlas, 3rd Edition. Springer-Verlag, Berlin, 1988

Noback, C.R., N.L. Strominger, R.J. Demarest: The Human Nervous System, Introduction and Review, 4th Edition. Lea & Febiger, Philadelphia, 1991

Nolte, J.: The Human Brain: An Introduction to its Functional Anatomy, 3rd Edition. C.V. Mosby Company, St. Louis, 1993

Nudo, R.J., D.P. Sutherland, R.B. Masterton: Inter- and intra-laminar distribution of tectospinal neurons in 23 mammals. Brain Behav. Evol. 42:1-23, 1993

Olszewski, J., D. Baxter: Cytoarchitecture of the Human Brain Stem, 2nd Edition. S. Karger, Basel, 1982

Pansky, B., D.J. Allen, G.C. Budd: Review of Neuroscience, 2nd Edition. Macmillan Publishing Company, New York, 1988

Parent, A., L. DeBellefeuille: The pallidointralaminar and pallidonigral projections in primate as studied by retrograde double-labeling method. Brain Res. 278:11-27, 1983

Patton, H.D., J.W. Sundsten, W.E. Crill, P.D. Swanson: Introduction to Basic Neurology. W.B. Sauders Company, Philadelphia, 1976

Platzer, W. (ed.): Pernkopf Atlas of Topographic and Applied Human Anatomy, 3rd Edition. Volume I, Head and Neck. Urban & Schwarzenberg, Baltimore, 1989

Poritsky, R.: Neuroanatomical Pathways. W.B. Saunders Company, Philadelphia, 1984

Rasmussen, A.T.: Atlas of Cross Section Anatomy of the Brain: Guide to the Study of the Morphology and Fiber Tracts of the Human Brain. Blakiston Division, McGraw-Hill Book Company, Inc., New York, 1951

Reddy, V.K., P. Cassini, R.H. Ho, G.F. Martin: Origins and terminations of bulbospinal axons that contain serotonin and either enkephalin or substance P in the North American opossum. J. Comp. Neurol. 294:96-108, 1990

Reddy, V.K., S.J. Fung, H. Zhuo, C.D. Barnes: Localization of enkephalinergic neurons in the dorsolateral pontine tegmentum projecting to the spinal cord of the cat. J. Comp. Neurol. 291:195-202, 1990

Roberts, M., J. Hanaway, D.K. Morest: Atlas of the Human Brain in Section, 2nd Edition. Lea & Febiger, Philadelphia, 1987

Romero-Sierra, C.: Neuroanatomy: A Conceptual Approach. Churchill Livingstone, New York, 1986

Rosenberg, R.N.: Neurology, Vol. 5 of The Science and Practice of Clinical Medicine, J.M. Dietschy, Editor-in-Chief. Grune & Stratton, New York, 1980

Rowland, L.P. (ed.): Merritt's Textbook of Neurology, 8th Edition. Lea & Febiger, Philadelphia, 1989

Rustioni, A.: Non-primary afferents to the nucleus gracilis from the lumbar cord of the cat. Brain Res. 51:81-95, 1973

Rustioni, A.: Non-primary afferents to the cuneate nucleus in the brachial dorsal funiculus of the cat. Brain Res. 75:247-259, 1974

Rustioni, A., A.B. Kaufman: Identification of cells of origin of non-primary afferents to the dorsal column nuclei of the cat. Exp. Brain Res. 27:1-14, 1977

Salt, T.E., R.G. Hill: Neurotransmitter candidates of somatosensory primary afferent fibres. Neuroscience 10:1083-1103, 1983

Sarnat, H.B., M.G. Netsky: Evolution of the Nervous System, 2nd Edition. Oxford University Press, New York, 1981

Schnitzlein, H.N., E.W. Hartley, F.R. Murtagh, L. Grundy, J.T. Fargher: Computed Tomography of the Head and Spine: A Photographic Color Atlas of CT, Gross, and Microscopic Anatomy. Urban & Schwarzenberg, Baltimore, 1983

Schnitzlein, H.N., F.R. Murtagh: Imaging Anatomy of the Head and Spine: A Photographic Color Atlas of MRI, CT, Gross, and Microscopic Anatomy in Axial, Coronal, and Sagittal Planes, 2nd Edition. Urban & Schwarzenberg, Baltimore, 1990

Schwerdtfeger, W.K., E.H. Buhl, P. Germroth: Disynaptic olfactory input to the hippocampus mediated by stellate cells in the entorhinal cortex. J. Comp. Neurol. 292:163-177, 1990

Shepherd, G.M.: Neurobiology, 3rd Edition. Oxford University Press, New York, 1994

Siegel, G., B.W. Agranoff, R.W. Albers, P.B. Molinoff: Basic Neurochemistry, Molecular, Cellular, and Medical Aspects. Raven Press, New York, 1989

Singer, M., P.I. Yakovlev: The Human Brain in Sagittal Section. Charles C Thomas, Springfield, 1964

Smith, C.G.: Serial Dissections of the Human Brain. Urban & Schwarzenberg, Baltimore, 1981

Smith, Y., J.P. Bolam: The output neurones and the dopaminergic neurones of the substantia nigra receive a GABA-containing input from the globus pallidus in the rat. J. Comp. Neurol. 296:47-64, 1990

Smith, Y., L.-N. Hazrati, A. Parent: Efferent projections of the subthalamic nucleus in the squirrel monkey as studied by the PHA-L anterograde tracing method. J. Comp. Neurol. 294:306-323, 1990

Snell, R.S.: Clinical Neuroanatomy for Medical Students, 3rd Edition. Little, Brown, Boston, 1992

Strata, P. (ed.): The Olivocerebellar System in Motor Control. Springer-Verlag, Berlin/New York, 1989

Sugiura, K., G.A. Robinson, D.G. Stuart: Illustrated Guide to the Central Nervous System. Ishiyaku EuroAmerica, Inc., St. Louis, 1989

Swash, M., J. Oxbury (Editors): Clinical Neurology, Volumes 1 and 2. Churchill Livingstone, New York, 1991

Terzian, H., G.D. Ore: Syndrome of Kluver and Bucy reproduced in man by bilateral removal of the temporal lobes. Neurology 5:373-380, 1955

Tieman, S.B., K. Butler, J.H. Neale: N-acetylaspartylglutamate: A neuropeptide in the human visual system. JAMA, 259:2020, 1988

Walker, J.J., G.A. Bishop, R.H. Ho, J.S. King: Brainstem origin of serotonin- and enkephalin-immunoreactive afferents to the opossums cerebellum. J. Comp. Neurol. 276:481-497, 1988

Walton, J.: Introduction to Clinical Neuroscience. Bailliere Tindall, London, 1983

Walton, L.: Essentials of Neurology. Churchill Livingstone, New York, 1989

Watson, C.: Basic Human Neuroanatomy: An Introductory Atlas, 4th Edition. Little, Brown, Boston, 1991

Werner, J.K.: Neuroscience: A Clinical Perspective. W.B. Saunders, Philadelphia, 1980

Westlund, K.N., S.M. Carlton, D. Zhang, W.D. Willis: Glutamate-immunoreactive terminals synapse on primate spinothalamic tract cells. J. Comp. Neurol. 322:519-527, 1992

Wicke, L.: Atlas of Radiologic Anatomy, 3rd Edition. Urban & Schwarzenberg, Baltimore, 1982

Willard, F.H.: Medical Neuroanatomy, A Problem Oriented Manual with Annotated Atlas. J.B. Lippincott Co., Philadelphia, 1993

Williams, P.L., R. Warwick, M. Dyson, L.H. Bannister: Gray's Anatomy, 37th British Edition. Churchill Livingstone, Edinburgh, 1989

Willis, W.D., Jr.: The Pain System: The Neural Basis of Nociceptive Transmission in the Mammalian Nervous System. Vol. 8, Pain and Headache. S. Karger, Basel, 1985

Willis, W.D., R.G. Grossman: Medical Neurobiology: Neuroanatomical and Neurophysiological Principles Basic To Clinical Neuroscience, 3rd Edition. C.V. Mosby Company, St. Louis, 1981

Witelson, S.F., D.L. Kigas: Sylvian fissure morphology and asymmetry in men and women: Bilateral differences in relation to handedness in men. J. Comp. Neurol. 323:326-340, 1992

Zuleger, S., J. Staubesand: Atlas of the Central Nervous System in Sectional Planes. Urban & Schwarzenberg, Baltimore, 1977

Index